tb
13
εt

Progress in
Cancer Research and Therapy
Volume 12

ADVANCES IN NEUROBLASTOMA RESEARCH

Progress in
Cancer Research and Therapy

Progress in
Cancer Research and Therapy
Volume 12

Advances in
Neuroblastoma Research

Editor

Audrey E. Evans, M.D.
Division of Oncology
The Children's Hospital of Philadelphia
Philadelphia, Pennsylvania

Raven Press ▪ New York

Raven Press, 1140 Avenue of the Americas, New York, New York 10036

Made in the United States of America

Great care has been taken to maintain the accuracy of the information contained in the volume. However, Raven Press cannot be held responsible for errors or for any consequences arising from the use of the information contained herein.

Library of Congress Cataloging in Publication Data

Symposium on Advances in Neuroblastoma Research, 2d,
   Children's Hospital of Philadelphia, 1979.
   Advances in neuroblastoma research.

   (Progress in cancer research and therapy; v. 12)
   Includes bibliographical references and index.
   1. Neuroblastoma—Congresses. 2. Neuroblastoma—
Research—Congresses. I. Evans, Audrey E.
II. Title. III. Series. [DNLM: 1. Neuroblas-
toma. W1 PR667M v. 12 / QA380 A244]
RC280.N4S95 1979   616.99′4   79–66513
ISBN 0–89004–459–7

Preface

The chapters in this volume are grouped according to five broad areas of investigation: (1) the problems of the disease and neuroblastoma, (2) genetics, (3) cell differentiation, (4) immunology, and (5) cytogenetics and chemotherapy models.

The introduction includes a presentation of the disease aspect in man citing some of the unique characteristics such as maturation, differentiation, and spontaneous regression. These relatively rare characteristics were recurring topics during the conference. New data are presented on the prognostic significance of the different patterns of catecholamine metabolism and a new excretion product, ferritin, which is also apparently a marker that can be used as an aid to determine the presence of disease.

The chapters in the section on genetics include new data on chromosomes from cultured human neuroblastoma lines and the relationship between the homologous staining region and double minute chromosomes. The major advance results from the use of neuroblastoma mouse hybrids and the ability to equate malignant growth with retention of specific human chromosomes.

The section on cell differentiation includes a presentation of neural oncogenesis induced by antinatal chemical carcinogens. The fact that the time of exposure strongly influences the resulting tumor type may have real significance in the etiology of neuroblastoma, the tumor most often diagnosed early in life and which is present at birth. In this section, preliminary studies are presented showing the growth of human neuroblastoma cells in serum-free media and the influence of changes in the media and on the patterns of the cell growth. The studies of cell membranes include data on the properties of the hybrids with their known chromosomal makeup and ability to form tumors.

The main advance in the field of immunology results from the new technique of using hybridomas and their production of monoclonal antibodies. Although there are still cross-reactivities among neuroblastoma, fetal brain and other tissues and some lymphoid malignant diseases, these monoclonal antibodies are coming much nearer to the ideal of tumor-specific antibodies. These have great implications regarding diagnosis and possible immunotherapy.

The final chapters deal with cytokinetics and models for the study of chemotherapy. Clinicians are in great need of data on which they can base a more rational approach to chemotherapy. Studies of the alteration in cell kinetics of marrow tumor cells during treatment can be helpful in deciding the sequence of drugs and their efficacy. Flow microfluorometric analysis demonstrates a wide variation between human tumors and within a single tumor. Such studies may provide a sensitive means of monitoring a therapeutic effect. Human tumors heterotransplanted in the nude mouse offer another attractive model for chemotherapy and preliminary data are presented, suggesting that the results in the mouse reflect the human response.

This volume will have the greatest interest for the clinician and basic scientist working in the field of human neuroblastoma. However, many of the chapters have a wider scope and deal with basic questions of cancer biology and therapy.

The Editor

Acknowledgments

The chapters which comprise this volume were presented at the Second Symposium on Advances in Neuroblastoma Research held at The Children's Hospital of Philadelphia in May 1979. The purpose of the meeting was to update the advances in current laboratory and clinical research that have occurred since the 1975 conference. In particular, the exchange of ideas between the clinician and laboratory scientist contributed to a better understanding of the problems of patients and the complexities in laboratory research. In addition, the organizers invited a small number of experts in various fields to provide insight into the biology of neuroblastoma and suggest tools for its study. The conference was successful, and the resulting volume is a unique collection on neuroblastoma research.

The editor wishes to thank all those who participated in the conference and regrets that much of the excellent discussion had to be curtailed. I would like to thank the members of the organizing committee, Drs. Green, Hummeler, and Seeger for their help in planning the program and moderating the sessions. The additional session chairmen, Drs. Knudson, Littauer, and Baserga, were invaluable for their leadership in the discussion and their syntheses of it for publication. Finally, I would like to thank Mrs. Goldberg for her assistance in organizing the conference and Mrs. Seelye for editing the manuscripts.

Contents

Contributors

Gloria Balaban-Malenbaum, Ph.D. *Division of Human Genetics, University of Pennsylvania, Philadelphia, Pennsylvania 19104*

Renato L. Baserga, M.D. *Division of Pathology, Temple University Health Sciences Center, Philadelphia, Pennsylvania 19140*

Kathleen B. Bechtol, Ph.D. *Wistar Institute of Anatomy and Biology, Philadelphia, Pennsylvania 19104*

William F. Benedict, M.D. *Department of Pediatrics, USC and Children's Hospital of Los Angeles, Los Angeles, California 90054*

Irwin D. Bernstein, M.D. *Division of Pediatric Oncology, Fred Hutchinson Cancer Research Center, Seattle, Washington 98105*

June L. Biedler, Ph.D. *Laboratory of Cellular and Biochemical Genetics, Sloan-Kettering Institute for Cancer Research, Rye, New York 10580*

Jane Bottenstein, Ph.D. *Department of Pediatrics, School of Medicine, UCLA, Los Angeles, California 90024*

Garrett Brodeur, M.D. *St. Jude Children's Research Hospital, Memphis, Tennessee 38101*

Mehroo Cooper, Ph.D. *Department of Pharmacology, University of Minnesota, Minneapolis, Minnesota 55455*

Giulio J. D'Angio, M.D. *Director, Children's Cancer Research Center, The Children's Hospital of Philadelphia, Philadelphia, Pennsylvania 19104*

Yehuda Danon, M.D. *Rogoff-Wellcome Medical Research Institute, Beilinson Medical Center, Petah-Tikva, Israel*

William L. Elkins, M.D. *Department of Pathology, University of Pennsylvania, Division of Oncology, The Children's Hospital of Philadelphia, Philadelphia, Pennsylvania 19104*

Martin B. Epstein, Ph.D. *Department of Radiological Sciences, UCLA School of Medicine, Los Angeles, California 90024*

Richard Epstein, M.D. *Department of Pathology, University of Pennsylvania School of Medicine, Philadelphia, Pennsylvania 19104*

Audrey E. Evans, M.D., *Division of Oncology, The Children's Hospital of Philadelphia, Philadelphia, Pennsylvania 19104*

Milligan C. Fossett, III. *Division of Hematology/Oncology, St. Jude Children's Research Hospital, Memphis, Tennessee 38101*

Esther Freier, M.S. *Laboratory Medicine and Pathology, University of Minnesota, Minneapolis, Minnesota 55455*

John T. Gallagher, M.D. *CRC Department of Medical Oncology, Christie Hospital, Manchester, England*

James M. Gerson, M.D. *Department of Pediatrics, Milton S. Hershey Medical Center, Hershey, Pennsylvania 17033*

Alfred Gilbert, M.D. *Division of Human Genetics, University of Pennsylvania, School of Medicine, Philadelphia, Pennsylvania 19104*

Beppino C. Giovanella, M.D. *The Stehlin Foundation for Cancer Research, Houston, Texas 77002*

Maria Y. Giovanni, B.A. *Division of Molecular Biology, The Children's Hospital of Philadelphia, Philadelphia, Pennsylvania 19104*

Mary Catherine Glick, Ph.D. *Division of Molecular Biology, The Children's Hospital of Philadelphia, Philadelphia, Pennsylvania 19104*

Nicholas K. Gonatas, M.D. *Department of Pathology, University of Pennsylvania, Philadelphia, Pennsylvania 19104*

John Graham-Pole, M.R.C.P., D. Ch. *Department of Pediatric Oncology, Rainbow Babies & Children's Hospital, Case Western Reserve University, Cleveland, Ohio 44106*

Melvin F. Greaves, Ph.D., M. R. Path. *Department of Membrane Immunology, Imperial Cancer Research Fund, Lincoln's Inn Fields, London WC2A 3PX, England*

Morris Gutenstein, M.S. *Department of Biochemistry, Children's Hospital of Los Angeles, Los Angeles, California 90054*

Ian N. Hampson, B.Sc. *Clinical Research, Christie Hospital & Holt Radium Institute, Wilmslow Road, Manchester M20 9BX, England*

Hie-Won L. Hann, M.D. *The Institute for Cancer Research, Fox Chase Cancer Center, Philadelphia, Pennsylvania 19111*

Paul J. Harlow, M.D. *Division of Hematology-Oncology, New York University Medical Center, New York 10016*

Ann Hayes, M.D. *St. Jude Children's Research Hospital, Memphis, Tennessee 38101*

Lawrence Helson, M.D. *Memorial Sloan-Kettering Cancer Center, New York, New York 10021*

Ronald B. Herberman, M.D. *Laboratory of Immunodiagnosis, National Cancer Institute, Bethesda, Maryland 20205*

Klaus Hummeler, M.D. *Director, Joseph Stokes Jr. Research Institute, The Children's Hospital of Philadelphia, Philadelphia, Pennsylvania 19104*

Shinsaku Imashuku, M.D. *Department of Pediatrics, Kyoto Prefectoral College of Medicine, Kyoto, Japan*

Tong Hyub Joh, Ph.D. *Laboratory of Neurobiology, Department of Neurology, Cornell University Medical College, New York, New York 10021*

Zdenka Jonak, Ph.D. *Wistar Institute of Anatomy and Biology, Philadelphia, Pennsylvania 19104*

John T. Kemshead, Ph.D. *The Hospital for Sick Children, London, England*

Roger Kennett, Ph.D. *Department of Human Genetics, University of Pennsylvania School of Medicine, Philadelphia, Pennsylvania 19104*

Alfred G. Knudson, Jr., M.D., Ph.D. *Director, The Institute for Cancer Research, Fox Chase Cancer Center, Philadelphia, Pennsylvania 19111*

William Krivit, M.D., Ph.D. *Department of Pediatrics, University of Minnesota, Minneapolis, Minnesota 55455*

Shant Kumar, Ph.D., M. Vet. Sci. *Clinical Research, Christie Hospital and Holt Radium Institute, Wilmslow Road., Manchester M20 9BX, England*

Lois A. Lampson, Ph.D. *Postdoctoral Fellow, Stanford University Medical School, Stanford, California 94305*

Benjamin Landing, M.D. *Department of Pathology, Children's Hospital of Los Angeles, Los Angeles, California 90054*

Walter E. Laug, M.D. *Department of Hematology/Oncology, Children's Hospital of Los Angeles, Los Angeles, California 90054*

Howard M. Levy, B.A. *The Institute for Cancer Research, Fox Chase Cancer Center, Philadelphia, Pennsylvania 19111*

Uriel Z. Littauer, Ph.D. *Department of Neurobiology, Weizmann Institute of Science, Rehovot, Israel*

Jack E. Maidman, M.D. *Department of Obstetrics and Gynecology, Charles R. Drew Postgraduate Medical School, Los Angeles, California 90059*

Bernard Minkin, M.D., Ph.D. *Department of Pediatrics, University of Minnesota, Minneapolis, Minnesota 55455*

Mariko Momoi, M.D. *Division of Biochemical Development and Molecular Diseases, The Children's Hospital of Philadelphia, Philadelphia, Pennsylvania 19104*

Paul Moorhead, Ph.D. *Division of Human Genetics, University of Pennsylvania and The Children's Hospital of Philadelphia, Philadelphia, Pennsylvania 19104*

Calvin P. Myers, M.S. *Department of Radiological Sciences, U.C.L.A. School of Medicine, Los Angeles, California 90024*

Mark Nesbit, M.D. *Department of Pediatrics, University of Minnesota, Minneapolis, Minnesota 55455*

Claudio A. Nicolini, Ph.D. *Division of Biophysics, Temple University Health Sciences Center, Philadelphia, Pennsylvania 19140*

Kedar N. Prasad, Ph.D. *Department of Radiology, University of Colorado Medical Center, Denver, Colorado 80262*

Jon Pritchard, M.D., MRCP. *Department of Haematology, The Hospital for Sick Children, Great Ormond Street, London WC1N 3JH, England*

Manfred F. Rajewsky, M.D. *Director, Institut fur Zellbiolgie, Universitat Essen, Essen, Germany*

Sylvia A. Raynar, B.S. *Department of Pediatrics, U.C.L.A. School of Medicine, Los Angeles, California 90024*

Donald J. Reis, M.D. *Laboratory of Neurobiology, Department of Neurology, Cornell University Medical College, New York, New York 10021*

Robert A. Ross, M.D. *Laboratory of Neurobiology, Department of Neurology Cornell University Medical College, New York, New York 10021*

R. Neil Schimke, M.D. *Department of Pediatrics, Kansas University and Medical Center, Kansas City, Kansas 66103*

Robert C. Seeger, M.D. *Divisions of Immunology and Hematology-Oncology, University of California Los Angeles, Los Angeles, California 90054*

Sara Shanske, Ph.D. *Department of Neurology, Columbia University College of Physicians and Surgeons, New York, New York 10032*

Kenneth N. F. Shaw, Ph.D. *Department of Biochemistry, Children's Hospital, Los Angeles, California 90054*

Michael M. Siegel, M.D. *Division of Hematology/Oncology, Children's Hospital of Los Angeles, Los Angeles, California 90027*

Stuart E. Siegel, M.D. *Division of Hematology-Oncology, Children's Hospital of Los Angeles, Los Angeles, California 90027*

John S. Stehlin, M.D. *Cancer Research Laboratory, St. Joseph Hospital, Houston, Texas 77002*

Paul M. Zeltzer, M.D. *Department of Pediatrics, University of Texas, San Antonio, Texas 78284*

Disease Characteristics in Man

Advances in Neuroblastoma Research,
edited by Audrey E. Evans.
Raven Press, New York © 1980.

Natural History of Neuroblastoma

Audrey E. Evans

The Children's Hospital of Philadelphia, Philadelphia, Pennsylvania 19104

The purpose of this chapter is to summarize the information currently available on the natural history of neuroblastoma. The presentation is divided into two broad areas: first, the more usual facets of the disease which often are similar to those of other tumors of childhood; and second, those which seem unique to neuroblastoma. Many of the points made and questions raised are addressed in greater depth elsewhere in this volume.

CHARACTERISTICS OF NEUROBLASTOMA

Incidence and Pathology

Neuroblastoma is one of the commoner solid tumors in the pediatric population, accounting for 7 to 10% of the cancers. The annual incidence is 10 per million children under the age of 15 years. Thus its incidence is similar to that of Wilms' tumors, and approximately 500 cases are diagnosed in the United States each year.

Neuroblastoma was first described in 1864 by Virchow (29), and in 1910 the appearance of the rosettes and fibrils was likened to the developing adrenal by Wright (32), who pointed out that the migration of primitive nerve cells explained the development of tumors with similar appearance in numerous sites in the body (32). Since these earlier reports, many pathologists have sought to refine the descriptions of cyto-histopathology in attempts to achieve a better understanding of the disease. It is clear there is a spectrum from a tumor composed of cells so incompletely differentiated that their distinction from the other small, round tumors of childhood is almost impossible, to the other end, where mature ganglion cells make up most if not all the tumor when it properly is called ganglioneuroma. Beckwith and Martin (2) have defined a method of grading tumors from I to IV depending on the degree of differentiation, grade I being predominantly differentiated and IV undifferentiated, i.e., without recognizable neurogenesis (2). They found an association between the lower or more mature grades and a better prognosis. However, the much larger proportion is made up of the undifferentiated or higher grade tumors, and here the varying cytologic proportions have not been found to be helpful by others in estimating the likelihood of relapse. It is interesting to note that children with IV-S disease usually have very undifferentiated tumors but a good prognosis.

Stage of Disease

Some years ago, a review of the records of a large number of patients entered on Children's Cancer Study Group (CCSG) studies was used to devise a staging system that has proved useful in estimating prognosis (14). Patients with localized disease were divided into three categories, and those with distant involvement into two. Stage I was used to designate tumors limited to the organ of origin; stage II included those with regional spread that did not cross the midline; and stage III, regional tumors crossing the midline. Stage IV included patients with metastases to distant discontinuous sites such as lymph nodes, bone, or lung. A special category termed IV-S was used for patients with small primary tumors and disseminated disease limited to the liver, the skin, the bone marrow, or their combinations—but without radiologic evidence of bone metastases. A more recent CCSG study attempted to refine the staging system using positive or negative lymph nodes as indices to see whether this would permit better prediction of outcome. Unfortunately, a problem arises when regional lymph node status is included as a staging system criterion because the lymph nodes are not sampled in one-third of patients with localized disease. Those patients in whom the lymph node status is not known lie at both ends of the staging spectrum; those with early stage disease have no visible lymph nodes to biopsy, and those with more advanced disease have large, unresectable tumors that obscure the regional nodes. It therefore is impractical to incorporate a factor missing in one-third of the patients as an index for staging purposes. Although not statistically significant because of small sample size, the presence of involved lymph nodes does appear to worsen the prognosis in a CCSG analysis (CCG-351) *(personal communication).* One suspects that the presence or absence of positive nodes would be a stronger prognostic variable than whether or not the disease crosses the midline, indeed, that the bilaterality of nodal disease often accounts for the worse outlook. The same study showed that there was a statistical difference in the survival by stage as originally defined, stages I and II being different from stage III. Therefore, until other criteria can be devised, the present staging system can still be used because it has value while recognizing that the presence of positive nodes probably has a deleterious connotation.

Site

It has long been recognized that patients with primary tumors arising in the cervical region or thorax have a better outlook than those with primaries located within the abdomen. The original analyses used to devise a staging system suggested that the difference in outcome for primary tumors originating above or below the diaphragm was due to the fact that the former were more often stage I or II at diagnosis, whereas the latter were usually stage III or IV. Thus, stage for stage, the outcome was not influenced by site. Other investigators have reported that the site of the primary tumor does influence the outcome when equivalent stages are compared, and more recently, our own studies have tended to confirm this impression (8,19).

Multiple Primary Tumors

On rare occasions, one encounters a patient who apparently has more than one primary tumor within the sympathetic nervous system (24). Tumors can appear either simultaneously or in sequence. As with bilateral Wilms' tumors, it is not always easy to be sure that these are simultaneous independent lesions rather than metastases. It is this investigator's belief, however, that when multiple neuroblastomas occur in metachronous fashion within the sympathetic nervous system, they are more likely to be multiple primary tumors. A good example of two primary tumors occurring at different times is the 9-year-old patient who remained well for 2½ years following excision of a stage II thoracic tumor. He then developed lower limb weakness and bladder dysfunction and was found to have a midline abdominal tumor at L4 with sacral plexus involvement. He remains well years later (V. Albo, *personal communication*) following surgery, irradiation, and chemotherapy. It does not seem likely that the thoracic primary tumor metastasized to the organ of Zukerkandl 30 months after the original excision. The age of this boy is exceptional since patients with multiple primary tumors tend to be younger than the average—usually under 1 year of age—at diagnosis (24).

Age

The median age of neuroblastoma patients is 2 years; indeed, neuroblastoma is the commonest cancer of early childhood. An analysis of factors predicting outcome showed age at diagnosis to be a strong, independent variable (separate from stage); it correlates inversely with survival (7). Younger children have a larger proportion of the more favorable stages, but stage for stage, age has an influence on the outcome. This is best illustrated by the survival experience of infants with stage IV disease. Of 69 infants under 1 year of age, 18 or 26% were stage IV at diagnosis and 5 (28%) of these survived; 93/130 (72%) of children 2 years or older were stage IV with a survival rate of 3%.

An interesting new observation emerging from continuing analyses of CCSG data is the better survival experience of the "older" child with metastatic neuroblastoma; i.e., over 5 years (20). The number of such patients is small, but there is a relatively good survival experience in some "older" stage IV patients with an overall 2-year survival rate of 50%. This number includes several patients alive with disease past the 2 year point; for example, 2 girls at our hospital, aged 12 and 8 when first seen, are surviving with disease 5 or more years from the time of diagnosis. Thus there appears to be a bimodal curve for age versus prognosis, the prognosis being excellent during the first year of life, to fall rapidly thereafter, only to rise again, apparently, at 5 years. The data to support this second peak are softer since some of the 2-year survivors will ultimately die. The improvement may be more one of prolonged survival rather than a difference in the cure rate. A better survival experience is also seen in the rare adult with neuroblastoma; MacKay et al. (26) report a more indolent course in 9 adults with regional and metastatic disease.

Pattern of Metastases

Like other tumors, neuroblastoma tends to metastasize to certain specific sites: the lymph nodes, bone marrow, and skeleton, less often the liver, and rarely the pulmonary parenchyma and brain. The tumor differs markedly from Wilms' tumor in this respect and mimics more nearly the lymphomas. One wonders what is so inhospitable about the lungs that neuroblasts do not lodge and grow in the pulmonary capillaries. Also, although there is commonly cranial bone involvement and at times extension into the meninges, intracerebral growth of the disease is rare. The sites of metastatic involvement found at autopsy are a little different from those seen clinically. Here, the number with pulmonary metastases is approximately 20%. There does not appear to be any correlation between histological appearance of the primary tumor and the sites of spread. This differs from Wilms' tumor where those with favorable histology tend to metastasize to the lung; the clear cell sarcoma, to bone as well as lung; whereas the rhabdoid variant (if indeed this is a true Wilms' tumor) has a predilection for brain along with lung (3).

Biochemical Activity

Neuroblastoma is an actively secreting tumor. Elevated levels of catecholamines are present in the urine of most patients (31). The commonest products seen are 3 methoxy-4-hydroxy mandelic acid (VMA) and homovanillic acid (HVA). A fuller discussion of the excretion of these two metabolites and their relationship to prognosis is found elsewhere in this volume. If all metabolites are tested, 90% of patients will be found to have secreting tumors. The small number of tumors that are not active are usually histologically primitive and presumably have not developed neurosecretory mechanisms. Voorhess (30) hypothesizes that tumors which arise near the midline are of dorsal root origin and are thus not expected to be catechol excretors.

Opsoclonus

There is an interesting association between the neurologic disorder opsoclonus seen in infants and the presence of neuroblastoma (28). This association is seen with sufficient frequency that any child developing the signs and symptoms should have a careful work-up for neuroblastoma. Since the neurologic disease is thought to be associated with a virus or an autoimmune disorder, Moe and Nellhaus (27) speculate that antigens common to cerebellar nuclei and neural crest structures are involved in antigen-antibody reactions which in turn produce cerebellar dysfunction. They also wonder whether a single virus could initiate both the cerebellar dysfunction and the tumor. This does not seem likely because the cerebellar effect becomes manifest some time after the presumed malignant transformation in the neural crest. The syndrome is probably not directly related to the elevated catecholamines because most neuroblastoma patients have elevated catechol levels but no opsoclonus, nor has an association between pheochromocytoma and opsoclonus been established.

It is interesting to note that children with opsoclonus and neuroblastoma have a good prognosis because the tumor is diagnosed at an early stage (1).

Results of Treatment

The development of an effective therapy for neuroblastoma has provided one of the major frustrations in pediatric oncology. The tumor is responsive to many chemotherapeutic agents and to radiation therapy, and the literature has been full of articles reporting the response of neuroblastoma both to phase II new agents and to multiple drug combinations since the first responses to nitrogen mustard were noted in 1946 (23). Yet the survival rate of these children has changed little if at all. Leikin et al. (25) reported the disappointing similarity in survival statistics in the years 1956 and 1967 for patients with metastatic disease. Perhaps there has been a slight improvement more recently; Finklestein et al. (20) comparing several multi-drug regimens for metastatic disease before and after 1972 show an improved 2-year survival, rising from 5 to 22%. The latter figure must be interpreted with caution since it includes some of the older children mentioned above who are living with disease. Static treatment results also pertain to those with localized disease. Two CCSG studies (11) using chemotherapy as an adjuvant to surgery and irradiation showed no changes in the survival rates, although in the second study more aggressive chemotherapy appeared to prolong the time to relapse slightly.

Why has this disease not followed the path of other pediatric cancers in which responses to treatment have been associated with significant increases in survival? Initially at least, this apparent lack of improvement was probably due to response rates being less than 50% and thus insufficient to influence the median survival; but now, many induction programs lead to response rates in excess of 50%; indeed, 70% has been reported. A combined CCSG and Southwest Oncology Group study of malignant hepatomas (17), by contrast, has yielded a response rate of 38%. This did not significantly affect the patients with more advanced disease, but for those patients in groups 1 and 2 where the chemotherapy could be considered adjuvant, there was a marked improvement in the DFS rates from 45% in control patients to 92% in study patients. Why, then, has this not occurred following treatment for neuroblastoma? Perhaps resistant clones develop early or cell kill is insufficient to prevent recurrence.

UNUSUAL ASPECTS OF NEUROBLASTOMA

Neuroblastoma in Situ

Beckwith and Perrin (4) examined the adrenals of infants dying suddenly of no obvious cause and observed that an unusual number contained nests of neuroblastoma cells. They coined the term "neuroblastoma in situ" to describe this finding (4). If one extrapolates from these necropsy data, the number of infants with neuroblastoma is much higher than that found clinically, the incidence being 40 to 50 times higher, depending on the data used for the calculation. Beckwith and others have proposed that the majority of these small tumors disappear spontaneously and never become manifest clinically. Others have suggested that the findings merely represent primitive adrenal tissue, and that the nests constitute a developmental abnormality rather than a malignant transformation. Beckwith has responded by saying that the tumors invaded the adjacent cortex in all cases reviewed, and that there was blood vessel invasion in some. These appearances are compatible with cancer, he contends, not a malformation of the adrenal tissue.

Maturation

One of the much quoted idiosyncrasies of the neuroblastoma is its ability to transform from the malignant to the benign state, when it looks and behaves like a ganglioneuroma. The classic case of Cushing and Wolbach (9) was the first report of this observation. Maturation can occur both spontaneously and as a result of treatment. It is difficult to determine how often maturation occurs, but it is certainly much less common than spontaneous disappearance of the tumor. The best evidence to substantiate the existence of spontaneous maturation are the reports of ganglioneuromas being found in the lymph nodes of patients at initial diagnosis. These are best explained as being the residue of malignant tumors metastatic to the node, where some change in the local or general environment induced the maturation. The alternate explanation is less likely; viz., that a benign tumor arose in a lymph node *de novo* while a malignant tumor was developing elsewhere. A more common occurrence is maturation following treatment. There is currently an interesting example of this phenomenon at The Children's Hospital of Philadelphia. A child with bone marrow infiltration with clumps of neuroblastoma cells was given cisplatinum. Repeated marrow biopsies thereafter have shown progressively more mature elements, and for the past year, all pathology reports read "ganglioneuroma metastatic to bone marrow." In some biopsies, as many as 75% of the cells seen were mature ganglion cells.

Spontaneous Regression

The most fascinating aspect of this tumor is the occurrence of spontaneous regression. In a monograph by Everson and Cole (18) on the topic, neuroblastoma was the tumor cited most as undergoing spontaneous regression. This is a remarkable fact, considering the low overall incidence of neuroblastoma among cancers of all types. Analysis of Children's Hospital of Philadelphia data shows an overall spontaneous regression rate of 7%. This occurred in both microscopic residual local disease and bulky lesions (15). The two factors that correlated best with spontaneous regression were low age and early stage of disease: 25 of 31 patients with well-documented spontaneous regression were under 1 year of age, 12 had stage II, and 15 had stage IV-S tumors. Spontaneous disappearance of skin nodules and liver tumors is described more often than for the primary site. This may be because most therapists treat the primary site if there is known residual disease.

Stage IV-S

Interest in this special pattern of involvement is based primarily on its known propensity to regress spontaneously (10). It is safe to say that most of these patients, who are usually infants, survive unless they develop some mechanical difficulty because of hepatomegaly, such as respiratory or renal compromise, or a complication of therapy (12). This is not to say that nothing need be done. Some of these patients develop progressive disease that requires some intervention. Rarely, the tumors continue to grow despite irradiation and chemotherapy, and kill. One example of this extraordinary complex will be given to illustrate the vagaries of the IV-S category.

A 6-week-old girl was seen initially in November 1975, because of a greatly enlarged liver. A right adrenal neuroblastoma was excised; and a lesion in the pancreas was noted but not biopsied. The marrow was positive for tumor.

The liver grew slightly for 1 month and extended 12 cm below the right costal margin and 8 cm below the left. No treatment was given; and 6 weeks after diagnosis, the liver started to regress while skin nodules made their appearance. The marrow aspirate was negative. Two lesions became evident in the pleura (one on each side) 3 months after diagnosis. The liver meanwhile continued to regress and skin lesions appeared and regressed. During all this time, there was a marked lymphocytosis with total lymphocyte counts ranging from 8,000 to 12,000/cu mm.

Four more pleural lesions appeared in the ensuing month, so that treatment was instituted with cyclophosphamide. The dose was 10mg/kg/day $\times$ 10 days. After one course, the pleural nodules partially regressed, and they disappeared after the second. No new skin lesions occurred after the initiation of treatment, which was discontinued after two courses. Marrow and liver biopsies at 9 months were negative for tumor as were the urinary catecholamines. At 3 years, she is alive and well, having developed normally.

The two aspects of her course which seem particularly interesting are (1) regression of the liver size while tumor was progressing in a second area—the pleura, and (2) association of non-IV-S sites; pancreatic and pleurae foci did not adversely affect the outcome in this infant who otherwise had the classic stigmata of the IV-S syndrome. The fact that the disease regressed after minor treatment we believe is typical for such patients.

The overall survival of IV-S patients under 1 year of age is 87%, compared with 42% in their age-cohorts with stage IV disease (13). Recently 31 prospectively staged IV-S children were reviewed, and 8 were found to have undergone spontaneous regression of disease distributed among a total of 12 sites. In an additional 6 patients, seven areas of disease, usually marrow, resolved untreated. [All known primary tumors were treated surgically or by irradiation.]

Immune or Host Responses

Host responses to this tumor are discussed in greater detail elsewhere in this volume. Cytotoxic activity of lymphocytes against neuroblastoma has been shown by the Hellstroms and others (21,22), but what is not clear is the role played by tumor-host interactions in the onset, progression, or regression of this neoplasm. It has been reported that tumors containing increased numbers of lymphocytes, and patients demonstrating a lymphocytosis have a better prognosis (5,6). In two studies of localized neuroblastoma conducted by investigators in CCSG, it was not possible to show an association between an initial absolute lymphocyte count greater than 3000/cu mm and an improved prognosis. Children with untreated IV-S neuroblastoma tend to have elevated total lymphocyte counts with numerous atypical or blast forms present (16). Such patients are usually infants, however, so that the high counts may be associated more with age than with a reaction to cancer. To see if the initial lymphocyte count reflected the stage of disease, the charts of 25 children in the first year of life seen at this institution were reviewed. The results given in Table 1 show no obvious

TABLE 1. *Neuroblastoma in infants under 1 year: initial lymphocyte count by stage*

Stage	No.	Total lymphs/mm³ × 10³		
		Mean	Median	Range
I–III	8	5.2	4.6	2.3–12.1
IV	7	5.5	5.6	3.3– 8.1
IV–S	10	7.2	5.6	4.0–16.8

The average count for each stage was elevated compared to that of older children. Thus, although the relative lymphocytosis does not account for the different prognosis between stages, it may be in some way associated with the overall better outcome seen in the young.

association between lymphocytosis and those stages that are predictive of a favorable outcome.

SUMMARY

The important "natural history" aspects of this tumor are that: (a) stage, age, histology, and primary site are prognostic variables; (b) the majority of tumors excrete catecholamines, and the ratio of the end-products relates to the prognosis; (c) multimodal treatment has to date altered survival little if at all; (d) stage O or "in situ" neuroblastoma occurs at a much higher incidence than the clinically diagnosed disease; (e) spontaneous regression occurs in 7% of patients, and less often, maturation to a benign ganglioneuroma; (f) the unusual disease pattern termed IV-S often undergoes spontaneous regression and has a good prognosis.

ACKNOWLEDGMENTS

This work has been supported in part by N.I.H. Grants CA-11796 and CA-14489.

REFERENCES

1. Altman, A. J., and Baehner, R. L. (1976): Favorable prognosis for survival in children with coincident opsomyoclonus and neuroblastoma. *Cancer,* 37:846–852.
2. Beckwith, J. B., and Martin, R. F. (1968): Observations on the histopathology of neuroblastoma. *J. Pediatr. Surg.,* 3:106.
3. Beckwith, J. B., and Palmer, N. F. (1978): Histopathology and prognosis of Wilms' tumor: Results of the First National Wilms' Tumor Study. *Cancer,* 41:1937–1948.
4. Beckwith, J. B., and Perrin, E. V. (1963): In situ neuroblastomas: A contribution to the natural history of neural crest tumors. *Am. J. Pathol.,* 43(6):1089–1100.
5. Bill, A. H. (1969): The implications of immune reactions to neuroblastoma. *Surgery,* 66:415–418.
6. Bill, A. H., and Morgan, A. (1970): Evidence for immune reactions to neuroblastoma and future possibilities for investigation. *J. Pediatr. Surg.,* 5(2):111–116.
7. Breslow, N., and McCann, B. (1971): Statistical estimation of prognosis of children with neuroblastoma. *Cancer Res.,* 31:2101.
8. Castleberry, R. P., Crist, W. M., Cain, W. S., Holbrook, P., and Salter, M. M. (1979): Thoracic neuroblastoma: Prognostic factors and approach to therapy. *Proc. ASCO,* 20:404 (abst. #C-464).
9. Cushing, H., and Wolbach, B. B. (1927): The transformation of a malignant paravertebral sympathicoblastoma into a benign ganglioneuroma. *Am. J. Pathol.,* 3:203–215.
10. D'Angio, G. J., Evans, A. E., and Koop, C. E. (1971): Special pattern of widespread neuroblastoma with a favourable prognosis. *Lancet,* 1:1046–1049.
11. Evans, A. E., Albo, V., D'Angio, G. J., et al. (1976): Cyclophosphamide treatment of patients with localized and regional neuroblastoma. A randomized study. *Cancer,* 38:655–660.
12. Evans, A. E., Chard, R., and Baum, E. (1978): Do children with IV-S neuroblastoma require treatment? *Proc. ASCO,* 19:367 (abst. #C243).
13. Evans, A. E., Chatten, J., D'Angio, G. J., Gerson, J. M., Robinson, J., and Schnaufer, L. (1979): A review of seventeen IV-S neuroblastoma patients at The Children's Hospital of Philadelphia. *Cancer (in press).*

14. Evans, A. E., D'Angio, G. J., and Randolph, J. (1971): A proposed staging for children with neuroblastoma. *Cancer,* 27:374–378.
15. Evans, A. E., Gerson, J., and Schnaufer, L. (1976): Spontaneous regression of neuroblastoma. *Natl. Cancer Inst. Mongr.,* 44:49–54.
16. Evans, A. E., and Hummeler, K. (1973): The significance of primitive cells in marrow aspirates of children with neuroblastoma. *Cancer,* 32:906–912.
17. Evans, A. E., and Land, V. (1979): Multiagent chemotherapy for primary liver tumors in children. *Proc. ASCO,* 20:425 (abst. #C555).
18. Everson, T. C., and Cole, W. H. (1966): *Spontaneous Regression of Cancer,* pp. 11–87. W. B. Saunders Company, Philadelphia.
19. Filler, R. M., Traggis, D. G., Jaffe, N., and Vawter, G. F. (1972): Favorable outlook for children with mediastinal neuroblastoma. *J. Pediatr. Surg.,* 7:136–143.
20. Finklestein, J. Z., Klemperer, M. R., Evans, A. E., et al. (1979): Multiagent chemotherapy for children with metastatic neuroblastoma: A report from the Children's Cancer Study Group. *Med. Pediatr. Oncol.,* 6:179–188.
21. Hellstrom, I., Hellstrom, K. E., Bill, A. H., Pierce, G. E., and Yang, J. P. S. (1970): Studies on cellular immunity to human neuroblastoma cells. *Int. J. Cancer,* 6:172–188.
22. Hellstrom, I., Hellstrom, K. E., Pierce, G. E., et al. (1968): Demonstration of cell bound and humoral immunity against neuroblastoma cells. *Proc. Natl. Acad. Sci. U.S.A.,* 60:1231–1238.
23. Jacobson, L. O., Spurr, C. L., Barron, E. S. G., et al. (1946): Nitrogen mustard therapy. *J.A.M.A.,* 132:263–271.
24. Leape, L. L., Lowman, J. T., and Loveland, G. C. (1978): Multifocal nondisseminated neuroblastoma. *J. Pediatr.,* 92(1):75–77.
25. Leiken, S., Evans, A. E., Heyn, R., and Newton, W. (1974): The impact of chemotherapy on advanced neuroblastoma. Survival of patients diagnosed in 1956, 1962, and 1966–68 in Children's Cancer Study Group A. *J. Pediatr.,* 84:131–134.
26. MacKay, B., Luna, M. A., and Butler, J. J. (1976): Adult neuroblastoma. Electron microscopic observations in nine cases. *Cancer,* 37:1334–1351.
27. Moe, P. G., and Nellhaus, G. (1970): Infantile polymyoclonia opsoclonus syndrome and neural crest tumor. *Neurology (Minneap.),* 20:756–764.
28. Solomon, G. E., and Chutorian, A. M. (1968): Opsoclonus and occult neuroblastoma. *N. Engl. J. Med.,* 279:475–477.
29. Virchow, R. (1865): Hyperplasie der Zirbel und der Nebenniern, *Die Krankhaften Geschwulste,* Vol. 11, pp. 149–150. August Hirshwald, Berlin.
30. Voorhess, M. L. (1971): Neuroblastoma with normal urinary catecholamine excretion. *J. Pediatr.,* 78:680–683.
31. Voorhess, M. L., and Gardner, L. S. (1961): Urinary excretion of norepinephrine and 3-methoxy-4-hydroxy mandelic acid by children with neuroblastoma. *J. Clin. Endocrinol. Metab.,* 21:321–335.
32. Wright, J. H. (1910): Neurocytoma or neuroblastoma, a kind of tumor not generally recognized. *J. Exp. Med.,* 12:556–561.

Advances in Neuroblastoma Research,
edited by Audrey E. Evans.
Raven Press, New York © 1980.

The Neurocristopathy Concept: Fact or Fiction

R. Neil Schimke

*Division of Metabolism, Endocrinology and Genetics, Kansas University Hospital,
Kansas City, Kansas 66103*

More than a century has elapsed since His first described the avian neural crest. His' pioneering investigation firmly established that the autonomic nervous system was derived from this tissue, a conclusion repeatedly confirmed over the intervening years. Later workers, notably Weston (29) and Pearse (19) have determined that the neural crest plays an extensive role in development, contributing wholly or in part to a variety of seemingly disparate tissues (Table 1). Not surprisingly, disordered development in the neural crest has been found to result in a number of clinical diseases, collectively referred to as neurocristopathies by Bolande (3). As the neural crest is embryologically almost ubiquitous, the use of the term usually has been confined to neoplastic alterations in the various derivatives (Table 2), since to do otherwise would render the concept too inclusive and therefore meaningless; e.g., strictly speaking, all facial cleft syndromes, of which there are many, would have to be considered neurocristopathies, since the membranous bones of the face ultimately come from the neural crest. Even with this restriction, there is some question as to how many of the tabulated conditions are actually pure, in the sense of involving neural crest development only. For example, although some components of the three recognized multiple endocrine neoplasia syndromes are clearly derived from neural crest—e.g., pheochromocytoma, medullary thyroid carcinoma—others such as the pancreatic islets and the parathyroid glands are likely not (22). By the same token, von Recklinghausen's disease certainly includes some elements that originate in the neural crest, but all the myriad facets of this condition cannot be easily fitted into this mold, particularly in light of the recently uncovered complex neoplastic potential of this syndrome (Fig. 1). In the final analysis,

TABLE 1. *Currently accepted derivatives of the neural crest*

Melanoblasts	Schwann cells
Autonomic, spinal, and some cranial ganglia	Some glial cells
	Part of the meninges
Paraganglia	Thyroid C cells
Odontoblasts	Adrenal medulla
Membranous bones	

TABLE 2. *Neurocristopathic conditions*

Neuroblastoma
Pheochromocytoma
Paraganglioma
Medullary thyroid carcinoma
Carcinoid
Melanoma
Neurocutaneous melanosis
Neurofibromatosis
Multiple endocrine neoplasias

perhaps if the term neurocristopathy is to be retained, it should be used in a restricted sense in conjunction with those conditions in which the tissue of origin of the tumor is not in doubt. Classic examples of such neoplasms pertinent to this volume include neuroblastomas and pheochromocytomas.

NEUROBLASTOMA

Roughly one in 10,000 live-born infants have or will develop one or more neuroblastomas. The tumors may be located in the adrenal or in the paravertebral area in conjunction with the autonomic ganglia. The presenting features and natural history of this tumor are dealt with elsewhere in this volume. Therapy has not been as effective when compared with that used with the other major embryonal neoplasms. In one series of approximately 500 patients, less than 25% survived 3 years (30). Thereafter, mortality tended to remain unchanged probably because of the tendency of the tumor to undergo maturation to ganglioneuroma or ganglioneurofibroma. Autopsy studies have suggested that *in situ*

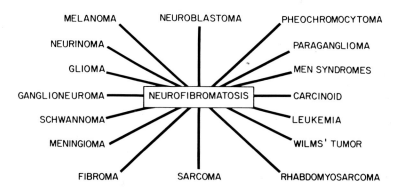

THE MALIGNANT FACE OF VON RECKLINGHAUSEN'S DISEASE

FIG. 1. Some neoplasms found to be significantly associated with von Recklinghausen's disease.

lesions are up to 50 times more common than the clinical disease, indicating that the tumor must undergo spontaneous regression a substantial part of the time (3). In addition to cytodifferentiation, tumor regression also occurs by cytolysis, perhaps on an immune basis, and hemorrhagic necrosis with dystrophic calcification. Late recurrences, even as long as 15 years after apparent cure, have been documented, although rarely (7).

Heritable Component of Neuroblastoma

The older literature tended to minimize the operation of genetic factors in the pathogenesis of neuroblastoma, despite the existence of scattered reports documenting familial aggregation. With earlier detection and some improvement in therapy, such reports are becoming somewhat more numerous. Knudson and Meadows (12) have summarized the current evidence in regard to the genetics of neuroblastoma elsewhere. The available family data are consistent with the postulate that, when heritable, the potential to develop neuroblastoma is inherited as an autosomal dominant trait with intermediate penetrance. The actual degree of penetrance may be nearly impossible to determine in view of two aforementioned factors: poor survival and spontaneous regression/maturation.

It is obviously of considerable importance to establish, first of all, which neuroblastomas are heritable, and second, if there exist criteria by which genetic tumors can be distinguished from the sporadic lesions. In general, it is known that inherited tumors occur at an earlier average age, and that they tend to be multifocal. Although these attributes of heritable tumors should apply to neuroblastoma, some difficulties arise, as patients with numerous tumors may have either multiple primaries or widely disseminated disease (stage IV). Some children with multiple tumors die in a very brief period of time because of disease, and for practical purposes have true stage IV disease. Others seem to have a better prognosis and are subclassified as IV-S. The usual clinical findings in the IV-S patients include small, frequently bilateral adrenal tumors with additional tumor nodules in liver, skin, and bone marrow. A recent report from The Children's Hospital in Philadelphia identified 17 such patients, six of whom had spontaneous regression of their tumor with neither chemotherapy nor irradiation (4). Six of the remaining patients died, but for the most part, it was difficult to ascertain whether the tumor or complications of therapy were responsible. In two of the six cases, the tumor so massively involved the liver that asphyxia was the likely cause of death, i.e., the deaths might be attributable to physical rather than physiologic factors. The ages of the 11 survivors ranged from 2 years to 33 years. None of the patients had a positive family history. However, Leape et al. (13) recently reported two brothers who presented with multifocal nondisseminated neuroblastoma who were treated conservatively; neither child had evidence of disease 4 years later. These authors reviewed the reports of similar cases and found that not only did all of them have a positive family history, but the clinical course of all the patients was relatively benign and not that expected of patients with disseminated disease.

It has been suggested that the gene mutation that gives rise to genetic neuroblastoma retards the usual tendency of the tumor to undergo spontaneous regression (12). A natural corollary to this hypothesis could be that inherited disease is more aggressive disease. Yet the lack of penetrance in most reported families, the evidence of tumor maturation in others, and the possibility that the gene defect may present initially in a benign fashion as Hirschsprung's disease or heterochromia all argue against such a supposition. In fact, genetic neuroblastoma may be relatively benign as indicated by the report of Leape et al. Moreover, in view of the clinical behavior of the tumor in patients with stage IV-S disease, it is not unreasonable to postulate that at least some of them have genetic neuroblastoma, despite the absence of a positive family history; i.e., they actually have multifocal rather than disseminated disease. To my knowledge, no systematic studies have been undertaken in the relatives of patients with IV-S disease to evaluate this possibility.

Problem of Multifocal Versus Disseminated Disease

Why some children with presumed IV-S disease do poorly while others do not is not known. As noted earlier, the physical effects of tumor mass or complications of therapy are obvious reasons. It would also be of considerable interest to correlate disease severity with perinatal factors including duration of labor, evidence of fetal distress, hypoxia, and low Apgar scores; with infant size and overall proportions, especially seeking mild degrees of asymmetry; and with gestational factors such as general maternal infection or drug ingestion. For example, two children with neuroblastoma and one with ganglioneuroblastoma have been described whose tumor may have been a complication of the fetal hydantoin syndrome (24). Obstetrical X-rays have already been suggestively incriminated (28).

In addition, it would be worthwhile to compare the cytogenetic findings from the tumors of patients with IV-S disease with those of children who have apparently sporadic disease with or without bone metastases. Differences in the incidence of chromosome breakage either spontaneous or in response to *in vitro* irradiation might provide a clue to underlying differences in tumor behavior. If available, tumors from patients with a definitely positive family history should be scrutinized with care. Genetic markers that may provide information on the clonal origin of the tumor might be employed. For example, two hereditary diseases, neurofibromatosis and multiple trichoepitheliomas, have been found to be multiclonal in origin in contrast to isolated neurofibromas or other acquired neuroplastic conditions such as chronic myelogenous leukemia (6). Another tumor derived from neural crest, medullary thyroid carcinoma, taken from patients with MEN type II, has recently been studied using glucose-6-phosphate dehydrogenase (G6PD) markers (2). Discrete tumor nodules from different areas in the affected thyroid gland showed either the A or B phenotype, indicating that the inherited mutation resulted in the production of multiple clones of cells susceptible to neoplastic change. Earlier studies of cells from a single thyroid tumor nodule and from a pheochromocytoma from only one patient suggested that both tumors were derived from only a single clone—hence the necessity of evaluating a number of such patients (1). Although the evidence is only suggestive, it is possible that hereditary tumors may be generally multiclonal. If tumors from patients with IV-S disease showed the same phenomenon, it would further support the contention that this form of neuroblastoma is also genetic.

Other studies that might be performed are shown in Table 3. Again, it must be emphasized that the tendency to pool the results from all neuroblastoma patients may well obscure underlying heterogeneity. Patients need to be carefully selected and perhaps a more extensive classification system devised to avoid this pitfall. It seems likely that neuroblastoma patients who have other congenital abnormalities could well have one or more chromosome anomalies in peripheral blood lymphocytes. Such has been found in some children with a retinoblastoma malformation syndrome (13q-) and in others with the Wilms' tumor-aniridia complex (11p-) (20,31). With both these embryonal tumors, the initial work suggests that the respective chromosomal regions containing the mutant genes may be readily locatable; e.g., a large deletion may give rise to retinoblastoma plus various anomalies, whereas a small one could result only in loss of that gene or those closely linked genes responsible for normal retinal differentiation. No specific pattern of congenital defects associated with neuroblastomas has yet been uncovered (17); however, this type of investigation should be pursued in some depth.

TABLE 3. *Features possibly useful in differentiating heritable from non-heritable neuroblastoma*

Cytogenetic studies
  Routine tumor karyotype
  Response to mutagens
  Sister chromatid exchange
Serologic markers
  Embryonic antigens
  Circulating growth-promoting factors
  HLA subtypes
Tissue culture
  Clonal markers
  Response to nerve growth factor
  Presence of NGF receptors
  Interaction with T and B cells
Other
  Immune profile of patients
    exhibiting spontaneous regression
  Careful search for congenital anomalies

Careful study should be made of patients under 1 year of age, who at the time of initial study are classified as stage I and within a few months develop lesions elsewhere, especially when these appear in the opposite adrenal or in the liver. It is possible that some of these children could be better classed as IV-S patients, the tumor development not being synchronous. There is precedence for this phenomenon in, for example, the MEN syndromes (22). Although therapy cannot at present be legitimately withheld from such patients, detailed history of their progress will be of considerable interest.

Long-Term Prognosis in Neuroblastoma

With improved therapy for all embryonal neoplasms has come the realization that second tumors develop with considerable frequency. One review of 36 patients revealed a 12% incidence of second tumors, all but one of which arose in tissues previously irradiated (14). Six of these children had neuroblastoma. Second tumor types in this group included thyroid carcinoma (2), basal cell carcinoma, osteogenic sarcoma, glioma, and renal cell carcinoma. In another larger series, 70 or 102 second malignancies developed in irradiated sites 5 months to 24 years post-therapy, but in one group of 21 patients neither radiation treatment nor genetic predisposition (familial retinoblastoma, neurofibromatosis, basal cell nevus syndrome, xeroderma pigmentosum) could be recognizably implicated (15). Knudson's two-hit hypothesis was originally conceived in the context of a single tissue which was directly at risk for malignancy because of a germinal mutation (11). Data from retinoblastoma survivors suggest an undue frequency of late-appearing osteosarcomas, both within and outside the radiation field (9). Most retinoblastoma patients who develop a second malignancy either have a positive family history or have bilateral, and hence by accepted definition, genetic disease (23).

Survival of patients with neuroblastoma has not been sufficiently prolonged for statistical assessment of the incidence of distinct "second-hit" malignancies whether the primary tumor is familial or not. If the original germinal mutation is pleiotropic and includes tissues other than neural crest, one might postulate that the greatest risk of second malignancies would be in patients with heritable neuroblastoma. This reasoning would apply whether or not the patients had recognizable genetic disease, i.e., some could be new mutations, others could be members of families harboring new, or perhaps better, hitherto unrecognized cancer syndromes (15). Particular attention should be paid to neuroblastoma patients who develop nonradiogenic malignancies and to their first-degree relatives. Current data would suggest that at least one type of cancer family syndrome does exist which includes among other tumors embryonal malignancies including neuroblastomas (23). It would be of considerable interest to study the families of patients with stage IV-S disease, looking for malignancies exclusive of the neural crest derivatives. It is conceivable that the neuroblastoma gene mutation might remain totally unexpressed until adult life, when an entirely different pattern of malignancy might occur. Exactly what type of adult malignancies might appear is difficult to predict, but one might expect an excess of those tumor types already reported as second malignant neoplasms in patients with neuroblastoma *(vide supra)*. A brief case report might usefully serve to illustrate the possibilities (5).

Case Report

A 26-year-old woman was first seen at the Kansas University Hospital at age 9 months for an abdominal mass which proved to be a neuroblastoma originating in the left para-aortic region near the bifurcation. The tumor was totally removed, no metastases were noted, and she received postoperative radiation therapy to the tumor bed. She was well until age 16 when readmission was necessitated by intractable headaches, left-sided seizures, and transient left hemiparesis. Her blood pressure was 145/120 and there was persistent tachycardia. Cerebral arteriograms showed no abnormalities, but an IVP revealed a calcified mass contiguous with the right kidney and a 24-hr urine VMA was markedly elevated. At laparotomy she was found to have an extra-adrenal tumor mass overlying the hilum of the right kidney to such an extent that total nephrectomy and partial adrenalectomy were necessary. Histologically, the tumor was a pheochromocytoma.

Over the next few years repeat urine VMA determinations were borderline and her diastolic blood pressure ranged between 90 and 100 mm Hg. At age 21 her diastolic pressure increased to 110 mm Hg, tachycardia recurred, and the VMA became clearly elevated. A liver scan showed a defect in the right lobe which was found to be highly vascular on arteriography. Hepatic wedge resection was performed and the lesion was identified as a pheochromocytoma. The left kidney, the right nephrectomy site, and the retroperitoneal area were visually examined at the time of surgery and were found to be normal. Abdominal lymph node biopsy revealed no evidence of metastatic disease. Postoperatively her blood pressure declined to normal, and over the next 4 years repeated VMA determinations were normal. When she was 24 a mass in her thyroid was detected and the possibility of MEN II was considered. The lesion was found to be a colloid nodule. At age 26, however, her pressure again rose, the urine VMA doubled, and repeat arteriography showed multiple areas of neovascularization both in the liver and in the remaining left kidney. Two of the accessible hepatic lesions were resected and were found to be pheochromocytomas. There were five separate lesions in the left kidney; all were hypernephromas. The kidney was removed and she is currently on chronic hemodialysis. An extensive metastatic survey performed prior to nephrectomy was negative.

To my knowledge this is the first description of neuroblastoma and pheochromocytoma occurring as discrete tumors, although a few early reports did note combined elements of both in a single lesion. The interesting feature of the case is the large time lapse between the detection of neuroblastoma and pheochromocytoma. One might postulate that the pheochromocytoma was metastatic to the liver at the time of initial detection, but for the patient to survive 10 years without evidence of more extensive disease would be distinctly unusual. It seems more likely that she had multiple primary foci of partially differentiated neural crest tissue in her liver that lay dormant for many years before the "second hit" triggered further differentiation, function, and hence detection.

The patient's family was extensively investigated and no abnormalities were found. In spite of this, I believe this patient has genetic disease and actually represents an extreme example of what is now termed stage IV-S neuroblastoma. The patients reported by Jaffe (7) who had so-called late recurrences of neuroblastoma may represent the same phenomenon. The hypernephromas could represent the late sequelae of irradiation received 25 years earlier. However, even if one accepts that explanation at face value, it is still necessary to account for the multiplicity of the renal lesions. It is quite possible that the kidney in this patient suffered from the same germinal mutation that affected the neural crest with either the earlier irradiation triggering eventual malignancy after a long latent period, or a "second hit," type unknown, stimulating neoplastic deterioration.

As noted previously, both hypernephroma and thyroid carcinoma have been described as second malignancies in patients with neuroblastomas. A number of thyroid nonmalignant nodules were reported, almost incidentally, in a series of patients with neuroblastoma studied as part of an earlier epidemiologic study (17). Furthermore, nonmedullary thyroid cancer has also been described as part of the same cancer family syndrome that includes neuroblastoma (23). Perhaps the thyroid and the kidney are two additional tissues that can suffer the potential ravages of the germinal mutation that leads to neuroblastoma in children; i.e., genetic neuroblastoma is not a "pure" neurocristopathy after all. If this hypothesis is correct, and indeed if patients with stage IV-S disease have genetic disease that is generally more benign and prone to spontaneous regression, it would be appropriate to avoid radiation and/or chemotherapy insofar as possible in order to minimize the risk of subsequent malignancy. Obviously, detailed longitudinal study will be required to either verify or refute these speculations.

PHEOCHROMOCYTOMA

Another neoplastic alteration in neural crest is the pheochromocytoma. This tumor is uncommon in childhood (about 10% of all cases), as it usually becomes clinically evident in the third decade or later (16). The incidence of pheochromocytoma has been estimated at approximately 1 per 1,000 individuals of both sexes, but the figure may be higher in a hypertensive population. The clinical symptomatology is well known and will not be recounted here; however, a few pertinent differences between the tumor in adults and in children are worthy of note (27). The associated hypertension is more likely to be sustained in children, the tumors are frequently extra-adrenal, and multiple tumors are more common with early-onset disease.

It has been estimated that about 20% of all pheochromocytomas are heritable, occurring in familial aggregates as an isolated tumor type, and with MEN II and III (10). They also develop occasionally in patients with neurofibromatosis and with von Hippel-Lindau syndrome. Each of these entities is a distinct autosomal dominant disorder, and in the first three conditions, the tumors are usually bilateral and often extra-adrenal. The overall incidence of true malignancy in the sense of metastasis is difficult to estimate because of the diffuse migratory behavior of the neural crest cells, but a figure of 10% would seem a reasonable approximation. A recent series of 107 tumors showed that only 2.4% of intra-adrenal lesions exhibited malignant behavior, whereas some 30% of extra-adrenal tumors did so (16). Whether familial tumors are more likely to become malignant is not known.

The recent literature provides evidence that pheochromocytoma, like neuroblastoma, is not always a simple neurocristopathy. Although the adrenal medulla itself is clearly of neural crest origin, many of the other tumors seen in greater than expected frequency with pheochromocytomas are not generally recognized as arising from this tissue (Fig. 2). The association of medullary thyroid carcinoma as in MEN II and III, or of neuroblastoma, neurofibroma, or paraganglioma with pheochromocytoma is not surprising in view of the common embryologic origin. The presence of pheochromocytoma in patients with the von Hippel-Lindau disease is less easy to explain from this limited developmental point of view. About 20% of patients with this syndrome suffer from hypernephromas, and sporadic cases of pheochromocytoma and hypernephroma also have been described. Curiously enough, one of the first collections of such cases was recorded by Sipple (26) in the same paper in which he noted the association of pheochromocytoma and thyroid carcinoma. The hemangioblastomas of the central nervous system characteristic of von Hippel-Lindau syndrome may be mistaken for metastatic renal cell carcinoma on frozen section, and on one occasion such an initial error led to the diagnosis of an asymptomatic hypernephroma in the index case of a von Hippel-Lindau family (21). It is conceivable that there is a fundamental relationship between oncogenesis in the neural crest

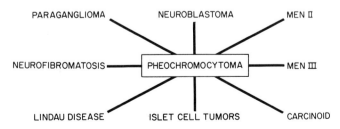

FIG. 2. Pheochromocytoma and its various associations.

and the metanephric blastema, the case report described earlier perhaps providing some additional evidence in this regard.

Carcinoid tumors likewise have been sporadically recorded with pheochromocytoma, but some workers feel that the carcinoid cell is directly descended from neural crest. Others, notably Pearse (19) and co-workers, contend that although the carcinoid tumor is composed of cells of the APUD series, it is ultimately derived from what he calls neuroendocrine-programed ectoblast. The pancreatic islet cells also reputedly come from this source, and it is noteworthy that pheochromocytomas have been recorded with islet cell tumors more frequently than would be expected by chance, at least once on a familial basis (Fig 3) (8). Parenthetically, an infant having congenital neuroblastoma and islet cell hyperplasia with intractable hypoglycemia also has been described (25). Both carcinoid and islet cell tumors are integral parts of MEN I, whereas pheochromocytoma is a component of the other two heritable endocrine tumor syndromes. Although in general the MEN syndromes can be considered as distinctive, there are obvious areas of known overlap; e.g., hyperparathyroidism. The family depicted in Fig. 3 might be an overlap family, for want of a better term. The findings in such a family do not necessarily imply any sort of basic relationship between MEN I and II, nor do they indicate that all the requisite tumors must come from neural crest as some clinicians would insist; certainly, there are substantive data to the contrary insofar as pancreatic islet cells are concerned. Moreoever, Odell and Wolfsen (18) have marshalled considerable evidence in support of the theory that virtually all neoplastic cells have the ability to elaborate peptides, only a few of which are biologically active in the production of hormonal syndromes. In other words, the tendency to become an APUD cell may be inherent in all malignant tissues, with the functional capacity dependent on the degree of dedifferentiation.

The pheochromocytomal-islet cell tumor family may provide evidence for the existence of a whole series of "endocrine tumor" genes that have some phenotypic features in common. A number of mutations early in embryogenesis could give rise to multiple clones of cells with malignant potential as exemplified by the various syndromes of colon polyposis. The various mutations would be

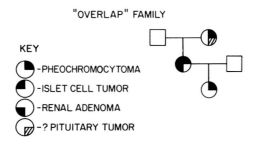

FIG. 3. A family showing both pheochromocytoma and islet cell tumors in a pattern consistent with autosomal dominant inheritance. Pedigree modified from ref. 8.

different, but perhaps only relatively restrictive in the sense that a single endocrine organ could undergo neoplastic change as the result of a variety of genetic insults. Some of the mutations might well involve other nonendocrine tissue, as appears true in the Gardner syndrome, to extend the polyposis analogy further. One member of the family shown in Fig. 3 had at least two renal adenomas in addition to bilateral pheochromocytomas and multiple islet cell lesions. Since pheochromocytomas are almost invariably treated surgically, the occurrence of a hypernephroma as a second tumor in such patients could hardly be considered a complication of therapy. Again, one is inclined toward the conclusion that more than a single embryonic tissue is unduly susceptible to malignancy in patients who develop tumors of the neural crest system. More specifically, it is possible that those sensitized tissues may be present only in individuals who have a genetic tumor syndrome.

CONCLUSIONS

It is apparent that the entire neurocristopathy concept has already undergone and will continue to undergo considerable modification. A "pure" syndrome totally due to neural crest malfunction may not exist; perhaps in the final analysis the term will be rejected in favor of more precise descriptive terminology. Nonetheless, tumors of neural crest tissue certainly exist as evidenced by neuroblastoma and pheochromocytoma, and a substantial portion of these are due to mutant genes. Data concerning the proportion of neuroblastomas that are heritable are scanty, but there is reason to believe that stage IV-S patients may have genetic disease. Moreover, this subclass may have tumors that are relatively benign in the sense that only surgical therapy is necessary except in unusual circumstances. This same group of patients may have the greatest risk of other malignancies later in life and the development of these second tumors may be accelerated by the overzealous use of radiation or chemotherapy. Similarly, the spectrum of conditions associated with pheochromocytoma has been considerably broadened in recent years and second tumors might be anticipated, especially in patients who are affected while comparatively young. The types of second tumors to be expected may eventually conform to a pattern predictively useful. More explicit study of both these neural crest tumors, particularly the hereditary varieties, may provide considerable insight in the mechanism and scope of genetic oncogenesis. Hard data, both from the laboratory and from epidemiological surveys, are urgently needed.

REFERENCES

1. Baylin, S. B., Gann, D. S., and Hsu, S. H. (1976): Clonal origin of inherited medullary thyroid carcinoma and pheochromocytoma. *Science,* 193:321–323.
2. Baylin, S. B., Hsu, S. H., and Gann, D. S. (1978): Inherited medullary thyroid carcinoma: A final monoclonal mutation in one of multiple clones of susceptible cells. *Science,* 199:429–431.
3. Bolande, R. P. (1974): The neurocristopathies. *Hum. Pathol.,* 5:409–429.
4. Evans, A. E., Chatten, J., D'Angio, G. J., Gerson, J. M., Robinson, J., and Schnaufer, L.

(1979): Review of seventeen IV-S neuroblastoma patients at The Children's Hospital of Philadelphia. *Cancer* (in press).

5. Fairchild, R. S., Kyner, J. L., Hermreck, A., and Schimke, R. N. (1979): Neuroblastoma, pheochromocytoma, and renal cell carcinoma occurring in a single patient. *J. Am. Med. Assoc.,* 242:2210–2211.

6. Fialkow, P. J. (1977): Clonal origin and stem cell evolution of human tumors. In: *Genetics of Human Cancer,* edited by J. J. Mulvihill, R. W. Miller, and J. F. Fraumeni, Jr., pp. 439–453. Raven Press, New York.

7. Jaffe, N. (1976): Recrudescence of neuroblastoma after apparent cure. *J. Natl. Cancer Inst.,* 57:731–732.

8. Janson, K. L., Roberts, J. A., and Varela, M. (1978): Multiple endocrine adenomatosis: In support of the common origin theories. *J. Urol.,* 119:161–165.

9. Kitchen, F. O., and Ellsworth, R. M. (1974): Pleiotropic effects of the gene for retinoblastoma. *J. Med. Genet.,* 11:244–246.

10. Knudson, A. G., Jr., and Strong, L. C. (1972): Mutation and cancer: Neuroblastoma and pheochromocytoma. *Am. J. Hum. Genet.,* 24:514–532.

11. Knudson, A. G. (1973): Mutation and human cancer. *Adv. Cancer Res.,* 17:317–352.

12. Knudson, A. G., Jr., and Meadows, A. T. (1976): Developmental genetics of neuroblastoma. *J. Natl. Cancer Inst.,* 57:675–682.

13. Leape, L. L., Lowman, J. T., and Loveland, G. C. (1978): Multifocal nondisseminated neuroblastoma. *J. Pediatr.,* 92:75–77.

14. Li, F. P. (1977): Second malignant tumors after cancer in childhood. *Cancer [Suppl.],* 40:1899–1902.

15. Meadows, A. T., D'Angio, G. J., Miké, V., Banfi, A., Harris, C., Jenkin, R. D. T., and Schwartz, A. (1977): Patterns of second malignant neoplasms in children. *Cancer [Suppl.],* 40:1903–1911.

16. Melicow, M. M. (1977): One hundred cases of pheochromocytoma (107 tumors) at the Columbia-Presbyterian Medical Center, 1926–1976. *Cancer,* 40:1987–2004.

17. Miller, R. W., Fraumeni, J. F., Jr., and Hall, J. A. (1968): Neuroblastoma: Epidemiologic approach to its origin. *Am. J. Dis. Child.,* 115:253–257.

18. Odell, W. D., and Wolfsen, A. R. (1978): Humoral syndromes associated with cancer. *Annu. Rev. Med.,* 29:379–406.

19. Pearse, A. G. E. (1977): The diffuse neuroendocrine system and the APUD concept: Related "endocrine" peptides in brains, intestine, pituitary, placenta and anuran cutaneous glands. *Med. Biol.,* 55:115–125.

20. Riccardi, V. M., Sujansky, E., Smith, A. C., and Franke, U. (1975): Chromosomal imbalance in the aniridia-Wilms' tumor association: llp interstitial deletion. *Pediatrics,* 61:604–610.

21. Richards, R. D., Mebust, W. K., and Schimke, R. N. (1973): A prospective study in von Hippel-Lindau disease. *J. Urol.,* 110:27–30.

22. Schimke, R. N. (1977): Tumors of the neural crest system. In: *Genetics of Human Cancer,* edited by J. J. Mulvihill, R. W. Miller, and J. F. Fraumeni, Jr., pp. 179–198. Raven Press, New York.

23. Schimke, R. N. (1978): *Genetics and Cancer in Man,* pp. 13–25. Churchill Livingstone, Edinburgh.

24. Seeler, R. A., Isreal, J. N., Royal, J. E., Kaye, C. I., Rao, S., and Abulabam, M. (1979): Ganglioneuroblastoma and fetal hydantoin-alcohol syndromes. *Pediatrics,* 63:524–527.

25. Shuangshoti, S., and Ekaraphanich, S. (1972): Congenital neuroblastomas and hyperplasia of islets of Langerhans in an infant. *Clin. Pediatr.,* 11:241–243.

26. Sipple, J. H. (1961): The association of pheochromocytoma with carcinoma of the thyroid gland. *Am. J. Med.,* 31:163–166.

27. Stackpole, R. H., Melicow, M. M., and Uson, A. C. (1963): Pheochromocytoma in children. *J. Pediatr.,* 63:315–330.

28. Stewart, A. M., and Kneale, G. W. (1970): Age-distribution of cancer caused by obstetric x-rays and their relevance to cancer latent periods. *Lancet,* 2:4–8.

29. Weston, J. A. (1970): The migration and differentiation of neural crest cells. *Adv. Morphol.,* 8:41–114.

30. Wilson, L. M., and Draper, E. J. (1974): Neuroblastoma, its natural history and prognosis: A study of 487 cases. *Br. Med. J.,* 3:301–307.

31. Yunis, J. J. (1978): Retinoblastoma and subband deletion of chromosome 13. *Am. J. Dis. Child.,* 132:161–163.

Advances in Neuroblastoma Research,
edited by Audrey E. Evans.
Raven Press, New York © 1980.

Patterns of Urinary Catecholamine Metabolite Excretion in Neuroblastoma

Stuart E. Siegel, Walter E. Laug, Paul J. Harlow, Kenneth N. F. Shaw, Benjamin Landing, and Morris Gutenstein

Departments of Pediatrics, Biochemistry and Pathology, University of Southern California School of Medicine; Department of Medicine, Divisions of Hematology-Oncology and Medical Genetics, and the Department of Pathology, Children's Hospital of Los Angeles, Los Angeles, California 90027

Tumors of neural crest origin, including neuroblastoma, commonly produce increased quantities of catecholamines and their metabolites which are detectable in urine and serum samples from patients with these malignancies (4–8). The relative ease of obtaining urine samples and the standardization of assay techniques have led to the use of these biological markers for diagnosis and monitoring of tumor response (5–8).

Several recent studies have suggested that the pattern of pretreatment urinary excretion of metabolites catecholamine may be of prognostic significance in patients with metastatic disease (5,8,12). At present, age and stage of disease at diagnosis remain the key "front-end" prognostic determinants (3,5,9). Unfortunately, a majority of children with neuroblastoma present with disseminated disease and only 20 to 30% of these survive 2 years from diagnosis (3,5,9). Gitlow et al. (5) found a significant correlation between good prognosis and lower initial levels of urinary homovanillic acid (HVA), and both they and LaBrosse (6) and co-workers noted the association of a good prognosis with a rapid return of catecholamine metabolism to normal with therapy. They did not, however, separate patients with localized disease from those with metastatic disease at onset (i.e., by stage of disease). Recently we reported that a favorable prognosis in disseminated neuroblastoma (stage IV) was associated with a higher ratio of vanilmandelic acid (VMA) to HVA, but not with the absolute levels of these metabolites (8). On the other hand, the presence of the DOPA metabolite vanillactic acid (VLA) correlated with a poor prognosis. A simplified schema for the synthesis of the catecholamines and their major metabolites indicating those measured in our studies is shown in Fig. 1. On the basis of the data from this analysis of initial urinary excretion patterns, we suggested that biochemically primitive neuroblastomas may be more virulent biologically than their more mature counterparts and that the biochemical excretion pattern of the tumor could be utilized to further define the "front-end" prognosis for children with disseminated disease.

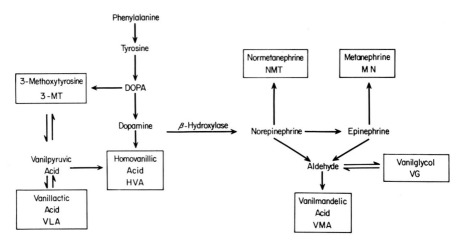

FIG. 1. Simplified schema for catecholamine metabolism in neuroblastoma. Framed metabolites represent compounds measured in our studies (Laug et al. 8).

The present chapter will further investigate this association in a larger series of patients as well as explore serial changes in urinary catecholamine metabolite excretion during therapy.

MATERIALS AND METHODS

These studies are based on a population of 113 children with histologically proven neuroblastoma seen at the Children's Hospital of Los Angeles from 1964 to 1978. The clinical and pathological correlates with known "front-end" factors for this study group have been reported previously (8).

Eighty of these patients had evaluation of urinary catecholamine metabolites prior to therapy. Single-voided urine specimens were obtained without prior dietary restrictions and metabolites measured by two-dimensional paper chromatography included vanilmandelic acid, homovanillic acid, vanilglycol (VG), normetanephrine (NMN), vanillactic acid, and 3-methoxytyrosine (3-MT) (8,11). All measurements were recorded in milligrams of metabolite per gram of urinary creatinine. Samples were chromatographed in replicate with a graded series of synthetic standards. The levels of VMA and HVA were then normalized by expressing them as multiples of the maximal normal value for the age of the patient. The maximum normal values for these compounds are shown in Table 1 and were obtained by evaluating single-voided urine samples from 150 healthy children ages 1 day to 15 years by the same methods. Since 3-MT and VLA are not normally detected in the urine of healthy children, only the presence (+) or absence (−) of these compounds is indicated in this chapter.

Serial urinary catecholamine metabolite determinations were available for 47 of these patients. All studies obtained following the pretreatment determination

TABLE 1. *Age-related maximum normal values for VMA and HVA*[a]

Age (Year)	VMA	HVA
0	12	16
0.5	10	14.5
1.0	8	13
1.5	6	11.5
2.0	4	10
> 2.0	3.5	9

[a] Values are expressed in milligrams per gram of urinary creatinine. From Laug et al. (8).

were derived from single-voided specimens collected after 48 hr of dietary restriction to eliminate competing materials, e.g., bananas, chocolate, vanilla, and nuts.

RESULTS

Clinical and Pathological "Front-End" Factors

Age and stage of disease at diagnosis by criteria of Evans et al. (3) continue to be the most important *independent* "front-end" clinical prognostic factors (Table 2). As in other large series, the majority of patients (57%) presented with stage IV disease and only 20% of these patients survived 2 years from diagnosis. Patients with stages I, II, and IV-S disease had a particularly

TABLE 2. *Relationship of survival to sex, age, and stage (N= 113)*

Characteristic	No. of patients	1-Year survival (%)	2-Year survival (%)
Sex			
M	54	51	42
F	59	57	47
Age (years)			
0–1	29	86	83
1–2	24	61	47
2–3	24	29	12
3–4	12	52	17
3–5	6	50	50
5+	18	61	44
Stage[a]			
I	9	100	100
II	16	100	91
III	12	66	37
IV	65	38	19
IV-S	10	100	100
(Stage unknown	1)		

[a] According to the criteria of Evans et al. (3).

good prognosis. All patients with stages I and IV-S disease in this series survived 2 years and all remain alive with a follow-up of 2 to 14 years.

Histologic grade of the tumor using the criteria of Beckwith and Martin (2) also correlated well with outcome (2). However, when these data were analyzed by stage of disease, no independent effect of histologic grade could be detected.

Pretreatment Urinary Catecholamine Excretion

Of the 80 patients with pretreatment studies available, only 3 patients (5%) failed to have increased levels of VMA or HVA, and these patients additionally had none of the other catecholamine metabolites elevated. Table 3 summarizes the distribution of metabolites by stage of disease at diagnosis.

As we have reported previously, markedly elevated levels of VMA and HVA were more common in disseminated disease (stages IV and IV-S) than in localized disease (stages I, II, and III), whereas no significant relationship between tumor burden and the VMA/HVA ratio was noted (8). The presence of any of the other metabolites did not appear to be related to extent of disease with the exception of VG.

TABLE 3. *Relationship between initial urinary excretion patterns and stage (N = 80)*

Metabolites	Normalized value[a]	No. of patients				
		Stage I	Stage II	Stage III	Stage IV	Stage IV-S
VMA	1	1	2	4	4	0
	2–4	2	3	0	13	0
	5–14	1	5	2	6	2
	15–49	1	2	0	7	3
	50+	0	0	1	16	5
HVA	1	0	3	2	4	0
	2–4	3	7	1	4	0
	5–14	1	1	3	15	7
	15–49	0	1	1	19	3
	50+	1	0	0	4	0
VMA/HVA	0–0.5	1	0	2	9	0
	0.5–1.5	2	5	3	13	0
	1.5–3.5	2	6	2	16	7
	3.5+	0	1	0	8	3
3-MT	−	4	12	6	30	8
	+	1	0	1	16	2
VLA	−	4	11	5	32	9
	+	1	1	2	14	1
VG	−	5	10	6	26	1
	+	0	2	1	20	9

[a] Levels of VMA, HVA are normalized by expressing them as multiples of the maximal normal value for age of the patient as shown in Table 1. Urinary 3-MT, VLA, and VG are either absent (−) or present (+).

TABLE 4. *Relationship between initial urinary excretion patterns and survival in patients with stage IV disease (N= 46)*

Metabolites	Normalized Value[a]	No. of patients	1-Year survival (%)	2-Year survival (%)	3-Year survival (%)
VMA	1	4	25	0	0
	2–4	13	31	15	15
	5–49	13	54	38	15
	50+	16	56	18	18
HVA	1	4	25	25	25
	2–14	19	42	10	10
	15+	23	50	27	18
VMA/HVA	0–0.5	9	22	12	12
	0.5–1.4	13	31	15	8
	1.5–3.5	16	52	21	21
	3.5+	8	66	33	25
3-MT	−	30	50	25	20
	+	16	6	0	0
VLA	−	32	51	23	23
	+	14	16	8	0

Levels of VMA, HVA are normalized by expressing them as multiples of the maximal normal value for the age of the patient as shown in Table 1. Urinary 3-MT and VLA are designated as either absent (−) or present (+).

Forty-six patients with stage IV disease were evaluated for the relationship of the pretreatment urinary pattern to survival (Table 4). Although no association between the absolute level of VMA or HVA and survival was detected, the ratio of VMA to HVA levels did correlate with outcome, a more favorable prognosis being associated with a higher (≥ 1.5) ratio. Of additional interest is the fact that all stage IV-S patients had a ratio ≥ 1.5 (Table 3). On the other hand, the presence of 3-MT and VLA was associated with a poorer prognosis, with no stage IV patients excreting either of these metabolites surviving more than 2 years from diagnosis. The absence or presence of VG or NMN failed to correlate with survival.

Relationship of Changes in Serial Catecholamine Levels and Course of Disease

Serial urinary catecholamine metabolite determinations were obtained in 47 patients, including 2 with stage I disease, 11 with stage II, 5 with stage III, 23 with stage IV, and 6 with stage IV-S disease. A total of 25 of 33 patients (76%) whose catecholamine metabolite levels fell to normal within 1 year of diagnosis survived 2 years, whereas only 3/14 (21%) of patients with persistently elevated levels at that time survived 2 years. One of these three patients subsequently noted a return to normal values 2 years after diagnosis and remains alive and free of disease 4 years after diagnosis. The second and third patients noted recurrent disease 3 and 4 years after diagnosis, respectively.

In 31 patients who achieved a complete response (CR) by clinical and radiographic examination (all stages), only 3 had persistently elevated urinary catecholamine levels at the time of CR. Urinary values were available at the time of disease recurrence in 19 patients who had attained an initial CR or partial response (PR). All 19 noted a rise in excretion of catecholamine metabolites at the time of relapse. We compared the pattern of excretion at recurrence of disease with that found in pretreatment samples from these same patients. In general, excretion patterns at relapse demonstrated the same characteristics as the initial studies. When patients were divided into groups on the basis of a VMA/HVA ratio greater or less than 1.5, only 2 of 19 patients noted a shift in the ratio of these metabolites at the time of relapse and both had "marginal" values initially (1.3 and 1.5, respectively). Similarly, only 3 of 19 patients had a change in the appearance of 3-MT and 2 of 19 in VLA.

DISCUSSION

These studies of initial and serial urinary catecholamine excretion patterns in childhood neuroblastoma have been designed to investigate the relationship of the biochemical activity of the malignant cell population to their biological and clinical behavior. We, as well as several other investigators, have demonstrated the sensitivity of these biochemical markers for diagnosis of neuroblastoma. In most large series 90% or more of patients with this tumor have had elevated levels of one or more catecholamines in pretreatment urine samples using a variety of biochemical techniques (5–8,12). In the present study, only 5% of patients with histologically proven neuroblastoma failed to demonstrate increased urinary excretion patterns.

Conflicting results have been noted in previous reports attempting to correlate the levels of VMA and HVA in pretreatment urine samples with ultimate outcome of the disease process. Two early studies of small patient populations failed to find any association between VMA or several other catecholamine metabolites and survival (1,10). Gitlow et al. (5) in a series of 54 patients found that low initial HVA levels were associated with a more favorable prognosis, but LaBrosse et al. (7) in a series of 239 patients confirmed the earlier studies, failing to find any correlation between survival and pretreatment values. Finally, Voute et al. (12) found that the presence of VLA in the urine indicated an unfavorable prognosis and the ratio of VMA + VG/HVA also had predictive value.

In the present study we took advantage of the staging criteria of Evans et al. (3) to compare clinical and biochemical activity in this tumor. As in every large series to date, stage of disease and age at onset were the most powerful clinical determinants of survival in our patient population. Although absolute amounts of VMA and HVA present were related to stage (tumor burden), we found no significant correlation between these levels and prognosis. On the other hand, prognosis correlated directly with the VMA/HVA ratio, independent of stage or age. In addition, the presence of VLA and/or 3-MT was associated with a poorer prognosis.

On the basis of the known pathways of catecholamine metabolism (Fig. 1), these results continue to suggest that a more primitive initial "biochemical phenotype" in this malignancy is associated with more aggressive biological activity and a poorer prognosis.

In contrast to the studies of initial urinary catecholamine patterns, our data agree completely with those of LaBrosse et al. (7) in indicating a high degree of correlation of disease course and serial changes in catecholamine metabolite excretion (7). Survival is clearly better in those patients experiencing a rapid fall to normal of these metabolites than in those with persistently elevated levels. Furthermore, 23 of 26 patients who achieved a CR had simultaneously normal catecholamine levels. Of particular interest to us was the pattern of excretion in patients experiencing disease relapse. Our data suggest that almost all patients retain the "biochemical phenotype" they demonstrated prior to initial treatment when their disease recurs.

It is increasingly apparent that neuroblastoma represents a heterogeneous neoplasm with varying biochemical, biological, pathological, immunological, and clinical expressions. Understanding the interaction of these factors may provide important new leads to the mechanisms involved in the etiology and regression of this tumor, as well as point to innovative therapeutic approaches. Our studies focus on only one of these determinants, but these results as well as previous investigations of biochemical markers in neuroblastoma have already given the clinician sensitive tools for diagnosis and monitoring of response as well as important "front-end" prognostic factors that may permit selection of high-risk patients for new treatment programs.

ACKNOWLEDGMENTS

This work has been supported in part by Grant CA-02649 awarded by the National Cancer Institute, DHEW. Walter E. Laug is a recipient of an American Cancer Society Junior Faculty Award, 1978–1979. Correspondence should be addressed to Stuart E. Siegel, M.D., Division of Hematology-Oncology, Children's Hospital of Los Angeles, 4650 Sunset Boulevard, Los Angeles, California 90027. The authors gratefully acknowledge the secretarial assistance of Ms. Ann McBride in the preparation of this manuscript.

REFERENCES

1. Barontini DeGutierrez Moyano, M., Bergada, C., and Becu, L. (1971): Significance of catecholamine excretion in the follow-up of sympathoblastomas. *Cancer,* 27:228–232.
2. Beckwith, J. B., and Martin, R. F. (1968): Observation on the histopathology of neuroblastoma. *J. Pediatr. Surg.,* 3:106–113.
3. Evans, A. E., D'Angio, G. J., and Randolph, J. (1971): A proposed staging for children with neuroblastoma. *Cancer,* 27:374–378.
4. Gerson, J. M., and Koop, C. E. (1974): Neuroblastoma. *Semin. Oncol.,* 1:35–46.

5. Gitlow, S. E., Dziedzic, L. B., Strauss, L., Greenwood, S. M., and Dziedzic, S. W. (1973): Biochemical and histologic determinants in the prognosis of neuroblastoma. *Cancer,* 32:898–905.
6. LaBrosse, E. H. (1974): Catecholamines in neuroblastoma. *Maandsch. Kindergeneestic.,* 42:407–417.
7. LaBrosse, E. H., Comay, E., Bohuan, C., Zucker, J., and Schweisguth, O. (1976): Catecholamine metabolism in neuroblastoma. *J. Natl. Cancer Inst.,* 57:633–638.
8. Laug, W. E., Siegel, S. E., Shaw, K. N. F., Landing, B., Baptista, J., and Gutenstein, M. (1978): Initial urinary catecholamine metabolite concentrations and prognosis in neuroblastoma. *Pediatrics,* 62:77–83.
9. Leikin, S., Evans, A., Heyn, R., and Newton, W. (1974): The impact of chemotherapy on advanced neuroblastoma. Survival of patients diagnosed in 1956, 1962 and 1966–68 in Children's Cancer Study Group. *J. Pediatr.,* 84:131–134.
10. Liebner, E. J., and Rosenthal, I. M. (1973): Serial catecholamines in the radiation management of children with neuroblastoma. *Cancer,* 32:623–633.
11. Shaw, K. N. F. (1976): Biochemical screening for metabolic disorders at Children's Hospital of Los Angeles. In: *Proceedings of the International Symposium on Laboratory Screening Techniques for Inborn Errors of Metabolism in Newborn and Selected High-risk Infants, Warsaw, Poland, September 3–6, 1972,* pp. 141–149. National Library of Medicine and National Science Foundation, Washington, D.C.
12. Voute, P. A., Van Putten, W. J., and Burgers, J. M. V. (1975): Tumors of the sympathetic nervous system. In: *Cancer in Children, Clinical Management,* edited by H. J. G. Bloom, J. Lemerle, M. K. Nerdhardt, and P. A. Voute, pp. 138–148. Springer-Verlag, New York.

Advances in Neuroblastoma Research,
edited by Audrey E. Evans.
Raven Press, New York © 1980.

Serum Catecholamine Metabolites in Stage IV Neuroblastoma

W. Krivit, B. L. Mirkin, E. Freier, M. Nesbit, and M. J. Cooper

Departments of Pediatrics, Pharmacology, Laboratory Medicine, and Pathology, Division of Clinical Pharmacology, University of Minnesota, Minneapolis, Minnesota 55455

Quantitation of catecholamine metabolites in urine is now widely accepted as an integral and critically important laboratory procedure for the diagnosis of neuroblastoma (2). An increase in the excretion of catecholamine metabolites has been observed in a highly significant proportion of patients with neuroblastoma (4). In addition, the prognosis and therapeutic response to chemotherapy, radiation, or surgery in patients with neuroblastoma have been correlated with urinary levels of specific catecholamine metabolites (5).

The prognosis of patients with stage IV neuroblastoma is extremely poor, and an 80% mortality has been reported 2 years after diagnosis. Consequently, there has been an increased interest in identifying those biological processes which may provide greater understanding of this neoplastic disorder (8). Furthermore, there is a need to quantitate changes in catecholamine metabolite patterns by more sensitive techniques to assess early response to therapy.

This study outlines the initial steps taken to develop methods for measuring serum catecholamine metabolites which appear to offer the advantages of ease of sampling and rapidity of measurement, and may offer increased sensitivity and a higher correlation with clinical status than with urinary analyses.

METHODS

Patient Population

Serum samples were taken from patients with stage IV neuroblastoma. Urines were collected for 24 hr and kept on ice with no preservatives added. These subjects had not received chemotherapy, radiation, or other drugs for more than 2 weeks prior to the study. Control subjects consisted of children with other malignancies.

Analytical Procedures

Urine. Catecholamine metabolites were analyzed by the following chemical methods: 3-methoxy-4-hydroxyphenylacetic acid (HVA) [Knight and Hay-

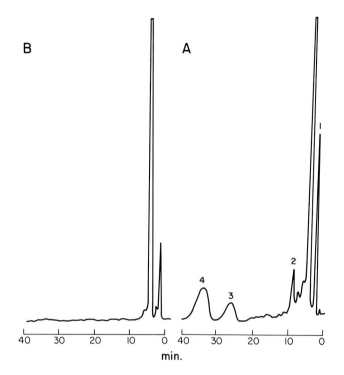

FIG. 1. HPLC of catecholamine metabolites. **A:** Patient serum containing 352 ng/ml VMA, 235 ng/ml MHPG, 240 ng/ml HVA. **B:** Normal serum. Peak 1, vanilmandelic acid; peak 2, 3-methoxy-4-hydroxy-phenylethlyene glycol; 3, vanillic acid (internal standard); 4, homovanillic acid. Conditions: column, microBondapak C_{18}; eluent, 50 mM KH_2PO_4; flow rate, 2 ml/min; electrochemical detection at 800 mV.

mond (3)] and 3-methoxy-4-hydroxymandelic acid (vanilmandelic acid; VMA) [Pisano, Crout, and Abraham (7)].

Serum. High-pressure liquid chromatography (HPLC) with electrochemical detection was used to assay serum for catecholamine metabolites. To 1 ml plasma 0.1 ml 2 N HCl and 5 ml ethylacetate were added. After mixing and centrifuging, the ethylacetate layer was taken to dryness *in vacuo* and redissolved with eluent for injection into the chromatograph. Standard curves were run concurrently with each analysis and vanillic acid was used as the internal standard. A typical chromatographic pattern is shown in Fig. 1. The detection threshold for VMA, HVA, and 4-hydroxy-3-methoxyphenylethylene glycol (HMPG) was 25 ng/ml.

RESULTS

Relationship Between Serum and Urinary Concentrations of VMA and HVA

Catecholamine metabolite levels were determined in sera and urine specimens obtained on the same day from patients with stage IV neuroblastoma (Table 1).

TABLE 1. *Urine and serum concentrates of VMA, HVA, and HMPG*

Patient No.	Age (years)	Stage of disease		VMA Serum ng/ml	VMA Urine μg/mg cr	HVA Serum ng/ml	HVA Urine μg/mg cr	HMPG serum ng/ml
		*A. Active disease stage IV neuroblastoma*						
1	2	Diagnosis		415	327	145	191	176
2	1	Diagnosis		400	280	520	368	236
3	1	Diagnosis		375	103	560	530	300
	2	Remission		25[a]	15	25[a]	35	120
		Postsurg.	1 d	50	13	25[a]	22	25[a]
		Postsurg.	2 d	60	15	90	28	25[a]
4	9	Diagnosis	1 d	60	43	25[a]	114	25[a]
		Diagnosis	2 d	55	14	25[a]	33	25[a]
		Diagnosis	3 d	25[a]	10	25[a]	18	—
5	16	Relapse		260	75	430	70	215
		Relapse		720	129	500	123	680
6	2	Relapse		100	42	280	35	125
		Remission		25[a]	13	25[a]	24	380
7	10	Relapse		60	15	200	65	75
8	2	Remission		25[a]	6	25[a]	46	25[a]
9	1	Relapse	1 d	230	283	390	—	280
		Relapse	2 d	—	—	74	14	25[a]
10	2	Diagnosis		352	266	240	254	235
11	1	Diagnosis		41	29	123	115	25[a]
12	2	Diagnosis		25[a]	—	25[a]	—	25[a]
13	3	Diagnosis		—	87	160	307	95
14	2	Diagnosis		—	8	67	37	31
15	1	Diagnosis		—	16	180	18	
		*B. Inactive disease stage IV neuroblastoma*						
16	4			25[a]	—	25[a]	20	25[a]
17	3			25[a]	22	25[a]	—	25[a]
18	6			52	5.0	90	—	130
19	1			25[a]	22	25[a]	39	25[a]
20	3			25[a]	Normal	—	—	25[a]
		*C. Controls*						
		Diagnosis						
21	3	Medulloblastoma		25[a]	—	25[a]	39	25[a]
22	2	Erythroleukoma		25[a]	8	25[a]	8	25[a]
23	3	Retinoblastoma		25[a]	7	25[a]	12	25[a]
24	52	Infection		25[a]	—	28	—	25[a]
25	24	CML		25[a]	—	25[a]	—	25[a]
26	16	Hodgkin's		25[a]	—	25[a]	—	25[a]
27	6	Wilms'		25[a]	—	25[a]	—	25[a]
28	18	CML		25[a]	—	25[a]	—	25[a]

Upper limits of controls of urinary/metabolites (U of M)/(μg/mg cr)

Age (years)	VMA	HVA
0–1	15	44
2–4	7	28
5–9	5	19
10–14	3	

[a] The number indicates that levels were nondetectable and are recorded at lower limits of sensitivity of 25 ng/ml for statistical analysis.

The statistical relationship between urinary VMA and serum VMA concentrations in patients with active stage IV neuroblastoma was shown to have a very high correlation coefficient (0.87), whereas a somewhat lower correlation coefficient was generated when HVA was compared in a similar fashion (0.74) (Table 1). Despite these correlations, discordance between serum and urinary metabolite concentrations was observed. HMPG concentrations are also recorded in Table 1.

Correlation Between Serum Concentrations of HMA, VMA, and HMPG

The serum concentrations of HVA, VMA, and HMPG are also presented in relationship to the clinical status of each patient (Fig. 2).

Comparison of serum HVA, VMA, and HMPG concentrations with each other demonstrated highly significant correlation coefficients when each variable was analyzed. The correlation coefficient for VMA when compared with HVA was 0.96 (Fig. 3), for VMA compared with HMPG was 0.88 (Fig. 4), and for HVA compared with HMPG was 0.81 (Fig. 5).

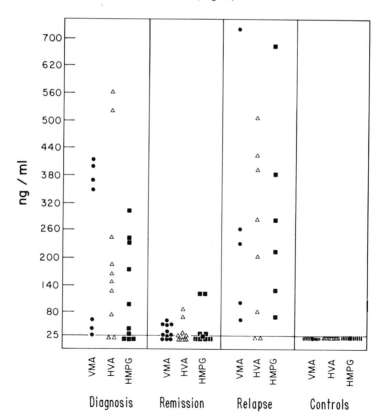

FIG. 2. Serum concentrations of HVA, VMA, and HMPG are presented according to activity of disease at time of serum sampling (at time of diagnosis, in remission, and in relapse and controls).

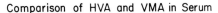

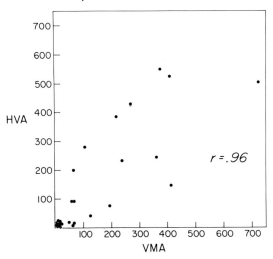

FIG. 3. Comparison of VMA and HVA concentrations in serum. Catecholamine metabolites (VMA, HVA, and HMPG) are recorded in ng/ml serum. The lower limit of sensitivity of this assay was 25 ng/ml. All nondetectable levels are noted as 25 ng/ml. For purposes of graphing, all levels of 25 ng/ml are recorded in figure at or below 25 ng/ml.

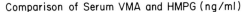

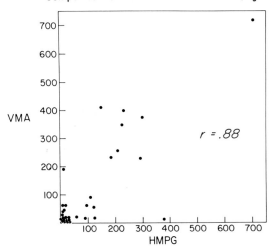

FIG. 4. Comparison of VMA and HMPG levels in serum. Same as Fig. 3.

Comparison of Serum HVA and HMPG (ηg/ml)

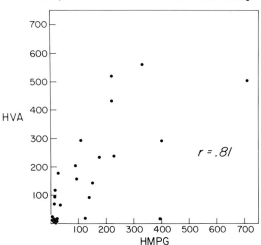

FIG. 5. Comparison of HVA and HMPG levels in serum. Same as Fig. 3.

Patterns of Catecholamine Metabolite Excretion in Serum and Urine Following Serial Determinations in Two Patients

In one patient with active stage IV neuroblastoma, a comparison was made between serum and urinary HVA and VMA concentrations (Fig. 6). Although a significant increase in serum HVA, VMA, and HMPG levels occurred over

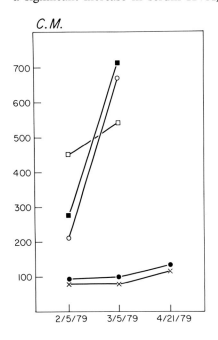

FIG. 6. This 16-year-old male patient with stage IV neuroblastoma had been in remission in stage IV for 6 months after receiving chemotherapy for 1 year. Clusters of neuroblastoma cells were noted in the bone marrow 2/5/79. Recurrence of skeletal system pain was also present. During the time intervals noted, no therapy was given (at patient's request). The urinary metabolites remained stable although elevated above the normal (5-fold). During this time, serum metabolites were elevated well above normal (10-fold) and continued to rise as noted (30-fold). The values for urine catecholamine metabolites are expressed as μg/mg creatinine excreted and for serum as ng/ml.

TABLE 2. *Serum and urine VMA/HVA ratios*

Serum VMA/HVA	Urine VMA/HVA
2.862	1.712
0.769	0.761
0.670	0.196
1.000	0.436
2.000	0.618
0.667	0.551
2.400	0.385
11.000	0.439
5.000	0.551
0.605	1.041
1.404	1.050
5.000	0.550
0.300	0.235
5.000	0.145
1.467	1.046
0.333	0.251
1.000	0.574
1.000	0.829
0.156	0.283
0.373	0.231
0.139	0.912

$r = 0.05$.

the time course noted, these were not paralleled by similar increments in the urinary VMA and HVA metabolite concentrations.

Ratio of VMA to HVA in Serum and Urine

The ratio of VMA to HVA was compared in urine specimens obtained 24 hr prior to the clinic visit and in serum specimen taken at time of examination. The coefficient correlation obtained was $r = 0.05$ (Table 2).

DISCUSSION

This preliminary investigation has established that serum catecholamine metabolite concentrations (HVA, VMA, and HMPG) are elevated in patients with stage IV neuroblastoma and that, in general, they tend to parallel urinary levels. The use of serum analyses offers the advantage of convenience, since a 24-hr urinary collection is not required. Serum analysis may offer a more sensitive and discriminating index of biogenic amine secretion by the tumor mass. Whether these data will provide an improved correlation with therapeutic response and prognostic assessment remains to be established by subsequent studies.

These data have demonstrated an increase in serum concentrations of catecholamine metabolites which are frequently 20-fold above those occurring in normal serum as compared to a several-fold increment usually noted in urinary metabolite concentrations when compared to control values. The higher discriminatory capacity provided by serum measurements may be of great significance in the detection of small neural crest tumors and may assist in clarifying the regulatory mechanisms which modulate biogenic amine synthesis and release.

The techniques employed in this investigation measure only unconjugated catecholamine metabolites. Since these substrates undergo conjugation to form sulfates and glucuronides, urinary analyses involving hydrolysis therefore measure total metabolite excretion. Discrepancies which may occur between serum and urinary concentrations of catecholamine metabolites may be due to this difference in analytical procedure. In addition, the capacities for sulfation and glucuronidation are age dependent; glucuronidation is generally diminished in infancy and early childhood, whereas sulfation is extremely active, continuing at this elevated level before decreasing at about age 12 years (6). Another maturational phenomenon which must be considered in this context is the age-dependent change in renal function, which also becomes rate limiting in terms of elimination of catecholamine metabolites, particularly those which are handled by the renal tubular acid transport system, i.e., HVA and VMA specifically. Consequently, the urinary excretion of these metabolites may be impaired in young infants since an active transport system is required.

These data have demonstrated a significant correlation coefficient between the serum and urinary concentrations of both HVA and VMA. Although this would generally be expected, there were several subjects in whom serum and urinary concentrations of these metabolites were clearly discordant, i.e., serum was elevated when urinary concentrations were normal and the converse. This discrepancy must be carefully investigated since false assessments of therapeutic response or tumor growth would be reached depending on which biological specimen was analyzed. Future studies in this area must establish whether serum or urinary analysis provide the better prognostic information on these processes. Serum analyses will probably prove useful in quantitative changes occurring over a shorter temporal period, whereas urinary analyses will tend to average out excretory patterns occurring over a longer period of time, and perhaps both should be used to provide the most accurate prognostic information.

The serum concentrations of VMA, HVA, and HMPG correlated well with one another utilizing linear regression analysis of the study population. Relationship between the stage of disease or clinical response and the VMA and HVA ratio was not apparent. As noted in Table 2, there was no significant correlation between serum VMA/HVA ratios and urine VMA/HVA ratios. The failure to find similar ratios in serum and urine may relate to factors mentioned previously which would tend to influence the urinary concentrations of these metabolites to a greater degree than serum. The physiologic meaning and importance of VMA/HVA ratios in urine and the prognostic significance imparted to these ratios by Siegel et al. (5) could not be substantiated by serum VMA/HVA ratios.

The most significant aspect of the present investigation will be the opportunity it offers to identify so-called front-end prognostic factors in patients with stage IV neuroblastoma (Siegel, *this volume*). Measurement of these serum metabolites and other metabolic profiling of urinary organic acids (1) along with antigen composition of bone marrow tumor cells or urinary and serum antigens may provide some important insights into the biologic characteristics of these tumors and perhaps lay the groundwork for establishing more selective chemotherapeutic approaches to the management of neuroblastoma.

SUMMARY

A highly specific and sensitive method for analyzing catecholamine metabolites in small serum volumes has been developed. Comparative studies were carried out in 24 patients with stage IV neuroblastoma in whom serum and urinary concentrations of HVA, VMA, and HMPG were determined. These data indicate that serum HVA and VMA and HMPG concentrations were elevated above levels observed in a control group. In addition, a very high correlation was shown between the serum and urinary concentrations of VMA ($r = 0.87$) and HVA ($r = 0.74$). Intragroup comparison of serum HVA, VMA, and HMPG concentrations utilizing linear regression analysis demonstrated highly significant correlation coefficients when concentrations of VMA were compared with those of HVA ($r = 0.96$), VMA with HMPG ($r = 0.88$), and HVA with HMPG ($r = 0.81$).

Sequential serum and urine determinations were completed in two patients with stage IV neuroblastoma. Concentrations of HVA, VMA, and HMPG in serum increased in one subject, whereas urinary VMA and HVA levels remained constant. In the second subject, serum and urinary concentrations of these metabolites followed a similar temporal pattern.

Catecholamine metabolite analysis of single serum samples appears to offer some advantages compared to urine methodology which requires collection over a 24-hr period. In addition, the concentrations of catecholamine metabolites in serum may constitute a more sensitive reflection of biogenic amine metabolism, and consequently may provide a more critical mechanism for studying the influences of specific chemotherapeutic interventions on tumor growth than is provided by analyses of urinary excretions.

ACKNOWLEDGMENTS

The authors acknowledge the technical assistance of Wilhelmina Ramos. This research was supported by the Training Program Grant in Pediatric Clinical Pharmacology (USPHS GM07466) and Pediatric Hematology-Oncology (USPHS HL07145; USPHS Grants CA21737 and CA07306; Leukemia Task Force and the Graduate School of the University of Minnesota).

REFERENCES

1. Gates, S. G., Sweeley, C. C., Krivit, W., Devitt, D., and Blaisdell, B. E. (1978): Automated metabolic profiling of organic acids in human urine. II. Analysis or urine simply from "healthy" adults, sick children, and children with neuroblastoma. *Clin. Chem.,* 24(10):1680–1689.
2. Gitlow, S., Dziedzic, L., and Dziedzic, S. (1976): Catecholamine metabolism in neuroblastoma. In: *Neuroblastoma,* edited by C. Pochedly, pp. 115–155. Publishing Sciences Group, Acton, Mass.
3. Knight, J. A., and Haymond, R. E. (1977): Improved colorimetry of urinary 3-methoxy-4-hydroxy phenylacetic and (homovanillic acid). *Clin. Chem.,* 23(11):2007–2010.
4. LaBrosse, E. H., Comoy, E., Bohuon, C., Zucker, J. M., and Schweisguth, O. (1976): Catecholamine metabolism in neuroblastoma. *J. Natl. Cancer Inst.,* 57:633–638.
5. Laug, W. E., Siegel, S. E., Shaw, K. N. F., Landing, B., Baptiste, J., and Gutenstein, M. (1978): Metabolite concentrations and initial urinary catecholamine. Prognosis in neuroblastoma. *Pediatrics,* 62:77.
6. Miller, R. P., Roberts, R. J., and Fischer, L. J. (1976): Acetominophen elimination kinetics in neonates, children, and adults. *Clin. Pharmacol. Ther.,* 19:284–294.
7. Pisano, J. J., Crout, J. R., and Abraham, D. (1962): Determination of 3-methoxy-4-hydroxy mandelic acid in urine. *Clin. Chem. Acta,* 7:285–291.
8. Siegel, S. E., et al. (1979): Children's Cancer Study Group Study #371 (Protocol available upon request from CCSG, Los Angeles, California).

Advances in Neuroblastoma Research,
edited by Audrey E. Evans.
Raven Press, New York © 1980.

Ferritin and Cancer: Study of Isoferritins in Patients with Neuroblastoma

*,** Hie-Won L. Hann, * Howard M. Levy, and **Audrey E. Evans

*Institute for Cancer Research, Fox Chase Cancer Center, Philadelphia, Pennsylvania 19111;
and **Children's Hospital of Philadelphia, Philadelphia, Pennsylvania 19104*

Ferritin is the major tissue iron binding protein. Small amounts of ferritin circulate in human serum in normal and pathological states (15,19), usually in proportion to the quantity of tissue iron stores (11,14). However, in patients with certain malignancies such as Hodgkin's disease (3,4,9,12), leukemia (12,18), breast cancer (5), and others (10,13,17), grossly elevated levels of serum ferritin have been observed without a corresponding increase in iron storage. Leukemic cells have been shown to contain a comparatively large amount of ferritin (24) and synthesize ferritin at a much higher rate than normal leukocytes (23). We attempted to see whether similar phenomena would occur in neuroblastoma and investigated the potential use of ferritin as a tumor marker in patients with this disease.

MATERIALS AND METHODS

Sera from 63 children with neuroblastoma and 31 normal children were tested for ferritin. As another control group for neuroblastoma, 22 patients with Wilms' tumor were also included. Six primary neuroblastoma tumors and cells from two established neuroblastoma cell lines, CHP-100 and CHP-134 (20), were studied. Supernatants from six different neuroblastoma cell lines grown in culture, the culture medium itself (RPMI 1640 with 10% fetal calf serum), and the supernatant from a human fibroblast cell line (IMR-90) (16) were also tested.

Serum ferritin levels were assayed by counterelectrophoresis (CEP) on 1.1% agarose plates in Veronal buffer, pH 8.2 (4), using antibody to human placental ferritin (Behring Diagnostics, Somerville, NJ). This antibody is shown to have a broad specificity against most of human isoferritins including those from HeLa cells which are the most acidic end of the human spectrum (8). In agreement with others (4), this method was found to give positive results with ferritin levels $\geq$ 400 ng/ml (as determined by radioimmunoassay) (10) in our laboratory. The normal range of serum ferritin levels in children (6 months to 15 years) is 7 to 142 ng/ml with a median 30 ng/ml (22). Therefore, a positive ferritin test by CEP represents an increase of 3 to 10 times that of normal value.

Ferritin was isolated from neuroblastoma tumors and purified according to the method described by Arosio et al. (2). Tumors were homogenized in 4 volumes of water and heated to 75°C for 10 min to precipitate heat-labile proteins. The supernatant fraction was then adjusted to pH 4.6 to remove other contaminants, and ferritin was subsequently recovered from the supernatant and precipitated in 50% ammonium sulfate. Ferritin was also extracted from neuroblastoma cells (CHP-100 and CHP-134) (20) grown in tissue culture. The purity of the ferritins was confirmed by polyacrylamide gel electrophoresis (2). The subunit composition of ferritins was analyzed by SDS gradient-pore gel electrophoresis as described by Arosio et al. (2).

RESULTS

Sera from 31 normal children ages 2 to 14 years were tested by CEP and all were negative (i.e., levels of ferritin < 400 ng/ml). All 22 patients with active Wilms' tumor were also negative. Sixty-three children with neuroblastoma at various stages and activity of disease were tested for the presence of elevated serum ferritin. Results are shown in Table 1. Among the 11 patients with stage I neuroblastoma, one had active disease and was positive for ferritin. The other 10 were free of disease and all were found to be negative. In stage II, 3 of 4 patients with active disease were positive for ferritin and 1 was negative. The 9 patients who were free of disease were all negative. In stage III, 4 had active disease. Two of these patients were positive while the other two were negative. One of the two negative patients was tested three times while her disease progressed and the ferritin results remained negative. In stage IV, all 22 patients had active disease and all but 4 were positive for ferritin. In stage IV-S, the association between active disease and positive ferritin was not apparent. Out of 6 patients with disease, 4 were negative. Table 2 summarizes the data from

TABLE 1. *Relation of serum ferritin test to stage and activity of disease*

Stage	N	Disease status[a]	Ferritin (+)	Ferritin (−)
I	11	Disease (+)	1	0
		Disease (−)	0	10
II	13	Disease (+)	3	1
		Disease (−)	0	9
III	7	Disease (+)	2	2
		Disease (−)	0	3
IV	23	Disease (+)	18	4
		Disease (−)	0	1
IV-S	9	Disease (+)	2	4
		Disease (−)	0	3
Total	63		26	37

[a] Disease (+) denotes active disease; disease (−) denotes clinical remission.

TABLE 2. *Relationship between disease activity and results of serum ferritin test*

Stages I – IV-S	Neuroblastoma	
	Serum ferritin	
	+	−
Disease(+)	26	11
Disease(−)	0	26

Correlation is significant ($p < 0.001$ by Fisher's exact 2×2 test). (+) = active disease; (−) = no evidence of disease.

Table 1. The correlation between active disease and positive ferritin and disease-free state and negative ferritin is significant at a p value < 0.001 by Fisher's exact 2×2 test (21).

In 39 of the 63 patients more than one serum sample was available and many were tested serially. The specimens had been collected during the course of disease and stored at $-70°C$. Twelve patients were disease free when first tested and remained so; all 25 specimens were negative. In 22 patients the disease activity fluctuated, in 19 the ferritin correlated with the patient's status, 50 specimens were positive when disease was active, and 30 were negative when in remission. In 2 of the 22, elevated ferritin levels lagged behind the clinical evidence of remission (measured by clearing of the bone marrow) and in 1 there was obvious disease progression before the ferritin level rose.[1] Five additional patients with clinical evidence of disease were repeatedly negative (15 samples). They represented all stages of disease (II, III, IV, and IV-S); the 2 IV-S patients contributed 8 of these discordant samples.

Since serum ferritin may increase in hepatic cell damage, we attempted to evaluate whether this played a role in our findings. Liver functions were available in the records of 24 of the 26 patients with elevated serum ferritin. Of these, 22 patients in various stages of neuroblastoma had normal serum transaminase levels; 1 of the 2 patients in stage IV-S with a positive ferritin had an elevated SGOT of 160 units, and 1 patient with stage IV had increased transaminase levels (SGOT 178 units, SGPT 118 units). When serial liver function tests were compared with simultaneous ferritin levels, there was no correlation.

Supernatant fluids were collected from six neuroblastoma cell lines grown in culture, concentrated 16 to 20 times, and tested for ferritin by CEP. All six were positive. The tissue culture medium, RPMI 1640 with 10% fetal calf serum, and the supernatant obtained from a human fibroblast cell line, IMR-90 (16), were used as controls. Both were concentrated 20 to 25 times and there were no detectable amounts of ferritin.

Extracted ferritins from neuroblastoma tumors and cells from neuroblastoma cell lines were characterized by subunit analysis on SDS gel. Ferritin, a spherical

---

[1] The first sample was not available for testing until 3 months after the patient relapsed, and at that time the results were positive.

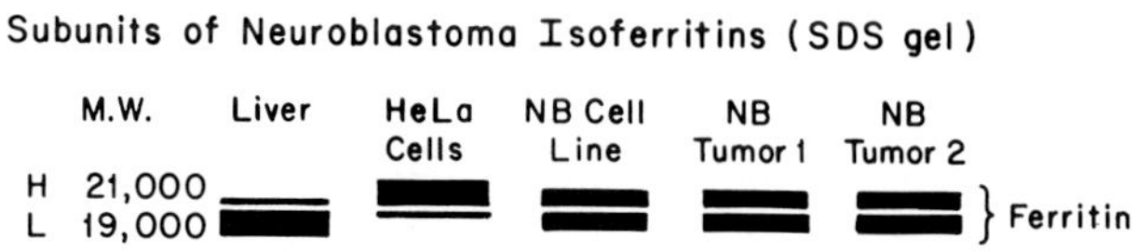

Subunits of Neuroblastoma Isoferritins (SDS gel)

	M.W.	Liver	HeLa Cells	NB Cell Line	NB Tumor 1	NB Tumor 2
H	21,000					
L	19,000					} Ferritin

FIG. 1. Subunits of ferritin were separated by electrophoresis on a SDS polyacrylamide gel (see Methods) from extracts of normal human liver tissue, HeLa cells, a neuroblastoma cell line, and two neuroblastoma tumors.

molecule, is composed of a total of 24 subunits (polypeptides), of which there are two different types, H (M.W. 21,000) and L (M.W. 19,000) (6). Different combinations of these two types of subunits account for the observed variation in isoferritins (6). Figure 1 shows the subunit composition of neuroblastoma ferritins. The most commonly seen isoferritin pattern in normal adults is that of liver or spleen. These ferritins consist of greater than 80% L and the remainder H (7). On electrofocusing, liver ferritin usually bands in the pH range of 5.4 to 5.8 (7). The other extreme is represented by the ferritins from HeLa cell, some hepatoma tumors, and fetal livers. They have 70 to 90% H with the remainder L (7). These ferritins usually band in the pH range of 4.8 to 5.3 (1). Subunit composition of three preparations (one neuroblastoma cell line and two primary tumors) contained at least 50% H (Fig. 1) and is, therefore, similar to the so-called carcinofetal isoferritins (1).

DISCUSSION

Our study indicates that elevated serum ferritin levels detected by CEP in patients with neuroblastoma correlate well with the presence of active disease. The associations between positive ferritin and active disease and between negative ferritin and disease-free status are statistically significant. A longitudinal study of 39 patients done retrospectively on stored sera also showed a similar correlation. Therefore, assaying ferritin levels during the illness could be of value in assessing disease activity.

With stage IV-S disease, this correlation is not apparent (Table 1); 4 of 6 patients with active disease are negative. Patients with stage IV-S constitute a unique group among children with neuroblastoma. They are usually infants (under 1 year of age) with a small primary tumor and disease spread to skin, bone marrow, or liver. Despite extensive disease, patients with IV-S spread have a good prognosis because of a high rate of spontaneous regression.

A similar poor correlation was noted in patients with ganglioneuroblastoma, a more mature form of neuroblastoma. Only 2 of 8 children with active ganglioneuroblastoma had elevated levels of serum ferritin. These children could have slightly increased levels which are not detected by CEP, or the presence of ferritin may simply be dependent on the proportion of neuroblastoma relative to the ganglioneuroma in the tumor.

Although we cannot identify with certainty the origin of increased ferritin in the serum of each patient with neuroblastoma, the elevated circulating ferritin does not seem to be due to liver damage or inefficient erythropoiesis. The presence of ferritin in cultured neuroblastoma tumor cells, as well as in the supernatant fluid and in neuroblastoma primary tumors, and the carcinofetal phenotype of these isoferritins suggest that the increased ferritin in sera of neuroblastoma patients comes from the tumor. Further research is needed to develop an assay for routine clinical use that would identify those elevated serum ferritins originating from tumor cells.

The results reported here suggest that the concentration of ferritin in serum could prove to be a valuable aid to diagnosis and serve as a guide to therapy for children with neuroblastoma.

SUMMARY

Elevated serum ferritin levels without corresponding increase in tissue iron storage have been observed in patients with certain cancers. Increased synthesis of ferritin by cancer cells has also been reported. In order to see whether similar phenomena would occur in patients with neuroblastoma, we have screened serum ferritin levels in 63 children with neuroblastoma by counterelectrophoresis (CEP) using antibody to human ferritin. Increased ferritin levels in serum, positive by CEP (≥ 400 ng/ml), correlated well with the presence of active disease ($p < 0.001$ by Fisher's exact 2×2 test). A longitudinal study of serum ferritin levels in 39 of the 63 patients showed the same association of elevated serum ferritin with active disease; a return of ferritin levels to the normal ranges coincided with remission. Primary neuroblastoma tumors and cells from neuroblastoma cell lines contained ferritins which had the electrophoretic characteristics of carcinofetal isoferritins. These findings suggest that the increased ferritin in the serum of patients is derived from the tumor. The serum ferritin level could be used as an aid to diagnosis and a guide to therapy.

ACKNOWLEDGMENTS

The authors wish to thank Dr. James W. Drysdale and Ms. JoAnn Eccher at Tufts University School of Medicine for their instruction and assistance in the chemistry of ferritin; Dr. H. Schlesinger at The Children's Hospital of Philadelphia for providing the neuroblastoma cell lines and supernatant fluids; Dr. L. Castor at The Institute for Cancer Research (ICR), Philadelphia, for culturing neuroblastoma cells and providing supernatant from IMR-90; Dr. Drysdale and Drs. W. T. London and B. Werner at ICR for their review and criticism of this chapter; and Ms. Maureen Walsh for her excellent typing of the manuscript. This work was supported by USPHS Grants CA-06551, RR-05539, CA-06927, CA-14489, and CA-13451 from the National Institutes of Health, by an appropriation from the Commonwealth of Pennsylvania, and by funds from the Elaine O. Weiner foundation trust.

REFERENCES

1. Alpert, E., Coston, R. L., and Drysdale, J. W. (1974): Carcinofetal human liver ferritins. *Nature,* 242:194–195.
2. Arosio, P., Adelman, T. G., and Drysdale, J. W. (1978): On ferritin heterogeneity, further evidence for heteropolymers. *J. Biol. Chem.,* 253:4451–4458.
3. Aungst, C. W. (1968): Ferritin in body fluids. *J. Lab. Clin. Med.,* 71:517–522.
4. Bieber, C. P., and Bieber, M. M. (1973): Detection of ferritin as a circulating tumor-associated antigen in Hodgkin's disease. *Natl. Cancer Inst. Monogr.,* 36:147–157.
5. Coombes, R. C., Powles, T. J., Gazet, J. C., Ford, H. T., Nash, A. G., Sloane, J. P., Hillyard, C. J., Thomas, P., Keyser, J. W., Marcus, D., Zinberg, N., Stimson, W. H., and Munro, N. A. (1977): A biochemical approach to the staging of human breast cancer. *Cancer,* 40:937–944.
6. Drysdale, J. W. (1977): Ferritin phenotypes: Structure and metabolism. Iron metabolism. *Ciba Found. Symp.,* 51:41–67.
7. Drysdale, J. W., Adelman, T. G., Arosio, P., and Yokota, M. (1976): Structural and immunological relationships of human isoferritins in normal and disease states. *Birth Defects,* 12:105–122.
8. Drysdale, J. W., and Singer, R. M. (1974): Carcinofetal human isoferritins in placenta and HeLa cells. *Cancer Res.,* 34:3352–3354.
9. Eshhar, Z., Order, S. E., and Katz, D. H. (1974): Ferritin, a Hodgkin's disease associated antigen. *Proc. Natl. Acad. Sci. U.S.A.,* 71:3956–3960.
10. Hazard, J. T., and Drysdale, J. W. (1977): Ferritinemia in cancer. *Nature,* 265:755–756.
11. Jacobs, A., and Worwood, M. (1975): Ferritin in serum: Clinical and biochemical implications. *N. Engl. J. Med.,* 292:951–956.
12. Jones, P. A. E., Miller, F. M., Worwood, M., Jacobs, A. (1973): Ferritinemia in leukemia and Hodgkin's disease. *Br. J. Cancer,* 27:212–217.
13. Kew, M. C., Torrance, J. D., Derman, D., Simon, M., Macnab, G. M., Charlton, R. W., and Bothwell, T. H. (1978): Serum and tumor ferritins in primary liver cancer. *Gut,* 19:294–299.
14. Lipschitz, D. A., Cook, J. D., and Finch, C. A. (1974): A clinical evaluation of serum ferritin as an index of iron stores. *N. Engl. J. Med.,* 290:1213–1216.
15. Mazur, A., and Shorr, E. (1950): A quantitative immunochemical study of ferritin and its relation to the hepatic vasodepressor material. *J. Biol. Chem.,* 182:607–627.
16. Nichols, W. W., Murphy, D. G., Cristofalo, V. J., Toji, L. H., Greene, A. E., and Dwight, S. A. (1977): Characterization of a new human diploid cell strain, IMR-90. *Science,* 196:60–63.
17. Niitsu, Y., Ohtsuka, S., Kohgo, Y., Watanabe, N., Koseki, J., and Urushizaki, I. (1975): Hepatoma ferritin in tissue and serum. *Tumor Res.,* 10:31–42.
18. Parry, D. H., Worwood, M., and Jacobs, A. (1975): Serum ferritin in acute leukemia at presentation and during remission. *Br. Med. J.,* 1:245–247.
19. Reissman, K. R., and Dietrich, M. R. (1956): On the presence of ferritin in the peripheral blood of patients with hepatocellular disease. *J. Clin. Invest.,* 35:588–595.
20. Schlesinger, H. R., Gerson, J. M., Moorhead, P. S., Maguire, H., and Hummeler, K. (1976): Establishment and characterization of human neuroblastoma cell lines. *Cancer Res.,* 36:3094–3100.
21. Siegel, S. (1956): The case of two independent samples. In: *Nonparametric Statistics,* pp. 96–104. McGraw-Hill, New York.
22. Siimes, M. A., Addiego, J. E., and Dallman, P. R. (1973): Ferritin in serum: Diagnosis of iron deficiency and iron overload in infants and children. *Blood,* 43:581–590.
23. White, G. P., Worwood, M., Parry, D. H., and Jacobs, A. (1974): Ferritin synthesis in normal and leukemic leucocytes. *Nature,* 250:584–585.
24. Worwood, M., Summers, M., Miller, F., Jacobs, A., and Whittaker, J. A. (1974): Ferritin in blood cells from normal subjects and patients with leukemia. *Br. J. Haematol.,* 28:27–35.

Advances in Neuroblastoma Research,
edited by Audrey E. Evans.
Raven Press, New York © 1980.

Discussion: Disease Characteristics in Man

The discussion was opened by *Dr. Krivit (Minneapolis)*, who pointed out that the response rates for children with the advanced stages of neuroblastoma have been rising steadily over the years as new therapeutic regimens are tested in the clinic. He therefore stressed that there was reason for optimism rather than a sense of pessimism that he thought he detected in the presentations. The neuroblastoma experience to date reminded him of the early days of clinical trials for acute leukemia, where it took some time for the better response rates to be manifest as better survival rates. He believed the same sequence might well be taking place in neuroblastoma.

There ensued an exchange among *Dr. D'Angio (Philadelphia)*, *Dr. Green (Memphis)*, and *Dr. Evans (Philadelphia)* with respect to staging criteria with special reference to stages III and IV-S. D'Angio thought that the multiple lesions in children with IV-S may represent multiple primary foci rather than metastases in the traditional sense. The distribution of the lesions and their clinical evolution were different from those seen with metastatic neuroblastoma. He therefore suggested that the term "disseminated disease" would be more apt in discussing the disease in IV-S patients; that the word *metastases* should at least be placed in quotation marks. Second, D'Angio discussed the significance of the midline when considering stage III disease. He believed that a poor prognosis is associated with tumors that cross the midline by direct extension of infiltrating tumor, or by metastases to the contralateral lymph nodes. Thus a tumor primary in the adrenal that infiltrates behind the great vessels to attain the opposite side would fit these criteria; one that overhangs the midline because of bulk would not have the same significance. The same concepts should be applied to tumors that are primary in the organ of Zuckerkandl. Even a small, well-encapsulated tumor arising in that organ would cross the midline; yet such a tumor would be expected to have a much better outcome than one that had infiltrated widely or had metastasized to contralateral lymph node chains. In short, aggressive tumors make clear their aggressive nature by their capacity to infiltrate or to metastasize distantly along lymphatic channels. Green was not prepared to consider stage IV-S disease as a multifocal process until evidence could be accumulated using cytogenetic or biochemical markers. He also believed that data from his institution demonstrated that widespread lymph nodal involvement, even on the ipsilateral side, was associated with a bad outlook. He made a plea for biopsy of lymph nodes in all patients so that the staging systems in use could be more precise.

Evans pointed out that it is extremely difficult to obtain lymph node biopsies in all patients because of the huge tumors that are sometimes encountered in these children. They are unresectable because of their size and friability, so that—desirable though it might be—it would be difficult to obtain systematic data regarding the pattern of lymph node metastases in all patients. Perhaps studies such as the one conducted at the Institut Gustave Roussy, where lymphangiograms were performed in patients with intra-abdominal neuroblastomas, could yield the necessary information. All three discussants were in agreement that more detailed information with respect to distribution of disease in these patients is needed to "fine tune" the staging system. They also agreed that some children with stage IV-S may be undertreated, whereas others are overtreated. What kind of therapy and when it should be used await better definition.

Individuals in the audience asked whether complete remission implied a return of the catecholamines to normal levels if they were elevated initially, and whether total healing of bone lesions was necessary. Green stated that complete remission implied a return of the catecholamine values to within 2 standard deviations of the normal values for the age; and that bone scans and skeletal radiographs must be normal. A persistent lytic lesion is considered a poor response, and reossification roentgenographically associated with a positive bone scan is called a partial response.

Dr. Evans (Philadelphia) was asked how she would stage a patient with the usual stigmata of IV-S disease, but who had a positive bone scan. She considers such patients as being stage IV, but believes that infants with such a constellation of finding probably have a better outlook than those with the usual stage IV pattern.

Dr. Voute (Amsterdam) discussed his results on the excretion of metabolites of catecholamines in 250 neuroblastomas. He emphasized the importance of the VMA/HVA ratio for prognosis provided that vanilglycol (VG) is added to the VMA. Under those circumstances, the excretion in the initial urine is a good prognostic criterion.

Dr. Siegel (Los Angeles) felt that the addition of VG to VMA in the ratio would not alter it significantly, but that appearance of early metabolites infers indeed a poor prognosis and that the VMA/HVA ratio is a prognostic factor independent from staging. Dr. Bernstein (Seattle) raised the question whether it is possible to correlate the excretion of early metabolites such as HVA with the state of differentiation of the tumor cells. Dr. LaBrosse (Maryland) said that there is no such correlation in his experience. He cautioned, however, that the VMA/HVA ratio in the early urine is not always a good prognostic tool. He demonstrated that with results of one patient on whom serial metabolite determinations were performed over a long period of time during the illness. The ratio changed frequently, especially during treatment, and had a very favorable high ratio a day before death. He cautioned against extrapolating from results on the initial urine specimens alone although, he emphasized, in general the results on early urines are indeed helpful in prognostication. Dr. Knudson (Philadelphia) commented on Schimke's presentation by discussing the question of single vs. multicellular origin of the neuroblastoma in stage IV-S cases. He pointed to a situation which might answer this question. Testing for glucose-6-phosphate dehydrogenase (G6PD) in IV-S neuroblastoma tumor lesions of different loci in black females who are heterozygous for this locus could reveal whether tumor cells found throughout the body arise from one or multiple doses and could thus be one-hit or two-hit tumor cells.

Genetics

Advances in Neuroblastoma Research,
edited by Audrey E. Evans.
Raven Press, New York © 1980.

Why the Genetics of Neuroblastoma?

Alfred G. Knudson, Jr.

Institute for Cancer Research, Fox Chase Cancer Center, Philadelphia, Pennsylvania 19111

This section of the proceedings is devoted to the genetics of neuroblastoma. As chairman I would like to say a few words about the reasons for being interested in the genetics of neuroblastoma.

We begin by stating that neuroblastoma, like many other tumors, does not fall equally on all members of a population; some persons are at greatly increased risk because of genetic predisposition. Knudson and Strong (4) estimated that 20% or so of cases might be individuals predisposed by a dominantly transmissible mutation. Arguing from an assumed parallel with retinoblastoma (3), we may hypothesize that all hereditary cases arise in individuals with a microscopic or submicroscopic chromosomal mutation present at conception, and that all nonhereditary cases are initiated by a somatic mutation at the same genetic locus in individuals who were normal at conception. Although the genetic site for such a mutation is apparently now known for retinoblastoma (6) and Wilms' tumor (5), it is not known for neuroblastoma, so we eagerly await new information bearing on this problem.

What might be done with such information? It is my contention that it could be used for the purposes of gene carrier identification and disease prevention, on the one hand, and for the purposes of physiological elucidation and disease treatment, on the other.

Chromosomal localization of a neuroblastoma gene might lead to the identification of the responsible segment of DNA in the human genome. New technology for the sorting of human chromosomes (1) might be employed to collect chromosomes from the fibroblasts of normal persons, from persons who carry in all cells of their bodies a chromosome from which the neuroblastoma gene has been deleted, and from persons who carry in all cells a chromosome rendered mutant by any of a variety of submicroscopic changes in the neuroblastoma gene (Fig. 1). By the appropriate analysis of nucleic acid products of restriction enzyme digestion and the cloning of appropriate nucleic acid sequences, it is theoretically possible to identify the DNA of the neuroblastoma gene and the alterations in it that are associated with various prezygotic forms of this tumor. Furthermore, it should then be possible to transcribe the normal gene and to identify its product.

If all classes of neuroblastoma mutations could be identified in all cells of

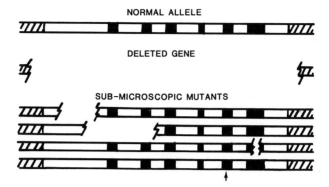

FIG. 1. A hypothetical tumor gene and its mutants. ▨▨, adjacent genes; ■, transcribed DNA sequences; □, untranscribed sequences; ↑, point mutation.

persons who carry a prezygotically determined mutation, there exists a potential to decrease the incidence of this tumor. All new hereditary cases could be identified as being at risk of transmitting the gene to their offspring. Fetal diagnosis would also be possible and might even lead to the identification of still unborn *new* hereditary cases. At present we can only offer empiric risk estimates, and these are very unsatisfactory, because so many variables are not known (Fig. 2). It would therefore be conceivable that all prezygotic cases could be prevented. Prevention of nonhereditary cases would not be accomplished, however, and we would necessarily look for other ways to modify this incidence. According to a genetic hypothesis, these cases could never be completely prevented, owing to spontaneous somatic mutation. The accumulated incidence,

Expectation of Tumor in Offspring

of Affected Individual

Fraction hereditary   = h

nonhereditary = 1-h

Relative fertility hereditary case = 1-a

Probability gamete carries gene   = 1/2

gamete survives   = 1-b

conceptus survives   = 1-c

tumor develops   = 1-d

Overall probability of affected child if

no genetic information on parent

$$= \frac{h(1-a)(1-b)(1-c)(1-d)}{2}$$

FIG. 2.

or prevalence (P), of a childhood cancer produced by mutations is the sum of the hereditary cases, which are dependent on germinal mutations that occur in the tumor gene at a rate μ_g, and the nonhereditary cases, which are dependent on somatic mutations that occur in that same gene at a rate μ_s (2):

$$P = a \cdot \mu_g + b \cdot \mu_s$$

Each of these mutation rates could be altered by environmental factors, and each of the constants, a and b, could be altered by various selective means. A corollary of this formulation is that in the absence of environmental modification of any of the processes, the incidence of such a tumor would be essentially the same in all parts of the world. Spontaneous nonhereditary cases will always be with us, and we therefore have great motivation for improving the tools of therapy.

The implications of a genetic model for the improvement of treatment are based on the hypothesis that the mutant gene can be replaced or that its expression can be modified. Is there a basis for hope that knowledge of the gene or its product could be useful therapeutically? Here we note that of all the tumors of man, neuroblastoma is the best known of those that can undergo spontaneous regression or differentiation to a benign state. Might this process be catalyzed and made general? We should begin by realizing that all cancers show some differentiation and cell death, and that it is not necessary to introduce a new process that never occurs spontaneously. In fact, there is the suggestion that many tumors live precariously. Perhaps the neuroblastomas that arise prenatally illustrate this best (Fig. 3). It is reasonable to suppose that the environment of a neuroblastoma is not the same prenatally and postnatally; some neuroblas-

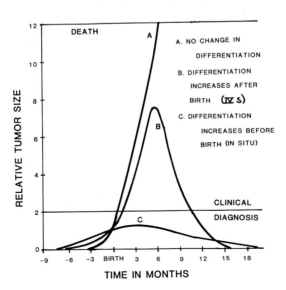

FIG. 3. Prenatal neuroblastoma. A schematic diagram of growth under different conditions.

toma mutations might thrive better under one condition than the other. Thus some mutations (A) that arise prenatally might continue their growth until death of the host ensues. Others (B) might fare less well and undergo more differentiation after birth than before; these could be the IV-S neuroblastomas. Still others (C) might even differentiate prenatally and be identified only incidentally as examples of neuroblastoma *in situ*. We ask, then, whether such a means as supplying the product of the normal allele of the neuroblastoma gene might convert examples of A to B and B to C.

We have much reason, therefore, to learn more about the genetics of neuroblastoma, and we look forward to the time when this knowledge can be applied to the prevention and treatment of this particularly fearsome cancer of children.

ACKNOWLEDGMENTS

This research was supported in part by an appropriation from the Commonwealth of Pennsylvania and by grants from the United States Public Health Service CA-22780 and CA-06927.

REFERENCES

1. Carrano, A. V., Gray, J. W., Langlois, R. G., Burkhart-Schultz, K. J., and Van Dilla, M. A. (1979): Measurement and purification of human chromosomes by flow cytometry and sorting. *Proc. Natl. Acad. Sci. U.S.A.*, 1382–1384.
2. Knudson, A. G. (1976): Genetics and the etiology of childhood cancer. *Pediatr. Res.*, 10:513–517.
3. Knudson, A. G. (1978): Retinoblastoma: A prototypic hereditary neoplasm. *Semin. Oncol.*, 5:57–60.
4. Knudson, A. G., and Strong, L. C. (1972): Mutation and cancer: Neuroblastoma and pheochromocytoma. *Am. J. Human Genet.*, 24:514–532.
5. Riccardi, V. M., Sujansky, E., Smith, A. C., and Francke, U. (1978): Chromosomal imbalance in the aniridia-Wilms' tumor association: 11p interstitial deletion. *Pediatrics*, 61:604–610.
6. Yunis, J. J., and Ramsay, N. (1978): Retinoblastoma and subband deletion of chromosome 13. *Am. J. Dis. Child.*, 132:161–163.

Advances in Neuroblastoma Research,
edited by Audrey E. Evans.
Raven Press, New York © 1980.

Genetic Regulation of Malignancy in Human Neuroblastoma Cell Hybrids

Fred Gilbert and Gloria Balaban-Malenbaum

Departments of Pediatrics and Human Genetics, University of Pennsylvania School of Medicine, Philadelphia, Pennsylvania 19104

Our approach to the study of the effects of individual genes on the development of cancer involves the use of tumor cells in culture and takes advantage of the technique of somatic cell hybridization for gene mapping (14). Hybrid cell lines formed from the fusion of any two cell types can be scored for the loss or retention of specific chromosomes and for the coordinate loss or retention of particular phenotypic characteristics. In this way genes responsible for specific functions can be assigned to individual chromosomes (20). If the fusion is between different malignant cell lines or between malignant and nonmalignant cells and the phenotype under investigation has the ability to form tumors in an appropriate host, then it is possible that one might be able to use such hybrids to gain insight into the genetic regulation of the expression of malignancy (14,27).

NEUROBLASTOMA

Certain tumors, e.g., neuroblastoma and retinoblastoma, offer special advantages in the proposed somatic cell studies in that they exist in both hereditary and nonhereditary forms (17). The hereditary form of each is dominantly inherited, although many hereditary cases of the childhood tumors result from new germinal mutations and do not present a positive family history. The neuroblastoma, which is the tumor on which we will focus, is a relatively common solid tumor of childhood with an estimated lifetime incidence of approximately one per 10,000 children (40). It is a particularly interesting tumor in that cases have been described which demonstrate spontaneous regression—through either cytolysis or hemorrhagic necrosis—or maturation of the tumor to a more benign form, the ganglioneuroma (10).

Several families have been reported in which more than one individual has had a neuroblastoma (6). When all of these cases are considered together, it becomes apparent that, although the familial cases do not fit the usual pattern of dominant inheritance, they do fit the pattern of a semilethal dominant gene in which most hereditary cases result from new mutations. However, only a small number of tumors arise in a gene carrier, suggesting that some further (somatic) event must occur. To explain these observations, Knudson and Strong (19) have advanced a two-mutation model, which proposes that two mutations are required before the malignant phenotype can be expressed. In the nonfamilial (sporadic) cases of neuroblastoma, the two mutations would occur in the somatic cell (the neuroblast) itself. In the familial neuroblastomas, Knudson and Strong hypothesize that the first mutation arises prezygotically in the germ line of an antecedent and that the second mutation occurs in the neuroblast. In the familial cases, the first mutation is present in all cells of the body but does not itself transform the cell to a cancer cell. The existence of the first mutation does, obviously, increase the likelihood that such transformation will occur in some cell within the target tissue. For any one cell, however, the probability of the transformation event is still low (approximately 5×10^{-6} per locus per cell generation) (23).

CHROMOSOMES AND MALIGNANCY

Any discussion of a genetic influence on the development of cancer must take into account the considerable literature which has accumulated over the last 20 years exploring the possible relationships between chromosomal aberrations and neoplasia. In the first such report, Nowell and Hungerford (29) showed (in 1960) that chronic myelogenous leukemia was associated with a distinctive abnormal chromosome, the Philadelphia chromosome. Since then, an association between chromosome abnormalities and malignant transformation has been seen with exposure to certain exogenous agents (radiation, viruses, and chemicals), in presumably sporadic tumors (e.g., meningioma, Burkitt's lymphoma, and seminoma), in recessively inherited disorders (e.g., xeroderma pigmentosum, Fanconi's anemia, ataxia-telangiectasia, and Bloom's syndrome), and in a number of dominant disorders (including the familial polyposes) (13).

The chromosomal aberrations may be random (as in the breakage and rearrangements reported in Fanconi's anemia) or specific (as in ataxia-telangiectasia, where translocations involving a particular region of chromosome 14 are found) (13). A number of malignancies, primarily leukemias and other myeloproliferative disorders, have been studied in which the chromosome abnormalities are not specific but tend to involve a limited number of chromosomes (i.e., numbers 1, 7, 8, 9, 14, 17, 20, 21 and 22) (28). Interest in this subject has increased in the last several years as the availability of newer staining techniques has made it possible to define chromosome rearrangements with greater precision (e.g., the Philadelphia chromosome, originally believed to be a deleted chromosome 22, is now known to involve a translocation between the long arm of chromosome 22 and another autosome, usually the 9) (32). Individuals have also been reported in whom clonal populations containing chromosome rearrangements are present for some time before a malignancy becomes apparent (24).

Several recent observations concerning chromosome abnormalities in two presumed genetic childhood tumors, retinoblastoma and Wilms' tumor, are also of interest. A number of individuals have now been reported with Wilms' tumor and aniridia who also carry a deletion involving a specific segment of the short arm of chromosome 11 (31). In addition, approximately 15 individuals have been described who have had a deletion of the long arm of chromosome 13 in all of their cells, a variable pattern of congenital defects, and retinoblastoma (either unilateral or bilateral) (18). If we accept the two-mutation hypothesis of Knudson and Strong which has been invoked to explain the origin of these tumors, then we can theorize that chromosomes 11p and 13q carry loci involved in the control of cell division and that deletion of these segments effectively constitutes the prezygotic first "mutations" predisposing these individuals to development of Wilms' tumor or retinoblastoma.

However, malignant proliferation of the retinal cells, for example, to produce a retinoblastoma—would only follow the second mutation, which might be at another position on the deletion chromosome, in the remaining intact chromosome 13, or at another site in the genome. The second possibility is particularly intriguing since it would imply that a cancer can result from mutations in a pair of genes at a single locus (a form of "homozygosity" at this locus).

No comparable deletion syndrome has yet been described in patients with neuroblastoma (for a discussion of chromosome abnormalities in neuroblastoma cases, see the chapter by P. Moorhead, p. 109 *this volume*). Tumors of the nervous system, including the neuroblastoma, have, however, been associated with two chromosome abnormalities, long marker chromosomes and double minute chromosomes (35). In 1974 Biedler and Spengler (4) showed that in two of four human neuroblastoma lines studied, the long marker chromosomes contained a region which did not demonstrate the usual banding pattern seen in trypsin-Giemsa stained preparations. The anomalous region stained a uniform gray and was termed the "homogenously staining region" (HSR). The cytological characterization of these two abnormalities and their possible relationship to each other are described in two chapters in this volume (J. L. Biedler, p. 81; G. Balaban-Malenbaum and F. Gilbert, p. 97).

Although it is clear that neoplasia is often associated with chromosomal changes, the exact relationship between these two phenomena is unknown. Whether the chromosomal changes reported are primary (i.e., responsible for malignant cell proliferation or responsible for predisposing the cell to a subsequent transformation event) or secondary (i.e., associated with continued division of an already neoplastic cell) remains an unanswered question in cancer biology.

In this regard, Rowley (33) has recently made an interesting observation. She has noted that the chromosomal abnormalities in the myeloproliferative disorders tend to involve a small group of chromosomes: chromosomes to which a number of gene loci responsible for nucleic acid metabolism have been assigned (by the study of somatic cell hybrids). It is possible, then, that these chromosome changes (translocations, duplications, etc.) affect the regulation of one or more genetic functions in such a way that they confer a proliferative advantage to the affected cell.

SOMATIC CELL HYBRIDIZATION AND THE STUDY OF MALIGNANCY

Cell hybridization as a tool for genetic analysis was initially introduced by Barski and co-workers in 1960 (3). After prolonged co-cultivation of two mouse lines differing both in morphology and in karyotype, these investigators noted the appearance of a third, morphologically distinct cell line in the same tissue culture dish. This new line was found to contain a total chromosome number approximately equal to the sum of the modal chromosome numbers of the two other cell lines (as well as containing the marker chromosomes found in each parental line). This was, in essence, a fusion product: a new cell line capable of continuous growth and division and containing the combined genomes of two other cell lines.

Ephrussi and Weiss (9) soon showed that hybrid combinations could also be produced from the fusion of cell lines of different species, and in 1967 Weiss and Green (39) first demonstrated the usefulness of somatic cell hybridization for gene mapping in man. They found that in human × rodent hybrid cell lines, human chromosomes were preferentially lost (or segregated) with time. The chromosome loss appeared to be largely random and was most rapid in the first cell divisions, then slowed with time. Hybrid clones could thus be generated that contained varying numbers of human chromosomes. Shortly thereafter, special staining procedures were introduced which made it possible to unambiguously identify each of the human and rodent chromosomes (5). It therefore became possible to analyze large numbers of human × mouse hybrid lines containing defined human chromosome complements for a variety of constitutive enzymes. If in such hybrids the presence or absence of a particular human enzyme activity was always associated with presence or absence of a specific human chromosome, one could assign a gene controlling the expression of the enzyme to that chromosome (34). At the present time over 200 genes have been mapped through a combination of cell hybrid analysis and family studies with at least one gene locus assigned to each of the 24 human chromosomes (26).

Cell hybrids have also been used in the study of malignancy (14,27). The results to date have been somewhat contradictory. The first experiments done in the early 1960s by Barski, Ephrussi, and co-workers demonstrated that hybrids formed from the fusion of highly malignant cells with less malignant or normal diploid cells produced tumors at high frequencies when injected into appropriate mouse strains (8). The hybrids thus appeared to inherit the malignancy potential of the more malignant parent, and it was concluded that malignancy acted as a dominant genetic trait.

In 1969, however, Harris (14) and Klein began a series of experiments that led these authors to the opposite conclusion. Using hybrids between highly malignant mouse ascites tumors and permanent mouse nonmalignant fibroblast lines, they found the frequency of tumors in susceptible mice to be low. In the few tumors that did develop, karyotypic analysis of the explanted cells indicated that there were fewer chromosomes contributed by the nonmalignant parent. These results implied that malignancy was recessive to nonmalignancy. The ability to produce tumors was suppressed in the majority of the hybrids formed between malignant and nonmalignant cells and could be re-expressed only in those hybrids that had lost one or more chromosomes from the nonmalignant parent.

The Harris-Klein group suggests that the earlier conclusion that malignancy acts as a dominant trait was based on an inadequate analysis of the chromosome complements of the hybrid cells and of the tumors they produced. They argue that extensive chromosome loss had occurred in the Ephrussi and Barski hybrids as they were passaged *in vitro* prior to inoculation into the test animals. They consider that malignancy is the result of a change in the genome (through mutation or chromosome rearrangement, for example) such that a normal gene product responsible for the suppression of malignancy is lost or an abnormal gene product is synthesized. Hybridization with a nonmalignant cell results in complementation (correction of the defect) with restoration of an effective level of the required normal gene product. With the loss of the gene (or genes) for suppressor activity as specific chromosomes are lost in successive divisions of the hybrid line, the malignant potential is re-expressed (14).

A large series of fusions involving different combinations of rodent with rodent, rodent with human, and human with human cell lines has since been performed by a number of investigators. The results of these studies have been interpreted as supporting one of the two seemingly contradictory conclusions: that malignancy acts as a dominant or recessive genetic trait (7,15,16,21,25,37).

It is, however, not unreasonable to assume that the different conclusions drawn from these studies reflect basic differences in the malignant cells participating in the fusions. Most of the previous studies have used highly aneuploid, permanent rodent lines as the malignant partner in the fusion. Those which have involved human malignant cells have used either virus-transformed cells or cells which have been in culture for many years (e.g., HeLa). It is therefore possible that in certain systems (virus transformation, for example) malignancy behaves as a dominant trait while in others it behaves as a recessive trait.

By using cells which have recently been isolated from tumors and are both stable and near diploid in karyotype, we hope to avoid at least some of the problems inherent in working with permanent lines (e.g., problems such as significant aneuploidy, unstable chromosome rearrangements, and altered metabolic requirements). By using cells for which no evidence of virus or chemical transformation exists, we avoid one other criticism of the previous cell hybrid studies. By using cell lines derived from human material, we avoid the obvious difficulty inherent in all of the rodent cell work, that of being able to relate our results directly to human tumor biology. By choosing to study tumors that occur in familial forms, we have perhaps enhanced our chances of identifying individual genes involved in the expression of the malignant phenotype.

METHOD OF PROCEDURE

Cells from two cell lines are fused using inactivated Sendai virus or polyethylene glycol (12). Hybrids are selected for their ability to divide and proliferate under conditions which kill the parent cells participating in the fusion.

Our protocol is as outlined in Table 1. The human neuroblastoma lines (described in detail in ref. 2) are fused with IT-22, a thymidine kinase deficient mouse line derived from 3T3 fibroblasts. The selection medium contains ouabain (to which the human cells are sensitive and the mouse cells are resistant) and hypoxanthine-aminopterin-thymidine (HAT; to which the mouse cells are sensitive while the human cells are resistant). Only complementing hybrids (those which contain thymidine kinase and are ouabain resistant) survive. Clones are allowed to grow up from single cells. The independent clones are screened for their ability to produce colonies in semisoft agarose, a property which correlates well but not absolutely with tumorigenicity (36,38). The agarose-positive and -negative clones are then tested for their ability to produce tumors in susceptible animals (immunologically deficient "nude" mice).

Karyotypes of the hybrid clones (using standard protocols: see G. Balaban-Malenbaum and F. Gilbert, p. 97 *this volume*) are prepared at the time the cells are placed in agarose, as well as when they are injected into the mice, and after the resulting tumor has been excised from the mouse. The human and mouse chromosome complements of the hybrids at different stages can then be compared with the karyotypes obtained from the original partners in the fusion.

RESULTS

Over 50 hybrid clones have now been isolated from fusions involving several human neuroblastoma sublines and the mouse line IT-22. The morphological appearance of the hybrids is quite variable: some are fibroblast-like while others resemble the neuroblastoma parent and extend small neuritic processes. Some of the hybrids also retain the capacity to synthesize neurospecific enzymes (11).

The results of our initial screen of the ability of the hybrid clones to produce colonies in semisoft agarose are given in Table 2. Agarose-positive and -negative

TABLE 1. *Method of procedure*

Fusion	Human Mouse
↓	neuroblastoma (IMR) × fibroblast (IT-22)
Selection	Complete medium + HAT/ouabain
↓	
Cloning	(From single cells)
↓	
Agarose screening	Agarose positive and negative lines
↓	
Injection into nude mice	

TABLE 2. *Colony formation in agarose*

Hybrid series	Lines positive	Lines negative
N4B (134B × IT-22)	1	4
N4D (134D × IT-22)	2	1
NR5 (IMR-5 × IT-22)	11	5
NR6 (IMR-6 × IT-22)	0	7
NB7 (NMB-7 × IT-22)	1	2
Totals	15	19

Agarose colony formation: 10^3 and 5×10^4 cells to each of three 60-mm agarose plates (0.26% agarose in complete medium). Positive lines produced visible colonies (containing at least 50 cells) within 2 weeks. Each line was tested at least twice.

clones have been identified in all but one of the hybrid series to date. (It is possible that agarose-positive hybrids will be found in the IMR-6 × IT-22 series once additional lines are tested.)

Each of the parent human neuroblastoma lines used in these fusions is capable of producing tumors in "nude" mice (Table 3). The mouse line IT-22 has consistently proved to be nontumorigenic in this test system in our laboratory. This has been observed in other laboratories as well (Carlo Croce, *personal communication*). Six representative hybrid lines were also injected into "nude" mice. Three agarose-negative lines proved to be nontumorigenic and three agarose-positive lines produced tumors in the mice.

The average length of time from the injection of cells to the detection of a palpable mass (the latency period) for IMR-5 and the hybrids is given in Table 4. The latency period is somewhat longer for the hybrids than it is for the parent neuroblastoma.

TABLE 3. *Tumor growth in nude mice*

Cell line	Tumors/mice
Human neuroblastoma lines	
IMR-6	1/3
IMR-5	7/8
134B	3/6
134D	4/6
Mouse fibroblast line	
IT-22	0/15
Hybrid cell lines	
N4BTP-8 (134B × IT-22)	0/15
NR6TV-1 (IMR-6 × IT-22)	0/15
NR6TV-7 (IMR-6 × IT-22)	0/4
NR5TP-3b(Ag) (IMR-5 × IT-22)	8/10
NR5TP-4a (IMR-5 × IT-22)	1/4
NR5TP-7b(Ag) (IMR-5 × IT-22)	4/4

10^7 cells injected s.c. into 2 sites per mouse. Line considered nontumorigenic is no growth apparent within 4 months after injection.

TABLE 4. *Latency period*

Cell line	Tumors	Latency period (days)
IMR-5	7/8	24 (16–38)
NR5TP-3b(Ag)	8/10	50 (45–55)
-3b(Ag)TC3	4/4	34 (30–39)
NR5TP-4a	1/4	45
-4aTC	5/5	36 (30–41)
NR5TP-7b(Ag)	4/4	82 (75–90)

Latency period: average time before tumors detected in nude mice.

Hybrid clone 4a was grown up soon after fusion and injected directly into "nude" mice. Only in one out of four test animals did a tumor develop. The tumor was explanted back into culture and the cell line which grew out was reinjected into "nude" mice. This line, designated 4aTC, produced tumors in five out of five test animals. Hybrid 4a was subsequently found to be agarose positive.

Hybrids 3b and 7b were initially screened for their ability to grow in agarose. They both proved to be agarose positive and colonies were picked from agarose, grown up in culture [3b(Ag), 7b(Ag)], and then injected into "nude" mice. Clones 7b(Ag) and 3b(Ag) produced tumors in four of four and eight of ten mice, respectively. Several 3b(Ag) tumors were excised and put back into culture. One such line, 3b(Ag)TC$_3$, when reinjected into "nude" mice, produced tumors in 100% of the test animals.

The results of our analysis of the karyotypes on the various cell lines and hybrids are given in Table 5. A comparison of the modal chromosome numbers of each parent line with those of the hybrid lines indicates that the hybrids are most likely the result of a 2:1 fusion (two mouse cells fused with one human cell).

Human chromosome 17 (the chromosome to which thymidine kinase has been assigned) is retained in virtually all of the cells of both tumorigenic and nontumorigenic hybrids. The nonmalignant hybrid lines each contain fewer than 20 human chromosomes, and the loss of individual chromosomes appears to be largely random. The double minutes or the HSR marker chromosome were, for the most part, not seen in these cells (the exception is described in the Discussion).

The chromosome complements were significantly different in the tumorigenic hybrids. The three lines resulting from the fusion and studied before passage through agarose or injection into the test animals—hybrids 3b, 4a, and 7b—each retain a small number of human chromosomes (including 17) as well as the HSR marker and double minutes. Sublines of hybrid 3b isolated after passage through agarose [3b(Ag)] and injection into "nude" mice [3b(Ag)TC$_3$], have lost virtually all intact human chromosomes (other than 17) but still retain the double minutes. Hybrid 7b and its derivative sublines behaved in a manner

TABLE 5. *Human chromosomes retained in hybrid lines*

Cell line	Avg. chromosome no.	Human chromosomes
N4BTP-8	100–130	15–20 total (#17, no HSR/DMS)
NR6TV-7	100–130	Under 10 (#17, no HSR/DMS)
NR6TV-1	90–100	Under 10 (see text)
NR5TP-3b	109 ± 20	#17, HSR/DMS
-3b(Ag)	104 ± 20	#17, HSR/DMS
-3b(Ag)TC$_3$	117 ± 15	#17, DMS (no HSR)
NR5TP-4a	159 ± 30	#17, HSR/DMS
-4aTC	129 ± 20	#17, DMS (no HSR)
-4aTCtc	109 ± 7	#17, DMS (no HSR)
NR5TP-7b	110 ± 20	#17, HSR/DMS
-7b(Ag)	94 ± 20	#17, DMS (no HSR)
-7b(Ag)TC	92 ± 10	#17, DMS (no HSR)
IMR-5	47 ± 1	All
IT-22	57 ± 3	0

Chromosome numbers in hybrid and parent lines (25–50 metaphases analyzed per cell line).

similar to 3b, with 7b(Ag)TC (cloned from agarose and then explanted from the "nude" mouse tumor) containing only human chromosome 17 and double minutes in addition to the mouse complement. Hybrid 4a was injected directly into "nude" mice, explanted back into culture (4aTC), and then reinjected into other "nude" mice. The second series of tumors which developed were excised and again explanted back into culture. One of the resulting lines (4aTCtc) was karyotyped and only human chromosome 17 and double minutes were identified along with the mouse chromosome complement.

DISCUSSION

We have demonstrated that the fusion of malignant human neuroblastoma cells with a nonmalignant mouse line can result in both tumorigenic and nontumorigenic hybrids. We have also found, in a small number of hybrids analyzed in detail, that the ability to form colonies in semisoft agarose and the retention of the HSR marker chromosome or double minutes appear to correlate with tumorigenicity to a sgnificant degree.

In previous hybrid studies, two diametrically opposed conclusions have been drawn concerning the genetic regulation of malignancy; it has been concluded that expression of the malignant phenotype can behave as either a dominant or recessive genetic trait. In the study we have described, it seems unlikely that the capacity of the neuroblastoma hybrids to grow as tumors in the "nude" mice is caused solely by the retention of a dominant "expressor" gene. This interpretation of our results is based on several lines of evidence.

In the reports advancing the hypothesis that malignancy acts in a dominant manner, virtually all of the hybrids analyzed were tumorigenic in appropriate test systems. This is presumed to result from the positive pressure exerted in favor of retention of a dominant gene by the test system (either passage through agarose or injection into a susceptible host). We did not find this to be the case in our system; both tumorigenic and nontumorigenic hybrids were produced in the fusions we have described.

The human chromosome complement in all of our analyzed hybrids is considerably reduced. No intact human chromosome (other than number 17, which was present in all hybrids whether tumorigenic or not) was retained in only the malignant hybrids and thus could be said to be required for tumorigenicity.

It is unlikely that the retention of an HSR is required to produce malignancy in the hybrids since a number of tumorigenic subclones have been isolated [e.g., NR5TP-4aTC and NR5TP-7b(Ag)] which have lost the HSR. That the retention of double minutes by themselves is also not sufficient to produce malignancy is suggested by an analysis of hybrid NR6TV-1 (Table 6).

Hybrid NR6TV-1 resulted from a fusion in September 1974. When initially karyotyped (May 1976), the HSR marker chromosome and double minutes were present in the hybrid cells. In August 1976, the cells were injected into 10 "nude" mice. Soon after injection, the cells were karyotyped and small numbers of double minutes were noted per cell: the HSR was no longer evident. In December 1976, an additional five mice were injected with the hybrid cells. The karyotypes of these cells (which had been in continuous culture since the fusion) demonstrated neither an HSR nor double minutes. In none of the 15 injected mice did a tumor develop within the period of observation (within 4 months from the time of injection).

Our results are similar to those reported by other investigators in studies which concluded that tumorigenicity in cell hybrids can be recessive to nontumorigenicity. This is because the increase in latency period of the hybrids (relative to that of the parent neuroblastoma) and the enhancement in tumorigenicity after passage through agarose (demonstrated in NR5TP-4a), as well as the production of both tumorigenic and nontumorigenic hybrids from similar fusions, all argue that the ability of the neuroblastoma hybrids to produce tumors is associated with the selective proliferation of a subpopulation of cells, presumably arising as the result of the loss of particular chromosomes (and, hence, particular genes) from the original hybrid.

TABLE 6. *NR6TV-1: time course in culture*

Fusion	9/24	
		5/5/76 Karyotype (HSR marker/DMS)
Injections	8/12/76 (3 mice)	
	8/19/76 (7 mice)	
		8/24/76 Karyotype (small number DMS; no HSR)
Injections	12/9/76 (5 mice)	
		12/15/76 Karyotype (no HSR or DMS)

Result: No tumors in any mouse within 4 months of injection (10^7 cells in each of 2 sites per mouse).

Since the nonmalignant partner in our fusions is a mouse cell, by this hypothesis it is a mouse chromosome (or chromosomes), carrying the gene(s) responsible for the suppression of tumorigenicity, which must be lost before the malignant phenotype can be expressed. Unfortunately, the hybrids involved in this study resulted from a 2:1 fusion (two mouse cells fused with one human cell), and the particular mouse line chosen for the fusion is aneuploid and contains numerous chromosome rearrangements. It is thus impossible either to identify individual mouse chromosomes with certainty or to draw any conclusions from the absolute number of mouse chromosomes retained in the hybrids. (Additional hybrids resulting from the fusion of the neuroblastoma cells with normal, diploid mouse cells will have to be analyzed before it can be established that a particular mouse chromosome is responsible for the suppression of malignancy.)

Although the loss of "suppressor" genes might be a necessary first step before these neuroblastoma hybrids are capable of producing tumors in appropriate animals, it is also possible that tumorigenicity might be enhanced by the presence of genes or extrachromosomal elements contributed by the malignant partner in the fusion. Obvious candidates for such "positive" effectors in our hybrids are the HSR and double minutes.

Evidence has already been presented from a number of laboratories which indicates that the HSR is a mechanism for the amplification of one or a small number of genes (1). If the gene(s) multiplied in such a segment play a role in cell division (perhaps by coding for a specific membrane component involved in cell-cell recognition or for an enzyme involved in nucleic acid biosynthesis), then the development of an HSR might confer a proliferative advantage to the cell in which it occurs.

We have also recently proposed that the double minutes are derived from the breakdown of the HSR (2; G. Balaban-Malenbaum and F. Gilbert, *this volume*, p. 97). In addition, it is known that the double minutes lack centromeres and, although it has been suggested that they can replicate independently, the number per cell tends to decrease over time in culture (22).

One might, then, speculate that an alteration in chromosome complement in the malignant hybrid might occur in several stages. After the fusion event, only those hybrids which lose the genes responsible for suppression of tumorigenicity are capable of malignant growth in an appropriate test animal. The hybrid subpopulation which also retains the HSR or double minutes might be at a proliferative advantage and, if so, would be expected to predominate in any tumor which ultimately develops.

If, however, the source of new double minutes were to disappear from the cell (either through the breakdown of the HSR or through the normal process of chromosome loss in hybrids) and the number of double minutes per cell were to decrease over time, then the division rate of the hybrid might decrease as well. This might result in a slowing in the rate of increase of tumor cells, and in the "nude" mouse model this might mean that no palpable tumor would be detected during the 4-month observation period after injection. Such a hybrid would be scored as negative for tumorigenicity (explaining, perhaps, what was found in hybrid NR6TV-1).

What insights have we gained into the possible roles played by individual genes in tumorigenesis? We have, unfortunately, not yet been able to identify genes on specific chromosomes which are responsible for the suppression or involved in the expression of malignancy. However, the results we have presented are most consistent with the conclusion that malignancy in the human neuroblastoma hybrid system (and, by extension, in the human tumor itself) behaves as a recessive trait. This is also consistent with the Knudson-Strong two-mutation hypothesis (which argues that no single dominant gene mutation would, under the conditions which normally apply *in vivo,* be sufficient to produce a neuroblastoma).

That the HSR does not represent one of the postulated primary gene changes responsible for production of a neuroblastoma is suggested by two observations: an HSR and/or double minutes have not been found in every neuroblastoma line in culture and the chromosomes carrying HSRs (although consistent within individual cells of the same line) have been different in each line examined to date. (It is, of course, possible that small HSRs may have been missed in these lines and that a single chromosome segment may develop into an HSR which, once formed, can translocate to other chromosomes within the genome.)

Our discussion of the possible significance of the HSR might be extended to the neuroblastoma itself. It can be hypothesized that after the primary gene changes have occurred which enable a neuroblast to continue to divide beyond its normal limits, an HSR might develop as a secondary event. By analogy to what we have already suggested for the hybrids, the presence of an HSR might confer a selective advantage on the population of tumor cells in which it is found. At some point in the evolution of the tumor, these cells might be able to continue in two possible directions. If the HSR is maintained intact, the cells would continue to proliferate as a neuroblastoma. If the HSR breaks down, double minutes appear which might ultimately be lost from the cell. This, in turn, might lead to alterations in the rate of increase of the tumor cell mass and in certain properties of individual cells (e.g., in the ability to metastasize) which might be more typical of a benign rather than of a malignant tumor.

A change in cellular characteristics, such as an alteration in cell membrane composition (dictated, perhaps, by the loss of the gene products specified by the HSR/double minutes), might also make the cells susceptible to attack by the host's immune surveillance system, resulting in regression of the tumor. As noted previously, both maturation (to produce a benign ganglioneuroma) and spontaneous regression of the tumor have been reported in patients with neuroblastoma.

Finally, it should be noted that the finding of an HSR is not limited to human neuroblastoma cell lines. HSRs have recently been reported in cell lines derived from a number of human and animal cancers. The formation of an

HSR may, then, represent a common occurrence in the clonal evolution of many tumors.

Whether the HSR does in fact play a role in cell proliferation, as we hypothesize, has yet to be established. Additional studies are therefore required to define the exact functional significance of both the HSR and double minutes and their relationship to malignancy.

ACKNOWLEDGMENTS

This research was supported by grants from the American Cancer Society VC-189A, the National Science Foundation PCM 76-82997, and The Children's Hospital Cancer Research Center CA-144898.

REFERENCES

1. Alt, F. W., Kellems, R. E., Bertino, J. R., and Schimke, R. T. (1978): Selective multiplication of DHFR genes in MTX-resistant variants of cultured murine cells. *J. Biol. Chem.*, 253:1357–1370.
2. Balaban-Malenbaum, G., and Gilbert, F. (1977): Double minute chromosomes and the homogeneously staining regions of a human neuroblastoma cell line. *Science*, 198:739–741.
3. Barski, G., Sorieul, S., and Cornefert, F. (1960): Production dan des cultures in vitro de deux souches cellulaires en association de cellules de caractere "hybride". *C.R. Acad. Sci. [D] (Paris)*, 251:1825.
4. Biedler, J. L., and Spengler, B. A. (1976): Metaphase chromosome anomaly: Association with drug resistance and cell-specific products. *Science*, 191:185–187.
5. Caspersson, T., and Zech, L. (eds.) (1973): *Chromosome Identification* (23rd Nobel Symposium). Academic Press, New York.
6. Chatten, J., and Voorhess, M. (1967): Familial neuroblastoma. *N. Engl. J. Med.*, 277:1230–1236.
7. Croce, C. M., Aden, D., and Koprowski, H. (1975): Somatic cell hybrids between mouse peritoneal macrophages and SV-40 transformed human cells II. *Proc. Natl. Acad. Sci. U.S.A.*, 72:1397–1400.
8. Ephrussi, B. (1972): *Hybridization of Somatic Cells*. Princeton University Press, Princeton, New Jersey.
9. Ephrussi, B., and Weiss, M. C. (1965): Interspecific hybridization of somatic cells. *Proc. Natl. Acad. Sci. U.S.A.*, 53:1040–1042.
10. Evans, A. E., Gerson, J., and Schnaufer, L. (1975): Spontaneous regression of neuroblastoma. *Natl. Cancer Inst. Monogr.*, 44:49–54.
11. Gilbert, F. (1976): The control of expression of differentiated functions in neuroblastoma hybrids. *J. Natl. Cancer Inst.*, 57:667–673.
12. Giles, R. E., and Ruddle, F. H. (1973): Production and characterization of proliferating somatic cell hybrids. In: *Tissue Culture*, edited by P. F. Kruse and M. K. Patterson, pp. 475–500. Academic Press, New York.
13. Harnden, D. G. (1977): Cytogenetics of human neoplasia. In: *Genetics of Human Cancer*, edited by J. J. Mulvihill, R. W. Miller, and J. F. Fraumeni, Jr., pp. 85–104. Raven Press, New York.
14. Harris, H. (1972): Cell fusion and the analysis of malignancy. *J. Natl. Cancer Inst.*, 48:851–864.
15. Jonasson, J., and Harris, H. (1977): The analysis of malignancy by cell fusion VIII. *J. Cell Sci.*, 24:255–263.
16. Jonasson, J., Povey, S., and Harris, H. (1977): The analysis of malignancy by cell fusion VII. *J. Cell Sci.*, 24:217–254.

17. Knudson, A. G. (1976): Genetics and the etiology of childhood cancer. *Pediatr. Res.,* 10:513–517.
18. Knudson, A. G., Meadows, A. T., Nichols, W. W., and Hill, R. (1976): Chromosomal deletion and retinoblastoma. *N. Engl. J. Med.,* 295:1120–1123.
19. Knudson, A. G., and Strong, L. (1972): Mutation and cancer: Neuroblastoma and pheochromocytoma. *Am. J. Hum. Genet.,* 24:514–532.
20. Kucherlapati, R., and Ruddle, F. H. (1976): Advances in human gene mapping by parasexual procedures. *Prog. Hum. Genet.,* 1:121–145.
21. Kucherlapati, R., and Shin, S. (1979): Genetic control of tumorigenicity in interspecific mammalian cell hybrids. *Cell,* 16:639–648.
22. Levan, A., and Levan, G. (1978): Have double minutes functioning centromeres? *Hereditas,* 88:81–92.
23. Matsunaga, E., and Ogyu, H. (1976): Retinoblastoma in Japan. *Jpn. J. Ophthalmol.,* 20:266–282.
24. McCaw, B. K., Hecht, F., Harnden, D. G., and Teplitz, R. L. (1975): Somatic rearrangement of chromosome 14 in human lymphocytes. *Proc. Natl. Acad. Sci. USA,* 72:2071–2075.
25. McDougall, J. K., et al. (1976): Mapping viral integration sites in somatic cell hybrids. *Cytogenet. Cell Genet.,* 16:206–210.
26. McKusick, V. A., and Ruddle, F. H. (1977): The status of the gene map of the human chromosome. *Science,* 196:390–405.
27. Minna, J. D. (1977): Genetic analysis of malignancy using somatic cell hybrids. In: *Genetics of Human Cancer,* edited by J. J. Mulvihill, R. W. Miller, and J. F. Fraumeni, pp. 243–354. Raven Press, New York.
28. Mitelman, F., and Levan, G. (1976): Clustering of aberrations to specific chromosomes in human neoplasms. *Hereditas,* 82:167–174.
29. Nowell, P. C., and Hungerford, D. A. (1960): A minute chromosome in human CML. *Science,* 132:1497.
30. Oxford, J. M., Harnden, D. G., Parington, J. H., and Delahanty, J. D. A. (1975): Specific chromosome aberrations in ataxia-telangiectasia. *J. Med. Genet.,* 12:251–252.
31. Riccardi, V. M., Sujansky, E., Smith, A. C., and Francke, U. (1978): Chromosomal imbalance in the aniridia-Wilms' association: 11p interstitial deletion. *Pediatrics,* 61:604–610.
32. Rowley, J. D. (1973): A new consistent chromosomal abnormality in chronic myelogenous leukemia identified by quinacrine fluorescence and Giemsa staining. *Nature,* 243:290–293.
33. Rowley, J. D. (1977): Mapping of human chromosomal regions related to neoplasia. *Proc. Natl. Acad. Sci. U.S.A.,* 74:5729–5733.
34. Ruddle, F. H. (1972): Linkage analysis using somatic cell hybrids. *Adv. Hum. Genet.,* 3:173–235.
35. Sandberg, A., Sakurai, M., and Holdsworth, R. N. (1972): Chromosomes and causation of human cancer and leukemia VIII. *Cancer,* 29:1671.
36. Shin, S., Freedman, V. H., Risser, R., and Pollack, R. (1975): Tumorigenicity of virus-transformed cells in nude mice is correlated specifically with anchorage independent growth in vitro. *Proc. Natl. Acad. Sci. U.S.A.,* 82:4435–4439.
37. Stanbridge, E. J. (1976): Suppression of malignancy in human cells. *Nature,* 260:17–20.
38. Stanbridge, E. J., and Wilkinson, J. (1978): Analysis of malignancy in human cells. *Proc. Natl. Acad. Sci. U.S.A.,* 75:1466–1469.
39. Weiss, M. D., and Green, H. (1967): Human-mouse hybrid cell lines containing partial complements of human chromosomes and functioning human genes. *Proc. Natl. Acad. Sci. U.S.A.,* 58:1104.
40. Young, J. L., and Miller, R. W. (1975): Incidence of malignant tumors in U.S. children. *J. Pediatr.,* 86:254–258.

Advances in Neuroblastoma Research,
edited by Audrey E. Evans.
Raven Press, New York © 1980.

Cytogenetic Studies of Primary Human Neuroblastomas

Garrett M. Brodeur, Alexander A. Green, and F. Ann Hayes

St. Jude Children's Research Hospital, Memphis, Tennessee 38101

The development of chromosome banding techniques has given added significance to the cytogenetic studies of cancer cells. Newer methods allow more detailed analysis of karyotypes, and subtle rearrangements can be detected which would have been missed with conventional techniques (15). Moreover, patterns of chromosome involvement are emerging which are nonrandom, and characteristic abnormalities have been identified in specific malignancies. Solid tumors have been less extensively studied than the hematologic malignancies, due to technical difficulties in obtaining and processing tumor tissue. Nevertheless, nonrandom patterns of involvement are becoming apparent as more cases are studied with banding.

We recently described a specific chromosomal abnormality, a deletion of the short arm of chromosome 1, in two primary neuroblastomas and in one of four neuroblastoma cell lines (4). There are no other reports of specific chromosomes involved in neuroblastoma, and there are no chromosomal syndromes with an increased incidence of neuroblastoma (5). Previously, the chromosomal anomaly most commonly associated with human neuroblastomas was the presence of double-minute sphere (dms) chromosomes (11), but they are also found in other neurogenic and non-neurogenic tumors (8,11). Giant marker chromosomes occur in neuroblastomas, but there are no chromosomes consistently involved in their formation (3,4). Possible mechanisms for the development of these markers are translocations or longitudinal duplication through exchange quadriradials (10). Another possible mechanism is by gene amplification with the formation of homogeneous staining regions (HSRs). Indeed, HSRs have been shown to develop in Chinese hamster lines coincident with the acquisition of drug resistance, and they have also been found in some neuroblastoma cell lines (3). An intriguing hypothesis has been proposed which attempts to further explain the development of the HSRs and relate them to the dms chromosomes (1). However, to date the HSRs have been reported only in cell lines.

Primary untreated tumors are the best source for cytogenetic analysis, since they are most likely to reflect the original stem line karyotype. About 80% of the tumors are diploid or near diploid and have relatively few rearrangements (4,13). Chromosomal damage is known to occur with certain drugs or with radiation treatment (6), and karyotypic rearrangements occur with time in long-term culture (2,14). Therefore, studies of primary tissue from untreated children should provide the most meaningful information concerning chromosomal rearrangements as they relate to malignant transformation.

The purpose of this prospective study was to examine tumor tissue from additional patients with neuroblastoma for cytogenetic abnormalities. We sought evidence for the nonrandom involvement of specific chromosomes, especially deletion or derangement of the short arm of chromosome 1. In addition we looked for the presence of dms chromosomes, as well as the HSRs in the samples where banding was successful. Finally, we looked for differences between the karyotypes at diagnosis and at relapse.

MATERIALS AND METHODS

Samples of neuroblastoma tissue were obtained from 12 patients over approximately a 1-year period. Cytogenetic analysis was unsuccessful in 3 patients, but two samples were obtained at different times from 3 other patients, so a total of 12 samples from 9 patients was analyzed. Tumor tissue was obtained from patients at the time of diagnostic surgery, bone marrow aspiration, or thoracentesis, or at the time of second-look surgery. Tissue was studied by direct preparation or short-term culture (7). In general, samples were harvested for chromosomal analysis after 2 to 4 days in culture, with one refeeding. Chromosomal analysis of neuroblastoma tissue was done using a modification of the technique of Moorhead et al. (9). Banding was done using a modification of the trypsin-Giemsa method of Seabright (12). Banding allowed complete analysis of the karyotypes of six samples (50 to 200 cells counted), whereas in the other six it was possible to determine only the mode and the presence or absence of dms chromosomes and giant markers (20 to 40 cells counted).

RESULTS

The patients from whom a single sample was obtained are listed in Table 1, along with the pertinent clinical information and the modal karyotypes. Patient

TABLE 1. *Neuroblastoma patients—single samples*

Patient	Age (years)	Site	Prior treatment	Karyotype
NGO	nb	Ab	—	46XY, normal
NMB$_2$	2	BM	CT, RT	45XY, 1p−, 14q+, −18
NRC	2	Ab	CT	72XXY, 1p−, other
NJH	9/12	Ab	—	44
NBW	6/12	Ab	—	70
NDH	3	PE	—	48

Clinical and cytogenetic data from 6 neuroblastoma patients from whom single tumor samples were obtained. Abbreviations: nb, newborn; Ab, abdominal; BM, bone marrow; PE, pleural effusion; CT, chemotherapy; RT, radiation therapy.

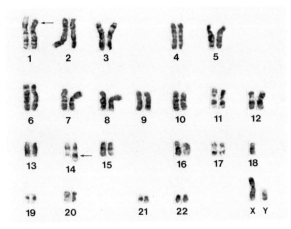

FIG. 1. Karyotype of the tumor from patient NMB$_2$. The modal karyotype is 45XY,1p−, 14q+,−18. The rearrangements of chromosomes 1 and 14 are described in Fig. 2.

NGO was a newborn, and his tumor cells had a normal karyotype, even with banding. Patient NMB$_2$ had received treatment prior to arrival, and his tumor had a mode of 45 chromosomes (Fig. 1). Abnormalities included a deletion of part of the short arm of chromosome 1, duplication of the long arm of chromosome 14, and monosomy for chromosome 18. Figure 2 is a partial karyotype showing the abnormal chromosomes 1 and 14 compared to the normal chromosomes from which they were derived. Only 1 of 100 cells counted had dms chromosomes, and no cells had HSRs. Tumor tissue was obtained from patient

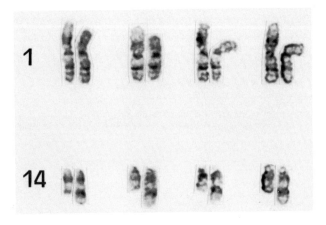

FIG. 2. Partial karyotype of the tumor from patient NMB$_2$, showing the chromosome 1 and chromosome 14 pairs from 4 cells. The abnormal chromosome 1 appears deleted beyond band 1p32 with an additional terminal dark band, possibly band 14q31 from the rearranged 14. The abnormal chromosome 14 appears to have lost the terminal dark band (14q31), with tandem duplication of bands q21→q24.

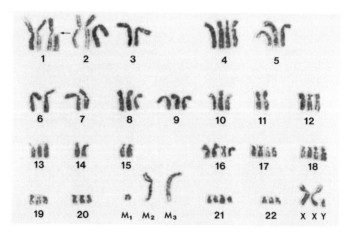

FIG. 3. Karyotype of the tumor from patient NRC. The mode is 72XXY, and there are multiple numerical abnormalities in this hypertriploid tumor. In addition, 4 marker chromosomes were consistently present, including a chromosome 1 with deletion of all of the short arm.

NRC at the time of second-look surgery, and his tumor had a mode of 72 chromosomes (Fig. 3). In addition to being hypertriploid, several marker chromosomes were present, including a chromosome 1 with deletion of all of the short arm. Banding was inadequate for complete analysis of the tumor karyotype from the other 3 patients, but 2 were in the diploid range; 1 was in the triploid range; and none of them had dms chromosomes or giant markers.

The patients from whom two samples were obtained are listed in Table 2, along with the pertinent clinical information and the modal karyotypes. In all cases a sample was obtained prior to therapy and at some later time during their course. The tumor from patient NBB had a normal karyotype at diagnosis (Fig. 4). Two percent of the cells had dms chromosomes, and no markers or HSRs were found. He was restudied at the time of bone marrow relapse, and the modal karyotype was 80 chromosomes. Banding was inadequate to com-

TABLE 2. *Neuroblastoma patients—2 samples*

Patient	Age (years)	Site	Prior treatment	Karyotype
NBB	2	BM	—	46XY, normal
		BM	CT	80
NKP	5	BM	—	53XX, ins(1p), other
		BM	CT	44XX, ins(1p), other
NCH	2	BM	—	102, mar × 2
		Ab	CT	49, mar

Clinical and cytogenetic data from 3 neuroblastoma patients from whom 2 tumor samples each were obtained. Abbreviations: Ab, abdominal; BM, bone marrow; CT, chemotherapy; mar, marker chromosome.

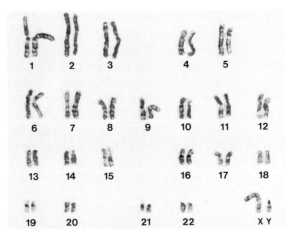

FIG. 4. Karyotype of the tumor from patient NBB. The modal karyotype is 46XY, with no apparent structural or numerical rearrangements.

pletely analyze the karyotype, but no dms chromosomes or giant markers were present.

The tumor from patient NKP had a mode of 53 chromosomes at diagnosis (Fig. 5). There were multiple rearrangements, including an insertion in the short arm of chromosome 1. This appeared to be a tandem duplication of bands 1p13→1p31. She was restudied at the time of relapse, and the mode was 44 chromosomes. Several of the same marker chromosomes were present, including the abnormal chromosome 1; no dms chromosomes or HSRs were present.

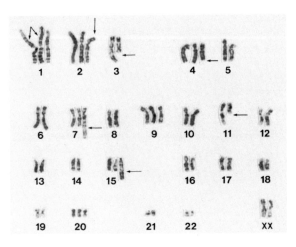

FIG. 5. Karyotype of the tumor from patient NKP. The modal karyotype is 53XX,+1,+2, +4,+7,+9,+15,+20,ins(1p),ins(1p),2p−,4q−,t(3;15),t(7,11). The insertion in the short arms of two number 1 chromosomes appears to be a tandem duplication of bands p13→p31.

Tumor cells from patient NCH were obtained from the bone marrow at diagnosis and from his abdominal primary at the time of second-look surgery, when his marrow was free of tumor. Only 30 metaphases were obtained in each case, and banding was unsuccessful. The initial sample had a mode of 102 chromosomes and there were two identical acrocentric markers. The second sample from the primary had a mode of 49 chromosomes, including one marker chromosome identical to the two seen in the earlier sample from the marrow.

The tumor from one patient (NCG) was not studied until it had become an established line. The modal karyotype was 45XY,del(1)(p13→pter),-15. It was included because it had only two abnormalities and because it was the only cell line which had been completely analyzed during the period of study.

DISCUSSION

In this prospective study of the cytogenetic features of primary neuroblastoma tissue, a deletion or derangement of the short arm of chromosome 1 was the most common abnormality. Two of the five tumors completely analyzed with banding had a deletion of part or all of chromosome 1, and an additional patient had derangement of part of the short arm. The regions of chromosome 1 involved in the primary neuroblastomas previously reported as well as those presented here are depicted in Fig. 6. Also depicted are the regions of involvement in two of five neuroblastoma lines studied.

Two of the five tumors examined with banding had a normal karyotype at diagnosis. Since the four tumors not completely analyzed with banding had abnormal modal chromosomal numbers, only two of the nine different tumors examined had a normal karyotype. This is similar to the finding of 10 of 39 previously reported cases having a normal karyotype (4). These tumors may

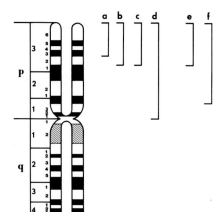

FIG. 6. Schematic representation of chromosome 1 as depicted at the Paris Conference (1971), with areas of deletion in several neuroblastomas represented by brackets: **(a)** NMB$_2$; **(b)** NTP (4); **(c)** NCC (4); and **(d)** NRC. Also shown are similar deletions in two neuroblastoma cell lines: **(e)** IMR (3,4,14); and **(f)** NCG.

have submicroscopic mutations or gene deletions which are undetectable with current techniques.

Two of the nine patients in this study had dms chromosomes in their tumor cells, but they were present in only 1 to 2% of the cells. None of the five tumors examined with banding had HSRs, and the four other tumors did not have giant marker chromosomes. More patients need to be studied to determine whether HSRs occur in primary neuroblastomas, either before or after therapy. It would be interesting if these regions develop in patients at relapse, similar to their development in drug-resistant Chinese hamster lines. However, thus far they have been observed only in cells in long-term culture.

Two samples were obtained at different times in 3 patients, and some interesting observations can be made. In 2 of the patients the tumor had a different karyotype at relapse, suggesting that a resistant clone developed in association with a change in the karyotype. The third patient had different karyotypes in the marrow tumor and the primary tumor. Although they were studied at different times, a single marker in the primary and two identical markers in the marrow tumor suggest that the cells which grew in the marrow were derived from the primary and had endoreduplicated.

Moreover, cytogenetic studies of human neuroblastomas have provided evidence that a specific chromosomal abnormality, a deletion of the short arm of chromosome 1, may be involved in malignant transformation. Also, serial studies of patients have shown different karyotypes in the tumor cells at relapse than at diagnosis, suggesting a cytogenetic mechanism for the evolution of a resistant clone. It is hoped that further study of the cytogenetics of primary neuroblastomas will give us a better understanding of the pathogenesis and behavior of this tumor.

ACKNOWLEDGMENTS

This work was supported in part by the Clinical Cancer Education Grant CA-23944, the American Cancer Society Grant ACS IN-99E (2046), the Program Project Grant from the National Cancer Institute CA-23099, the Ruby Levi Research Fund, and by ALSAC. We wish to thank Ms. Nancy Olson-Irussi and Ms. Sharon Nooner for technical assistance.

REFERENCES

1. Balanban-Malenbaum, G., and Gilbert, F. (1977): Double minute chromosomes and the homogeneous staining regions in chromosomes of a human neuroblastoma cell line. *Science,* 198:739–741.
2. Biedler, J. L., Helson, L., and Spengler, B. A. (1973): Morphology and growth, tumorigenicity, and cytogenetics of human neuroblastoma cells in continuous culture. *Cancer Res.,* 33:2643–2652.
3. Biedler, J. L., and Spengler, B. A. (1976): A novel chromosome abnormality in human neuroblastoma and antifolate-resistant Chinese hamster cell lines in culture. *J. Natl. Cancer Inst.,* 57:683–697.

4. Brodeur, G. M., Sekhon, G. L., and Goldstein, M. N. (1977): Chromosomal aberrations in human neuroblastomas. *Cancer,* 40:2256–2263.
5. Knudson, A. G., and Strong, L. C. (1977): Neuroblastoma and pheochromocytoma. *Am. J. Hum. Genet.,* 24:514–532.
6. Koller, P. C. (1972): Chromosomes and the treatment of cancer. In: *The Role of Chromosomes in Cancer Biology. Recent Results in Cancer Research,* Monograph 38, pp. 97–118. Springer-Verlag, Berlin.
7. Kotler, S., and Lubs, H. A. (1967): Comparison of direct and short-term tissue culture technics in determining solid tumor karyotypes. *Cancer Res.,* 27:1861–1866.
8. Mark, J. (1974): Chromosomal patterns of benign and malignant tumors in the human nervous system. In: *Chromosomes and Cancer,* edited by J. German, pp. 484–495. John Wiley and Sons, New York.
9. Moorhead, P. S., Nowell, P. C., Mellman, W. J., Battips, D. M., and Hungerford, D. A. (1960): Chromosome preparations of leukocytes cultured from human peripheral blood. *Exp. Cell. Res.,* 20:613–616.
10. Oshimura, M., Kakati, L., and Sandberg, A. A. (1977): Possible mechanisms for the genesis of chromosome abnormalities including isochromosomes and the Philadelphia chromosome. *Cancer Res.,* 37:3501–3507.
11. Sandberg, A. A., Sakurai, M., and Holdsworth, R. N. (1972): Chromosomes and the causation of human cancer and leukemia. VIII. DMS chromosomes in a neuroblastoma. *Cancer,* 29:1671–1679.
12. Seabright, M. (1971): A rapid banding technique for human chromosomes. *Lancet,* 2:971–972.
13. Sonta, S., Oshimura, M., Evans, J. T., and Sandberg, A. A. (1977): Chromosomes and causation of human cancer and leukemia. XX. Banding patterns of primary tumors. *J. Natl. Cancer Inst.,* 58:49–59.
14. Tumilowicz, J. J., Nichols, W. W., Cholon, J. J., and Greene, A. E. (1970): Definition of a continuous human cell line derived from neuroblastoma. *Cancer Res.,* 30:2110–2118.
15. Yunis, J. J., and Chandler, M. E. (1977): The chromosomes of man—Clinical and biologic significance. *Am. J. Pathol.,* 88:466–495.

Advances in Neuroblastoma Research,
edited by Audrey E. Evans.
Raven Press, New York © 1980.

Human Neuroblastoma Cytogenetics: Search for Significance of Homogeneously Staining Regions and Double Minute Chromosomes

*June L. Biedler, **Robert A. Ross, *†Sara Shanske, and *Barbara A. Spengler

*Laboratory of Cellular and Biochemical Genetics, Memorial Sloan-Kettering Cancer Center, New York, New York 10021; and **Laboratory of Neurobiology, Department of Neurology, Cornell University Medical College, New York, New York 10021 †Present address: Department of Neurology, Columbia University College of Physicians and Surgeons, New York, N.Y. 10032

It is becoming increasingly clear that human neuroblastoma cell lines established in cell culture share basic biological features that may serve to distinguish them from many other types of human tumor cells. We have examined and compared nine different cell lines derived from 8 patients with the diagnosis of neuroblastoma in respect to several specific features. The most uniform of these is a capacity to express neurotransmitter-synthesizing enzyme activities (e.g., 7,13,21,26). Another distinguishing feature of the cell lines that we have studied is their sodium dodecyl sulfate-polyacrylamide gel (SDS-PAGE) protein patterns when compared to those of other tumor and normal cell types. A less consistent characteristic is a near-diploid karyotype which makes the cell lines useful for cell genetic studies. However, still another set of phenomena now appears to be common among human neuroblastoma cells in continuous culture, and less common or uncommon in human tumor cells of different tissue origin, and is the focus of the studies reported here. Most human neuroblastoma lines are characterized by one or both of two unusual metaphase chromosome anomalies: a long, nonbanding, homogeneously staining region (HSR), and small, paired chromatin bodies known as double minutes (DMs). We first described HSRs in antifolate-resistant Chinese hamster cells characterized by highly increased levels of target enzyme dihydrofolate reductase activity (4) and demonstrated a quantitative relationship between presence and length of HSRs and degree of target enzyme overproduction (10). Just as we initially suggested on the basis of our cytological findings (8), by analogy with experimental evidence obtained with methotrexate-resistant mouse tumor cells (1,3,20), and in view of the demonstration that HSR-like regions in CHO cells contain dihydrofolate reductase genes (17), we may now conclude that the HSRs of the drug-resistant Chinese hamster cells are sites of amplified genes encoding the folate-reducing enzyme. The similarity between these HSRs and the HSRs of human neuroblastoma cells has been emphasized (8,9). The presence of HSRs in independently derived human neuroblastoma lines was reported by Balaban-Malenbaum and Gilbert (2) and also by Seeger et al. (23). Of particular pertinence to the present study is the observation that DMs appear to be derived from HSRs, as reported by Balaban-Malenbaum and Gilbert (2). We, too, suggested earlier that HSRs and DMs are alternative manifestations of the same genetic phenomenon (12) and in the present report provide further evidence on this point. Whether HSRs and DMs of human neuroblastoma cells in culture represent sites of amplified, transcriptionally active genes is a current consideration.

MATERIALS AND METHODS

Cells and Culture Methods

The human neuroblastoma lines included in the present study are listed in Table 1, and initial reports describing the lines are cited. The NAP line was provided by Dr. B. W. Ruffner and the LA-N-1 and LA-N-2 lines by Dr. R. C. Seeger. The IMR-32 line was obtained from the American Type Culture Collection (Rockville, Md.). The SMS-KAN line, established recently, was provided by Drs. C. P. Reynolds and G. Smith (Department of Internal Medicine, Southwestern Medical School, Dallas, Texas); it will be described in detail elsewhere.

Cells were grown in Eagle's MEM or MEM and Ham's F-12 (1:1) supplemented with 15% heat-inactivated fetal bovine serum, nonessential amino acids (Eagle's formulation), 100 IU penicillin/ml, and 100 μg streptomycin/ml.

TABLE 1. Clinical history

Cell line	Patient age (years)	Sex	Tissue source	Treatment[a]	Reference
SK-N-SH	4	F	Bone marrow	Radiotherapy Chemotherapy	6
SK-N-MC	15	F	Metastatic tumor	Radiotherapy Chemotherapy	6
SK-N-BE(1)	2	M	Bone marrow	None	5,7
SK-N-BE(2)			Bone marrow	Chemotherapy Radiotherapy	5,7
NAP		F			19
SMS-KAN	3	F	Primary tumor	None	Unpublished
IMR-32	1	M	Primary tumor	None	25
LA-N-1	2	M	Bone marrow	Chemotherapy	23
LA-N-2	3	F	Primary tumor	None	23

[a] Treatment received by patient prior to cultivation of biopsy material.

Karyotype Analysis

For preparation of metaphase chromosomes, cell suspensions were exposed to a hypotonic salts solution, fixed in methanol-acetic acid (3:1), applied to slides, and stained by a modification of the trypsin-Giemsa banding technique of Seabright (22).

RESULTS

General Characteristics of Human Neuroblastoma Cell Lines

Information concerning the age and sex of the patient from whom the human neuroblastoma cell lines included in the present studies were established, the source of the biopsy material, and the therapy received prior to cell culturing are summarized in Table 1. All cell lines with the exception of SMS-KAN have been described in previous publications. One objective has been to characterize and compare human neuroblastoma lines in respect to neurotransmitter-synthesizing enzyme activities. Results, detailed in the accompanying report (R. A. Ross et al., *this volume*), are summarized in Table 2. The data show that several of the lines [SK-N-SH, SK-N-BE(1), SK-N-BE(2), LA-N-1] express only the enzyme activities of adrenergic cells; several (NAP, SMS-KAN, LA-N-2) have both adrenergic and cholinergic traits; and one line (SK-N-MC) has the marker enzyme for cholinergic cells. In general, the kind and degree of neurotransmitter enzyme activity expression have been stable features of these cell lines during their cultivation in our laboratory. The enzyme data further document the relatedness between the SK-N-BE(1) and SK-N-BE(2) cell lines established in culture 5 months apart from the same patient (5,7).

Chromosomal Characteristics: HSRs and DMs

Results of karyotype analysis are presented in Table 3. The major finding is that all cell lines, with the clear exception of SK-N-SH, have either HSRs

TABLE 2. *Neurotransmitter-synthesizing enzyme activities of human neuroblastoma cell lines[a]*

Cell line	Tyrosine hydroxylase	Dopa-de-carboxylase	Dopamine-β-hydroxylase	Choline acetyl-transferase
SK-N-SH	0.017 ± 0.002	5.7 ± 0.42	14.66 ± 0.42	0
SK-N-MC	0	0	0	3.52 ± 0.28
SK-N-BE(1)	42.8 ± 2.8	6.5 ± 0.7	10.54 ± 0.64	0
SK-N-BE(2)	54.1 ± 1.9	22.9 ± 1.6	5.79 ± 0.45	0
NAP	0.76 ± 0.003	0	4.97 ± 0.24	1.72 ± 0.20
SMS-KAN	3.68 ± 0.34	8.39 ± 0.11	14.04 ± 1.72	2.63 ± 0.29
IMR-32	1.47 ± 0.32	1.26 ± 0.7	0	0
LA-N-1	3.05 ± 0.053	0	0	0
LA-N-2	0.23 ± 0.002	0.16 ± 0.05	3.69 ± 0.12	9.40 ± 1.04

[a] Enzyme activity is expressed as nmoles/hr/mg cell protein ± SEM.

TABLE 3. Chromosomal characteristics of human neuroblastoma cell lines: Frequency of cells with HSRs, DMs, and ring chromosomes

Cell line	Months in culture[a]	Modal chromosome no.	Frequency (%) of cells with:		Number of DMs per cell (%)			DM size	Frequency (%) of cells with rings
			HSRs	DMs	1–50	51–100	>100		
SK-N-SH	2	47	0	0					0
	7	47	0	0					0
SK-N-MC	1	47	?	70	97	0	3	Faint to small	0
	14	43–45	54	38	100	0	0		0
SK-N-BE(1)	11	46	0	100	97	0	3	Barely visible to very small	0
	18	47	0	100	90	7	3		0
SK-N-BE(2)	4	44	100	0					0
	18	42,43	100	0					0
NAP	(14)	45	0	99	68	20	12	Faint to large	5
	(32)	46	78	22	94	0	6		3
SMS-KAN	(1)	46	0	100	0	16	84	Barely visible to small	0
IMR-32	(2)	48,49	100	0					0
LA-N-1	(2)	86–89	100	0					0
LA-N-2	(3)	70	1	100	67	19	14	Faint to small	2

[a] Months of continuous in vitro cultivation are given. Numbers in parentheses refer to months in culture after cells were received in our laboratory.

or DMs in many or all cells. As previously reported (6), the number of SK-N-MC cells with DMs declined with time in culture. In late passage cells of this line we recently observed the presence of comparatively short HSRs. Whether HSRs were present and not detected in early passage cells remains to be clarified. SK-N-BE(1) cells consistently possess DMs (Fig. 1a), whereas

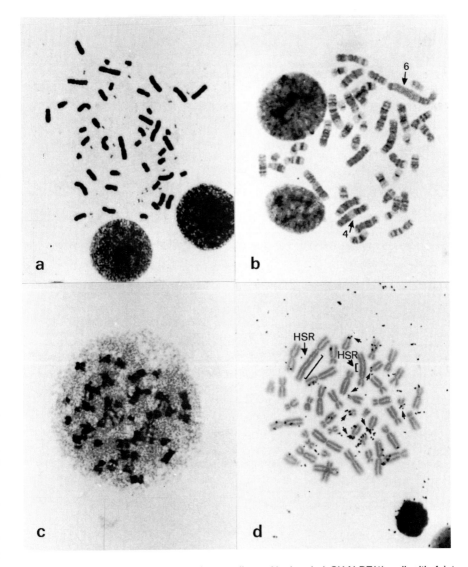

FIG. 1. Human neuroblastoma metaphase cells. **a:** Nonbanded SK-N-BE(1) cell with faint DMs. **b:** G-banded SK-N-BE(2) cell with HSRs on chromosomes 4 and 6. **c:** G-banded cell of the SMS-KAN line with hundreds of DMs. **d:** SK-N-BE(2) cell after *in situ* hybridization with human rRNA showing silver grains at known nucleolar organizer sites and no grains over HSR.

SK-N-BE(2) cells, as described earlier (8,9), consistently possess HSRs (Fig. 1b) and no DMs. These lines share several marker chromosomes indicative of their origin from a common cell precursor. Cells of the NAP line contained DMs (Fig. 2a and b) when examined during the first year of cultivation. After

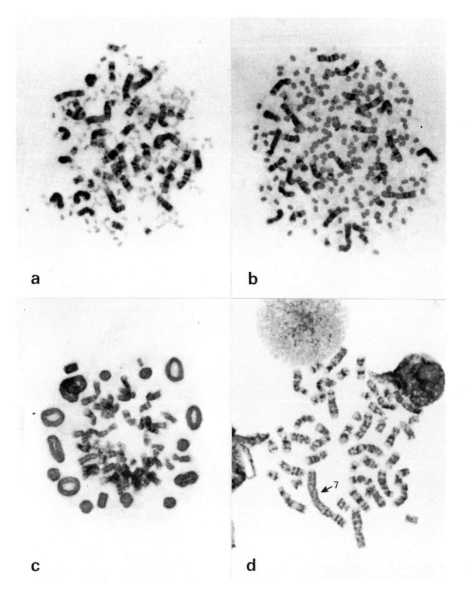

FIG. 2. G-banded metaphase cells of the NAP line. **a:** Small DMs; **b:** medium DMs; **c:** large rings; **d:** long HSR on chromosome 7.

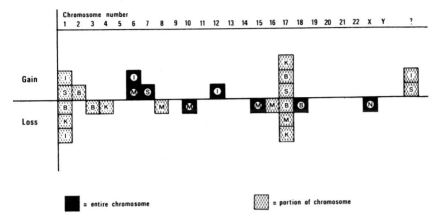

FIG. 3. Net gains and losses of chromosomes in the near-diploid human neuroblastoma lines. Each square represents the net numerical deviation from normal found in 50–100% of cells examined. Within each square a letter identifies the cell line: S, SK-N-SH; M, SK-N-MC; B, SK-N-BE(1) and SK-N-BE(2); N, NAP; K, SMS-KAN; I, IMR-32.

approximately 3 years of continuous culture, a large proportion of cells now exhibit HSRs (Fig. 2d). SMS-KAN and LA-N-2 are characterized primarily by the presence of DMs, and IMR-32 and LA-N-1 cells by HSRs. Only rarely were HSRs and DMs found in the same cell.

Within a given cell line the size of DMs varies. Nevertheless, as described in Table 3, cell lines are distinctive in respect to size, class, and range. For example, as shown in Fig. la, DMs of SK-N-BE(1) cells are often barely visible. Most cells contain fewer than 50. NAP cells, in contrast, exhibit the largest DMs seen in this group of neuroblastoma lines (Fig. 4). At the same time that HSR-containing cells (Fig. 2d) had not yet appeared, there was a high number of DMs per cell. Cells containing the greatest number of DMs are those of the newly established SMS-KAN line; 84% of cells were observed to contain more than 100 up to uncountable numbers of DMs (Fig. 2c). Another feature of NAP cells is the presence of ring chromosomes (Table 1, Fig. 2c), in addition to DMs, in 3 to 5% of cells. The rings depicted in Fig. 2c are unusually large; this cell, however, serves to illustrate that the ring chromosomes, like the large DMs, are HSR-like in that they are nonbanded.

Correlation Between Chromosomal Characteristics and the Neuronal Phenotype

The data of Tables 2 and 3 indicate that there is no obvious relationship between presence or type (HSR versus DM) of chromosomal abnormality and expression of neurotransmitter enzyme activity. In a further attempt to ascertain the possible function of HSRs in the SK-N-BE(2) line, we isolated clonal sublines with different sets of HSR-bearing chromosomes. Clones consisted of cells with either a long HSR on chromosome 10 or two shorter HSRs on chromosomes

HUMAN CHROMOSOME 1

CHINESE HAMSTER CHROMOSOME 2

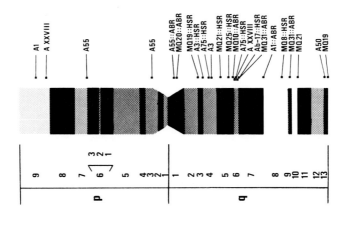

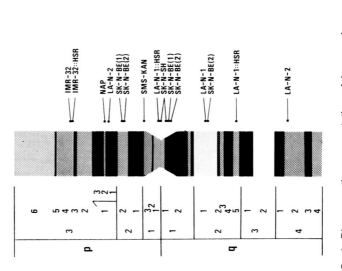

FIG. 4. Diagrammatic representation of human chromosome 1 and Chinese hamster chromosome 2. Consistent sites of deletions and of HSRs are indicated. ABR, abnormally banding regions.

TABLE 4. *Numerical and structural abnormalities of chromosome 1: Net gain and loss of chromosome regions and chromosomal location of deletion sites and HSRs*

Cell line	Net quantitative change from normal diploid[a]				Chromosomal location		
	Gain	Frequency	Loss	Frequency	Break[b]	HSR	Frequency
SK-N-SH	cen→qter or	70%	None		cen or		
	q12→qter	50%			q12		
SK-N-MC	None		None		None		
SK-N-BE(1)	q12→qter	0–30%	pter→p22	100%	p22		
					q12		
SK-N-BE(2)	q12→qter	0–50%	pter→p22	50–100%	p22		
					q12,q21		
NAP	None		None		p31.2		
SMS-KAN	None		pter→p21	100%	p21		
IMR-32	p34→qter	100%	pter→p34	100%	p34	p34	100%
LA-N-1	q21→qter	100%	None		q21	p11	46%
						q25	4%
LA-N-2	p31.1→q42	100%	None		p31.1		
					q42		

[a] The data for the near-tetraploid LA-N-1 and LA-N-2 lines are based on the diploid chromosome number.

[b] Site of chromosome break associated with deletion and translocation.

4 and 6. Enzyme assay revealed differing but stable levels of tyrosine hydroxylase and dopamine-β-hydroxylase activities, ranging from 0 to approximately those levels found in SK-N-BE(2) cells (R. A. Ross et al., *this volume*). There was no apparent correlation between chromosomal location of HSRs and neurotransmitter enzyme activity.

Net Gain and Loss of Chromosomes: Involvement of Chromosomes 1 and 17

The "diploid" chromosome constitution (Table 3) of many of the neuroblastoma lines permitted assessment of net gain and loss of whole or parts of chromosomes. Results of analysis of the seven near-diploid lines are diagrammed in Fig. 3. Only two chromosomes showed numerical abnormality, in the form of either trisomy or partial trisomy or monosomy or partial monosomy, in more than two of the cell lines, viz., chromosome 1 and chromosome 17.[1] An extensive analysis of chromosome 1 in all nine lines is presented in Table 4. As shown by the data, five lines exhibited a gain of part or all of the long (q) arm in some proportion of cells; in two lines there was also gain of a portion of the short (p) arm. There was no instance of net loss of q arm material. In those four lines exhibiting net loss of a portion of chromosome 1, only short arm material was deleted from the cell. The results indicated, furthermore, that a particular region of chromosome 1 (q12→q42) was consistently trisomic in

---

[1] See also Brodeur p. 73.

affected cells of the five lines. A similar analysis was performed for chromosome 17 (data not shown). Of the nine lines, five exhibited a net gain in long arm material. About 5 to 40% of NAP cells were trisomic for the entire chromosome, one line (SMS-KAN) was trisomic for the q arm in at least 50% of cells, and three lines [SK-N-SH, SK-N-BE(1), LA-N-1] were trisomic for a distal portion of the q arm. Therefore, the region of chromosome 17 that was consistently trisomic in affected cells was q21→qter. Net loss of chromosome 17 was seen in three of the nine lines and involved short arm material as well as, in one instance, a proximal region of the long arm (cen→q21). Just as for chromosome 1, that region of chromosome 17 that tended to be gained (q21→qter) was never found in a monosomic state. The chromosomal locations of consistent break points in chromosome 1, in addition to those involved in the deletions and translocations resulting in net gain or loss of chromosome segments, are listed in Table 4. The deletion at band p31.2 for the NAP line, for example, is associated with a reciprocal exchange between chromosome 1 and chromosome 12. The location of HSRs is also noted. There is approximately equal involvement of the long and short arms. Further, the distribution of deletion sites along chromosome 1, shown in Fig. 4a, indicates that there is no preferential site of chromosome breakage.

Comparisons of Human Neuroblastoma and HSR-Containing Chinese Hamster Cells

We previously reported the presence of HSRs in antifolate-resistant Chinese hamster cells (4,8,9) as well as in human neuroblastoma cells (8,9); in fact, the recognition of HSRs in an experimental system aided in their detection and appraisal in the human tumor cells. In 16 independently derived drug-resistant hamster sublines, there are distinctive, abnormally banding chromosome regions including HSRs that are associated with overproduction of target enzyme dihydrofolate reductase (J. L. Biedler, P. W. Melera, and B. A. Spengler, manuscript submitted for publication). These regions are located on the long arm of Chinese hamster chromosome 2 in 12 out of the 16 sublines and very likely represent sites of amplified dihydrofolate reductase genes (8,17). However, despite their preferential location, HSRs as well as the other specifically abnormal regions of the less-resistant sublines (11) are positioned at different sites on the chromosome 2q arm (Fig. 4b).

The chromosomal location of HSRs observed in the six HSR-containing neuroblastoma lines is given in Table 5. It is apparent that there is no consistent involvement of a particular chromosome. Further, there is no consistent positioning of the HSR when the same chromosome is involved, with the possible exception of chromosome 18. In one regard, these results clearly differ from those obtained with the drug-resistant hamster cells, in that the latter show nonrandom location of HSRs. However, the lack of specificity of HSR sites as well as deletion sites on Chinese hamster chromosome 2 is similar to the

TABLE 5. *Chromosomal location of HSRs in human neuroblastoma cell lines*

Cell line	1	2	3	4	5	6	7	8	9	10	11	12	13	14	15	16	17	18	19	20	21	22	X	Y
SK-N-BE(2)				q25	q35	p21				p13							921	q23	q13.3			p13[a]		
SK-N-MC																			q13.4			q13[a]		
IMR-32	p34										p13[a]		p11											
NAP							p22	p23																
LA-N-1	p11 q25	p23			q33											q13		q23	p13.3				p22	
LA-N-2											q24													

[a] Identification as an HSR is uncertain because of the small size of the region.

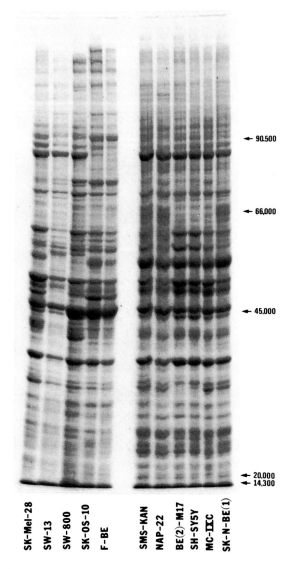

FIG. 5. A 10% polyacrylamide slab gel of SDS-treated cytosol fractions (135,000 *g* supernatants) stained with Coomassie blue. SK-Mel-28 is a human melanoma line obtained from Dr. L. J. Old (Sloan-Kettering Institute). SW-13 is a line established from an adenocarcinoma of the adrenal cortex, SW-800 from a bladder carcinoma, and SK-OS-10, an osteogenic sarcoma line; these lines were obtained from Dr. J. Fogh (Sloan-Kettering Institute). F-BE is a fibroblast-like strain isolated from biopsy material giving rise to the SK-N-BE(1) neuroblastoma line. The human neuroblastoma lines SMS-KAN and SK-N-BE(1) are described in the text. NAP-22 was clonally derived from the NAP line, BE(2)-M17 from SK-N-BE(2), SH-SY5Y from SK-N-SH, and MC-IXC from SK-N-MC. Molecular weight markers used were lysozyme, 14,300 d; dihydrofolate reductase, 20,000 d; ovalbumin, 45,000 d; albumin, 66,000 d; phosphorylase B, 90,500 d.

situation obtaining for human chromosomes 1 (Fig. 4a) and 17, in particular.

In an approach parallel to that taken with the drug-resistant Chinese hamster cell system (24), we have begun to look at the protein complement of neuroblastoma cells with the technique of SDS-PAGE. Cells are fractionated into nuclear, mitochondrial, microsomal, and cytosol fractions and each fraction analyzed electrophoretically. Dihydrofolate reductase-overproducing hamster cells display a prominent band with an apparent molecular weight of 20,000 daltons that is not present in cytosols of control cells. A similar preliminary analysis of neuroblastoma cell cytosols has not revealed a prominent band that could be correlated with presence of an HSR, for example. In fact, as shown by the electrophorogram in Fig. 5, there is considerable identity between the various neuroblastoma cell lines irrespective of presence or absence of HSRs and DMs. As a further comparison, we displayed cytosol proteins from several other near-diploid human tumor lines and also from fibroblast-like cells (F-BE) derived from the bone marrow specimen that gave rise to the SK-N-BE(1) cell line. There are evident differences among these cell lines and between this group and the neuroblastoma lines as a group. These preliminary results suggest that even though the putative protein product(s) associated with HSRs and DMs may not be able to be detected by this method, the distinct electrophoretic patterns based on relative amounts of Coomassie blue-staining polypeptides of neuroblastoma cytosols may serve as a useful method of cell and tissue identification (16).

In an attempt, by another approach, to determine the nature of the HSR, ^{125}I-iodinated human rRNA, provided by Dr. Wolff Prensky of the Sloan-Kettering Institute, was hybridized *in situ* to HSR-containing Chinese hamster and human cells. In autoradiograms, such as shown in Fig. 1d, preferential localization of silver grains to known nucleolus organizer regions of the human cells and, less clearly, of the Chinese hamster cells (not shown) was discerned. There was no labeling of HSRs. This result was substantiated by the observation of negative staining of HSRs and positive staining (not shown) of nucleolar organizers by the silver staining technique (15).

Retention of HSRs by Human-Mouse Neuroblastoma Cell Hybrids

With the ultimate objective of assigning a human chromosomal location for the tyrosine hydroxylase gene, a collaborative project with Dr. Xandra O. Breakefield (Department of Human Genetics, Yale University, New Haven, Conn.) was initiated. SK-N-BE(2) cells were fused with a tyrosine hydroxylase-negative clone of C-1300 mouse neuroblastoma cells, and cell hybrids were selected in tyrosine-deficient growth medium. Over a year's time eight hybrid clones have gradually lost human chromosomes until the average number per cell hybrid ranges from 6 to 19; the average number of mouse chromosomes is 135. Karyotype analyses by Dr. T. D. Chang have demonstrated a selective retention, so far, of two different chromosomes in all or most cells. Furthermore, each clone, except one that is now tyrosine hydroxylase negative, has retained an HSR-bearing chromosome in all or nearly all cells. The SK-N-BE(2) cells used as a fusion partner consistently possessed two HSRs, one on a chromosome 4 and the other on a chromosome 6 (see Fig. 1b). The hybrid clones have one or the other of these chromosomes and not both. It is anticipated that this experiment will enable us to map the tyrosine hydroxylase-encoding gene and to assess the role of the HSR in the expression of this gene.

SUMMARY AND DISCUSSION

1. All lines except SK-N-SH have either HSRs or DMs. The prevalence of these two abnormalities in human neuroblastoma cells, as well as various cytological characteristics, suggests that HSRs and DMs are alternative manifestations of the same basic phenomenon. The finding of DMs in SK-N-BE(1) and HSRs in SK-N-BE(2) cells derived from the same patient and the gradual evolution in cell culture of DM- to HSR-containing cells manifested by the SK-N-MC and NAP lines support this contention.

2. There is preferential involvement of chromosomes 1 and 17 in the form of net gain of long arm material and loss of short arm material of both chromosomes. These results bear a striking similarity to those reported by Rowley (18) for malignant cells of the myeloid system. The apparent preferential deletion of chromosome 1p is consistent with the finding of Brodeur et al. (14; and p. 73, *this volume*). However, involvement (numerical gain) of 1q is no less frequent, and deletion (break) sites are distributed about equally and apparently nonspecifically in both arms.

3. There is no discernible correlation between expression of neurotransmitter enzyme activity and presence of HSRs and DMs.

4. Analysis of a large series of antifolate-resistant Chinese hamster sublines characterized by excessive synthesis of target enzyme dihydrofolate reductase has indicated that specific, abnormally banding regions including HSRs are located preferentially on the long arm of chromosome 2. However, the abnormal regions are positioned at different sites along the arm, and in the HSR-containing cells the normal terminal portion of 2q has been deleted and translocated at random to another chromosome within the cell. On the basis of these observations, to be published in detail elsewhere, we hypothesize that the dihydrofolate reductase gene (and possibly flanking sequences) is excised, amplified extrachromosomally, and reinserted usually near but sometimes distant from its permanent location. We favor the speculation that a similar process may occur in human neuroblastoma cells. Thus, one or several genes may be excised, amplified, and inserted more or less at random within the chromosome complement. There are, of course, alternative possibilities to explain the ubiquity of the 25 or so HSRs of the six different neuroblastoma lines (Table 5). The notion that a gene may be amplified outside of the chromosome and reintegrated at many

different sites is consistent with current knowledge of transposable genetic elements in bacteria and lower eukaryotes.

ACKNOWLEDGMENTS

This work was supported in part by NCI Core Grant CA-08748 and NIH Grants CA-18856, NS-06911, HL-18974, and T32 CA-09055.

REFERENCES

1. Alt, F. W., Kellems, R. E., Bertino, J. R., and Schimke, R. T. (1978): Selective multiplication of dihydrofolate reductase genes in methotrexate-resistant variants of cultured murine cells. *J. Biol. Chem.*, 253:1357–1370.
2. Balaban-Malenbaum, G., and Gilbert, F. (1977): Double minute chromosomes and the homogeneously staining regions in chromosomes of a human neuroblastoma cell line. *Science*, 198:739–741.
3. Biedler, J. L., Albrecht, A. M., and Hutchison, D. J. (1965): Cytogenetics of mouse leukemia L1210. I. Association of a specific chromosome with dihydrofolate reductase activity in amethopterin-treated sublines. *Cancer Res.*, 25:246–257.
4. Biedler, J. L., Albrecht, A. M., and Spengler, B. A. (1974): Non-banding (homogeneous) chromosome regions in cells with very high dihydrofolate reductase levels. *Genetics*, 77:s4–5.
5. Biedler, J. L., and Helson, L. (1974): Human neuroblastoma cells maintained in continuous culture: Morphological, tumorigenic, cytogenetic, and biochemical characteristics. *Maandschr. Kindergeneesk.*, 42:423–427.
6. Biedler, J. L., Helson, L., and Spengler, B. A. (1973): Morphology and growth, tumorigenicity, and cytogenetics of human neuroblastoma cells in continuous culture. *Cancer Res.*, 33:2643–2652.
7. Biedler, J. L., Roffler-Tarlov, S., Schachner, M., and Freedman, L. (1978): Multiple neurotransmitter synthesis by human neuroblastoma cell lines and clones. *Cancer Res.*, 38:3751–3757.
8. Biedler, J. L., and Spengler, B. A. (1976): Metaphase chromosome anomaly: Association with drug resistance and cell-specific products. *Science*, 191:185–187, 1976.
9. Biedler, J. L., and Spengler, B. A. (1976): A novel chromosome abnormality in human neuroblastoma and antifolate-resistant Chinese hamster cell lines in culture. *J. Natl. Cancer Inst.*, 57:683–695.
10. Biedler, J. L., and Spengler, B. A. (1976): Quantitative relationship between a chromosome abnormality (HSR) and antifolate resistance associated with enzyme overproduction. *J. Cell Biol.*, 70:117a.
11. Biedler, J. L., and Spengler, B. A. (1977): Abnormally banded metaphase chromosome regions in cells with low levels of resistance to antifolates. *In Vitro*, 13:200.
12. Biedler, J. L., Spengler, B. A., and Ross, R. A. (1977): Chromosomal and biochemical properties of human neuroblastoma lines and clones in cell culture. In: *International Symposium on Neuroblastoma, Genoa, Italy, 1977. Biological Bases and Therapeutic Perspectives*, p. 4. Abstr. (Milano, Antonio Cordani, 1977).
13. Biedler, J. L., Spengler, B. A., and Ross, R. A. (1978): Expression of catecholamine-synthesizing enzymes in human neuroblastoma lines with unique chromosomal abnormalities. In: *4th International Catecholamine Symposium, Pacific Grove, California. Catecholamines: Basic and Clinical Frontiers; Proceedings*, edited by E. Usdin, I. J. Kopin, and J. Barchas, 1:192–194. New York, Pergamon Press.
14. Brodeur, G. M., Sekhon, G. S., and Goldstein, M. N. (1977): Chromosomal aberrations in human neuroblastomas. *Cancer*, 40:2256–2263.
15. Howell, W. M., Denton, T. E., and Diamond, J. R. (1975): Differential staining of the satellite regions of human acrocentric chromosomes. *Experientia*, 31:260–262.
16. Irwin, D., and Dauphinais, I. D. (1979): A tissue-specific code based on the abundance of SDS-solubilized proteins. *Anal. Biochem.*, 92:193–198.
17. Nunberg, J. H., Kaufman, R. J., Schimke, R. T., Urlaub, G., and Chasin, L. A. (1978): Amplified

dihydrofolate reductase genes are localized to a homogeneously staining region of a single chromosome in a methotrexate-resistant Chinese hamster ovary cell line. *Proc. Natl. Acad. Sci. U.S.A.,* 75:5553–5556.

18. Rowley, J. D. (1977): Mapping of human chromosomal regions related to neoplasia: Evidence from chromosomes 1 and 17. *Proc. Natl. Acad. Sci. U.S.A.,* 74:5729–5733.

19. Ruffner, B. W., Jr. (1976): A cholinergic permanent cell line from a human neuroblastoma (Na). *Proc. Am. Assoc. Cancer Res.,* 17:219.

20. Schimke, R. T., Alt, F. W., Kellems, R. E., Kaufman, R. J., and Bertino, J. R. (1978): Amplification of dihydrofolate reductase genes in methotrexate-resistant cultured mouse cells. *Cold Spring Harbor Symp. Quant. Biol.,* 42:649–657.

21. Schlesinger, H. R., Gerson, J. M., Moorhead, P. S., Maguire, H., and Hummeler, K. (1976): Establishment and characterization of human neuroblastoma cell lines. *Cancer Res.,* 36:3094–3100.

22. Seabright, M. (1971): A rapid banding technique for human chromosomes. *Lancet,* 2:971–972.

23. Seeger, R. C., Rayner, S. A., Banerjee, A., Chung, H., Laug, W. E., Neustein, H. B., and Benedict, W. F. (1977): Morphology, growth, chromosomal pattern, and fibrinolytic activity of two new human neuroblastoma cell lines. *Cancer Res.,* 37:1364–1371.

24. Shanske, S., Melera, P. W., and Biedler, J. L. (1978): Overproduction of dihydrofolate reductase by antifolate resistant Chinese hamster cells. *J. Cell Biol.,* 79:345a.

25. Tumilowicz, J. J., Nichols, W. W., Cholon, J. J., and Greene, A. E. (1970): Definition of a continuous human cell line derived from neuroblastoma. *Cancer Res.,* 30:2110–2218.

26. West, G. J., Uki, J., Herschman, H. R., and Seeger, R. C. (1977): Adrenergic, cholinergic and inactive human neuroblastoma cell lines with the action-potential Na^+ ionophore. *Cancer Res.,* 37:1372–1376.

Advances in Neuroblastoma Research,
edited by Audrey E. Evans.
Raven Press, New York © 1980.

Relationship Between Homogeneously Staining Regions and Double Minute Chromosomes in Human Neuroblastoma Cell Lines

Gloria Balaban-Malenbaum and Fred Gilbert

Departments of Human Genetics and Pediatrics, School of Medicine, University of Pennsylvania, Philadelphia, Pennsylvania 19104

The vast majority of the karyotypic abnormalities—aneuploidies and rearrangements—seen in malignant cells are qualitatively the same as those seen in constitutionally abnormal individuals or in experimentally induced chromosome aberrations *in vitro.*

There are, however, two chromosome abnormalities which are largely limited to tumors: double minutes and homogeneously staining regions (HSRs) (12).

The HSRs and double minutes have each been separately reported in multiple cases of human neuroblastoma (5,6,12,13,16), and Biedler (*this volume,* p. 81) has discussed her hypothesis that they are altered phases of the same phenomenon in these tumors.

This discussion will be confined to the further hypothesis that in human neuroblastoma the double minutes originate from the HSR.

This hypothesis is based on three lines of evidence: first, the pattern of segregation of HSRs and double minutes in subpopulations of neuroblastoma cell lines; second, the quantitative determination that the HSR represents additional DNA, linearly integrated into the chromosome (providing a source of the double minute DNA); and finally, that the fusion of a human neuroblastoma cell line containing two HSRs with a mouse line resulted in the breakdown and disappearance of the HSR concomitant with the appearance of double minutes.

DOUBLE MINUTES

Double minutes are small, paired chromatin bodies whose number and size vary from cell to cell. They were first reported in 1962 (Spriggs et al.) in a direct preparation from the pleural effusion of a patient with an untreated carcinoma of the lung. Double minutes were reported in experimental animal tumors by Mark (14) in 6 Rous virus-induced mouse sarcomas. They have since been reported in at least 70 cases of human and animal tumors (12). Their origin, method of propagation in the tumor cell population, and function have remained obscure.

The human tumors containing double minutes have most often been of neurogenic origin (e.g., neuroblastoma and glioblastoma), although they have also been reported in an embryonic rhabdomyosarcoma (7) and in breast cancer cell lines (4) among others.

The most informative reports include those of Cox et al. (7), Lubs et al. (13), and Sandberg et al. (15), all of whom concluded that the double minutes seen in direct preparations of cells from human tumors were not viral or bacterial contaminants, but were chromosomal of unknown origin.

Although they have no centromeres, double minutes have been shown by Levan and Levan (11) in a mouse tumor cell line and by Barker and Hsu (4) in a human breast tumor line to be transported through mitosis, loosely attached to the ends of chromosomes by adhering nucleolar material. Some double minutes are lost with each cell division and may appear in micronuclei in association with interphase cells. Double minutes in human neuroblastomas show the same staining characteristics as do the HSRs. They stain with an intermediate intensity when treated with trypsin-Giemsa or "Q" banded; they do not contain constitutive heterochromatin by "C" banding; they are Feulgen positive and incorporate BUdR.

CHARACTERIZATION OF CELL LINES AND SEGREGATION OF HSRs AND DOUBLE MINUTES

Karyotypes were prepared from uncloned cell lines which were recently derived from several human neuroblastomas, as well as from IMR-32, which has been shown to have two HSRs (5). Trypsin-Giemsa banded karyotypes of IMR-32 confirmed the HSRs. This line has been in continuous culture since 1967 and the long marker chromosome has been present since at least the tenth subculture (18). "C" banding revealed that the HSR regions were not heterochromatin.

Analysis of four recently established, uncloned neuroblastoma lines showed three to have an HSR and one, CHP-166, to have only double minutes. In those lines with an HSR, the HSR-containing chromosome differed in each line.

One line, CHP-134, is pseudo-diploid (modal chromosome number, 46) and contains one HSR in the short arm of chromosome 7 and another in the long arm of chromosome 6.

Another line, NMB, is hypotetraploid (modal chromosome number, 83) and most cells contain HSRs in the short arm of three copies of chromosome 13. Each cell had a normal 13. The chromosome with HSRs which are characteristic of each line were found in virtually every cell of that line.

Examination of the remaining neuroblastoma line, CHP-126 (modal chromosome number, 46), in passage 8, revealed the presence of two classes of cells: one with an HSR, the other with double minutes. One class had a marker chromosome 5 with an HSR in its long arm and the other class of cells had

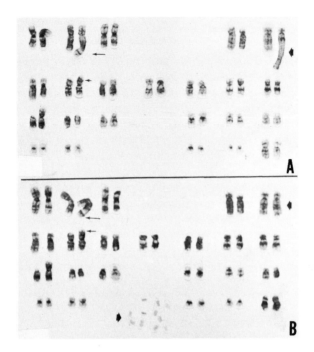

FIG. 1. CHP-126—two classes of cells. **A:** Karyotype of cell with HSR on one number 5 chromosome *(large arrow)* and two additional marker chromosomes *(small arrows).* **B:** Karyotype of cell of other subpopulation with double minutes *(large arrow),* two normal number 5 chromosomes *(large arrow),* and same additional marker chromosomes *(small arrows).* From Balaban-Malenbaum and Gilbert (2).

no HSR, but did contain two normal number 5 chromosomes and a varying number of double minutes (Fig. 1). Analysis of 110 cells from CHP-126 showed 66 with the HSR and 44 with the double minutes. Scanning of many more metaphases demonstrated that each cell had only one of these chromosome abnormalities; no cell had both. All of the cells examined also had two additional marker chromosomes (one with an extra band on the long arm of chromosome 2 and another with an extra band on the short arm of chromosome 7), indicating that both subpopulations had a common precursor (2).

Multiple subpopulations were also identified in a clone of NMB (NMB-7), which has a wide range of chromosome counts and demonstrates continuous remodeling of the karyotype. Cells were found with four HSRs and no double minutes whereas other cells containing three or fewer HSRs with varying numbers of double minutes were also evident. The pattern of segregation of these two chromosome abnormalities appears to be similar to that already described in CHP-126.

Another line examined, CHP-166, had double minutes in every cell. It was not analyzed in detail.

In addition to the HSRs and double minutes, three of the lines contained other consistent chromosome rearrangements: IMR-32 ($11q^-$, $16q^+$, $19q^+$); CHP-134, [t(1p; ?), $6p^+$, $7p^-$, $19q^+$)]; CHP-126 ($2q^+$, $7p^+$).

These initial studies confirm the original report of HSRs in human neuroblastoma and describe three additional lines with HSRs. They further demonstrate, for the first time, the segregation of HSRs and double minutes in a neuroblastoma cell line (CHP-126). The pattern of segregation of the HSR and double minutes (individual cells contain one or the other abnormality, not both) and our finding that the HSR marker chromosome is replaced by an intact normal chromosome (without HSR) in the cells which contain double minutes suggest that the HSR is a region of additional DNA, that the double minutes could originate from preexisting chromosome material, and that in CHP-126, at least, the specific chromosome segment involved is the HSR.

DNA MEASUREMENTS

The unique characteristics of the HSR and the fact that it is larger than any band in the normal karyotypes indicate that the HSR is not a normal segment translocated from another chromosome. In order to determine that this segment is not simply an uncoiled or stretched chromosome segment, the relative DNA content of homologous chromosomes with and without an HSR has been measured (3). This was done by means of scanning cytophotometry which, when used in conjunction with histochemical procedures specific for DNA—such as Feulgen stain—makes it possible to determine quantitatively the DNA content of whole cells or single chromosomes (9). Using this technique, standard values for the DNA content of each chromosome in the normal human karyotype have been generated. Three lines, each with an HSR on a different chromosome, were analyzed (in collaboration with Dr. Gary Grove). For each cell line, the DNA content of one HSR marker chromosome was compared to that of a normal homologue without HSR—a chromosome 1 in the case of IMR-32 and a chromosome of group B for CHP-126 or group D for NMB.

The metaphases and individual chromosomes from each cell line stained with trypsin-Giemsa and Feulgen are illustrated below (Fig. 2). The Feulgen stain demonstrated that the HSR is linearly integrated into the chromosome. The DNA content of each marker chromosome with an HSR is significantly greater than that of its normal homologue without an HSR (Table 1). The DNA content of the chromosomes with HSRs in the three lines was increased between 50 and 250%.

This finding—that the HSR-containing chromosomes contain more DNA than do their normal homologues and thus provide a potential source for the double minute DNA—is consistent with our hypothesis that breakdown of the HSR gives rise to the double minutes.

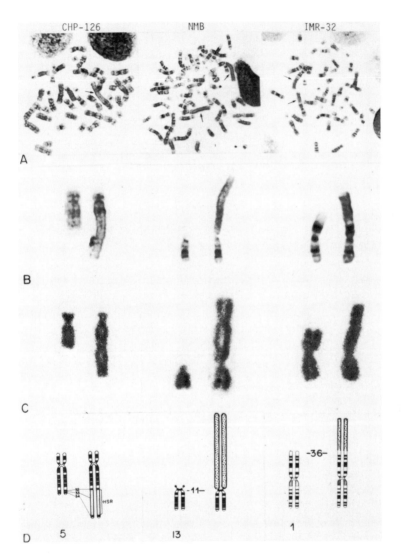

FIG. 2. A: Trypsin-Giemsa stained metaphases of cells from 3 human neuroblastoma lines (*arrows* mark the HSR chromosomes). **B:** Trypsin-Giemsa stained homologous chromosomes with and without HSR. **C:** Feulgen-stained homologous chromosomes with and without HSR. **D:** Diagrammatic representations of chromosomes (using Paris classification) showing position of HSR. From Balaban-Malenbaum and Gilbert (3).

TABLE 1. *Comparative DNA content of HSR and normal homologous chromosomes*

	Human neuro-blastoma	Cell no.	HSR chromo-some	DNA content	Normal chromo-some	DNA content	Δ%[a]
A)	CHP-126	1	5	12.07 ± 9.93	B	6.51 ± 0.37	85.4%
		2		11.28 ± 1.08	group	5.58 ± 0.16	102.3
		3		9.68 ± 1.01		5.40 ± 0.35	79.3
		4		11.46 ± 0.55		5.81 ± 0.26	97.3
		5		9.69 ± 0.38		4.72 ± 0.13	105.3
		6		13.60 ± 0.80		6.16 ± 0.48	120.8
		7		13.08 ± 0.58		6.59 ± 0.54	98.5
					Average	98.4% ± 13.5%	(SD)
B)	NMB	1	13	6.03 ± 0.20	D	1.34 ± 0.24	350.0%
		2		4.24 ± 0.26	group	1.30 ± 0.11	226.2
		3		4.97 ± 0.24		1.52 ± 0.11	227.0
		4		4.97 ± 0.61		1.65 ± 0.19	201.2
		5		5.58 ± 0.55		1.31 ± 0.08	326.0
		6		6.26 ± 0.36		1.30 ± 0.06	381.6
		7		5.62 ± 0.36		1.67 ± 0.13	236.5
					Average	278.2% ± 72.2%	(SD)
C)	IMR-32	1		17.02 ± 1.20	1	12.84 ± 0.91	32.55%
		2		15.48 ± 1.32		11.52 ± 1.48	34.38
		3		20.20 ± 3.68		11.16 ± 2.12	81.00
		4		21.32 ± 1.68		13.00 ± 1.72	64.00
		5		15.69 ± 1.85		11.56 ± 1.13	35.73
					Average	49.5% ± 21.8%	(SD)

[a] Δ% (DNA content $\frac{\text{HSR chromosome} - \text{normal chromosome}}{\text{Normal chromosome}} \times 100\%$) determined by cyto-photometric analysis of Feulgen-stained metaphases comparing HSR marker chromosome and normal chromosome of the same group without HSR within the same metaphase. DNA content values are expressed in arbitrary machine units of integrated optical density. Each value is the average of 6 measurements.
From Balaban-Malenbaum and Gilbert (3).

SOMATIC CELL HYBRID STUDIES

Our hypothesis concerning the relationship between the HSR and double minutes is strengthened by somatic cell hybrid studies. When IMR and CHP-134 were passaged through nude mice, chromosome analysis of the tumors and of cells which grew out when the tumors were explanted into tissue culture showed that the HSRs were retained. No double minutes or micronuclei were ever seen.

IMR-5, a cloned human neuroblastoma line (Fig. 3), has been fused with a nonmalignant, permanent mouse fibroblast line, IT-22 (thymidine kinase deficient). IT-22 has been used in many hybrid studies (8). Double minutes have never been reported in IT-22 or in any of the previous hybrid studies. When injected into nudes, IT-22 is not tumorigenic (Gilbert and Balaban-Malenbaum, *this volume*).

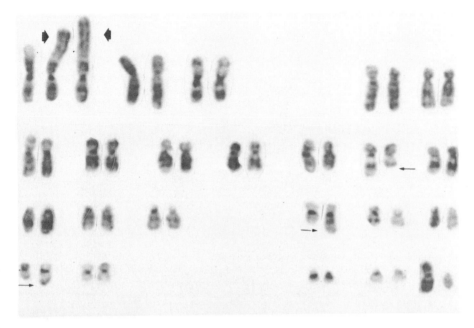

FIG. 3. IMR-5—karyotype with two HSRs *(large arrows)*.

Double minutes did, however, appear in three of the hybrid cloned cell lines resulting from the fusion of the IMR and IT-22.

Clone NR5TP-3b (hereafter referred to as 3b), examined as soon as possible after hybridization, showed the same pattern of segregation of HSRs and double minutes as did CHP-126: cells with HSRs, other cells with double minutes (Fig. 4)—no cell had both. In all cells the human number 17 chromosome, to which the enzyme thymidine kinase has been assigned, was present. The number 17, along with the few other nonconsistent human chromosomes present, were intact and showed no breakage or other evidence of chromosome damage. The IT-22 marker was present and all of the mouse chromosomes were intact. Although the banding in some cells identified the HSR containing chromosome as the number 1 from IMR-5, the banding was not definitive in every cell. The identification of the human origin of the submetacentric chromosome was confirmed by the formamide "C" technique which distinguishes between mouse and human centromeric heterochromatin (10). The hybrid clone 3b was then tested for its capacity to produce colonies in semisoft agar, a property which has been found to correlate well but not absolutely with tumorigenicity (17). Analysis of cells from NR5TP3bAg (hereafter referred to as 3bAg), an agar positive clone, showed only double minutes. No HSRs were seen. The 17s, still evident, were normal. Many interphases had micronuclei associated with them, a phenomenon closely associated with the presence of double minutes in metaphase cells (11). This clone was expanded and when injected into nudes

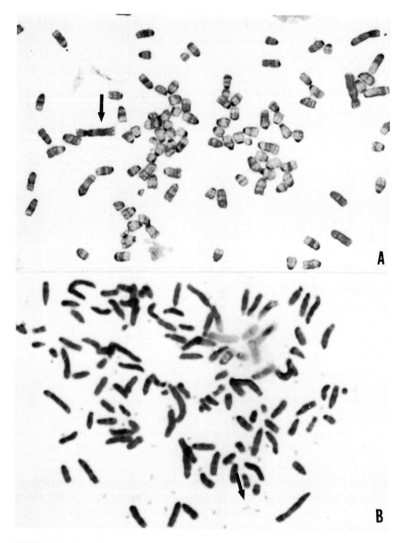

FIG. 4. NR5TP-3b—hybrid clone (IMR5 × IT22). **A:** Metaphase with HSR *(arrow)*. **B:** Metaphase with double minutes *(arrow)*.

proved to be tumorigenic. Cells from one of the resulting tumors (3bAgTc), explanted back into culture, were analyzed as soon as possible. Almost every cell has double minutes (Fig. 5), normal human 17s, and very few other human chromosomes. The IT-22 marker was retained.

Cells from this culture were tumorigenic when injected into nude mice. Cells with micronuclei, indicative of double minutes, were associated with interphase nuclei in a direct preparation of one of these tumors.

Two other clones NR5TP-7b and NR5TP-4a arising from the same

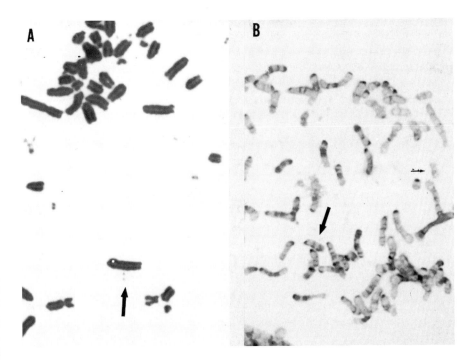

FIG. 5. 3bAgtc. **A:** Metaphase (partial) from 3bAg tumor explanted back into culture: all cells had double minutes *(arrows)*. **B:** Metaphase (partial), double minutes *(large arrow)*, normal human 17 *(small arrow)*.

fusion (IMR-5 × IT-22) confirmed these results. The hybrid clones had cells with HSRs and other cells with double minutes. Again, no cell had both. The other chromosomes, human and mouse, were normal and interphases had associated micronuclei. Cells from these clones were also tumorigenic in the nude mouse and cells from the resulting tumors, when explanted back into culture, contained only double minutes.

The pattern of segregation of HSRs and double minutes in these hybrid lines is consistent with our hypothesis concerning the origin of double minutes. The fusion of cells of different species here appears to have led to the breakdown of the HSR to form double minutes.

DISCUSSION

The chromosomes of five uncloned neuroblastoma cell lines, derived from independent human tumors, have been analyzed in this study. The project was undertaken to characterize two chromosome abnormalities in human neuroblastoma—the HSR and double minutes—using modern cytological and histochemical techniques, to define the relationship existing between them, and to gain insight into the possible roles they play in the function of the tumor cell.

In one neuroblastoma line, CHP-126, the segregation of HSRs and double minutes in two subpopulations of cells was demonstrated for the first time. A normal intact chromosome replaced the HSR marker in those cells containing double minutes. Another line, NMB, showed a similar segregation of HSRs and double minutes. Based on these findings, we propose that the double minutes originate from the breakdown of the HSR.

The Feulgen stain, specific for DNA, demonstrated that the HSR contains DNA which is linearly integrated into the chromosome. DNA measurements, by scanning cytophotometry, of the Feulgen-stained chromosomes showed the DNA content of each marker chromosome with an HSR to be significantly greater than that of its normal homologue without an HSR.

Our hypothesis that double minutes are derived from the HSR is supported by the results of fusions between a neuroblastoma cell line (IMR-5) containing an HSR-marker chromosome and a mouse fibroblast line. Neither double minutes nor micronuclei have ever been identified in metaphase spreads of either of the two cell lines participating in these fusions.

Double minutes have, however, been found in three of the resulting hybrid clones, and the pattern of segregation of the HSR and double minutes is consistent with our hypothesis concerning the origin of double minutes. These hybrid lines were tumorigenic in "nude" mice. When explanted back into tissue culture, the hybrid tumor cells contained only double minutes; the HSR marker chromosome was no longer apparent. The remaining human and mouse chromosomes in the hybrids were unchanged. The fusion of cells of different species, then, appears to have led to the breakdown of the HSR to produce double minutes (1).

This study therefore concludes that in human neuroblastoma (and, perhaps, in other tumors as well) the HSR represents a region of amplified, transcriptionally active DNA, coding for one or a few genes which confer a selective advantage to these cells at some stage in the evolution of the tumor. It further concludes that the origin of the double minutes in CHP-126 and in the IMR5 × IT-22 hybrids is from the breakdown of the HSR, and that this could be a model for the origin of double minutes in other tumors.

It is also possible that the breakdown of the HSR into double minutes and their subsequent loss from the cell might be involved in the spontaneous regression sometimes seen in these tumors.

ACKNOWLEDGMENTS

This work was supported by grants from the American Cancer Society VC-189A, the National Science Foundation PCM 76–82997, and The Children's Hospital Cancer Research Center CA-144898.

REFERENCES

1. Balaban-Malenbaum, G. (1979): Homogeneously staining regions and double-minute chromosomes in human neuroblastoma cell lines. Thesis, Department of Pathology, University of Pennsylvania, Philadelphia (for discussion of possible mechanisms).

2. Balaban-Malenbaum, G., and Gilbert, F. (1977): Double-minute chromosomes and the homogeneously staining regions of a human neuroblastoma cell line. *Science,* 198:739–741.

3. Balaban-Malenbaum, G., Grove, G., and Gilbert, F. (1979): Increased DNA content of HSR-marker chromosomes of human neuroblastoma cells. *Exp. Cell Res.,* 119:419–423.

4. Barker, P. E., and Hsu, T. C. (1979): Are double minutes chromosomes? *Exp. Cell Res. (in press).*

5. Biedler, J. L., and Spengler, B. A. (1976): Metaphase chromosome anomaly: Association with drug resistance and cell-specific products. *Science,* 191:185–187.

6. Brodeur, G. M., Sekhon, G. S., and Goldstein, M. N. (1977): Chromosomal aberrations in human neuroblastomas. *Cancer,* 40:2256–2264.

7. Cox, D., Yuncken, C., and Spriggs, A. I. (1965): Minute chromatin bodies in malignant tumors of childhood. *Lancet,* 2:55–58.

8. Croce, C. (1976): Loss of mouse chromosomes in somatic cell hybrids between HT-1080 human fibrosarcoma cells and mouse peritoneal macrophages. *Proc. Natl. Acad. Sci. U.S.A.,* 73:3248–3252.

9. Deitch, A. D. (1966): Cytophotometry of nucleic acids. In: *Introduction to Quantitative Cytochemistry,* edited by G. L. Wied, pp. 327–354. Academic Press, New York.

10. Dev, V. G., Miller, D. A., Allderdice, P. W., and Miller, O. J. (1972): Method for locating the centromeres of mouse meiotic chromosomes and its application to T163H and T70H translocations. *Exp. Cell Res.,* 73:259–262.

11. Levan, A., and Levan, G. (1978): Have double-minutes functioning centromeres? *Hereditas,* 88:81–92.

12. Levan, A., Levan, G., and Mitelman, F. (1977): Chromosomes and cancer. *Hereditas,* 86:15–30.

13. Lubs, H. A., Salmon, J. H., and Flanigan, S. (1966): Studies of a glial tumor with multiple minute chromosomes. *Cancer,* 19:561–599.

14. Mark, J. (1967): Double-minutes—A chromosomal aberration in Rous sarcomas in mice. *Hereditas,* 57:1–21.

15. Sandberg, A. A., Sakurai, M., and Holdsworth, R. N. (1972): Chromosomes and causation of human cancer and leukemia. VIII. DMS chromosomes in a neuroblastoma. *Cancer,* 29:1671–1979.

16. Seeger, R. C., Rayner, S. A., Banerjee, A., Chung, H., Laug, W. E., Neustein, H. B., and Benedict, W. F. (1977): Morphology, growth, chromosomal pattern, and fibrinolytic activity of two new human neuroblastoma cell lines. *Cancer Res.,* 37:1364–1371.

17. Shin, S., Freedman, V. H., Risser, R., and Pollack, R. (1975): Tumorigenicity of virus-transformed cells in nude mice is correlated specifically with anchorage independent growth in vitro. *Proc. Natl. Acad. Sci. U.S.A.,* 82:4435–4439.

18. Tumilowicz, J. J., Nichols, W. W., Cholon, J. J., and Greene, A. E. (1970): Definition of a continuous human cell line derived from neuroblastoma. *Cancer Res.,* 30:2110–2118.

Advances in Neuroblastoma Research,
edited by Audrey E. Evans.
Raven Press, New York © 1980.

Chromosomal Findings in Patients with Neuroblastoma

*Paul S. Moorhead and **Audrey E. Evans

*Department of Human Genetics, and **Department of Pediatrics, University of
Pennsylvania and The Children's Hospital of Philadelphia,
Philadelphia, Pennsylvania 19104

Most human cancers appear to have both hereditary and nonhereditary forms (7). Knudson has hypothesized that as few as two successive mutational events may account for this with the distinction between these forms reflecting whether the initial mutation is germinal or somatic. This genetic concept of cancer has provided a stimulus for genetic and cytogenetic studies concerned with various childhood tumors. The facts for retinoblastoma are the most convincing, making this neoplastic disease the prototype for the hypothesis (6). Similar elements of support are emerging from the body of information on other tumors, such as Wilms' and neuroblastoma. Parallels among these rare embryonal tumor conditions as emphasized by Knudson include a similar worldwide incidence, a tendency for the hereditary form to be multifocal in origin, and an earlier age of detection for the hereditary form.

The general view is that for these childhood tumors and certain other cancers an increased susceptibility to neoplastic disease can be inherited in a dominant fashion. The hereditary or familial forms of these conditions contrast with the rare conditions termed the "breakage syndromes" that show patterns of recessive inheritance of increased sensitivity to certain classes of environmental carcinogenic agents. The hereditary form of neuroblastoma may thus be due to the transmission of a dominant gene with low penetrance. However, there is a unique difficulty in assessing penetrance for neuroblastoma since neither spontaneous regression nor maturation to ganglioneuroma is uncommon (14). In addition, very few familial cases are known. In one remarkable instance of familial neuroblastoma, each parent of the affected propositus had previously had a child with neuroblastoma by a different spouse (12).

Greater susceptibility to both retinoblastoma and Wilms' tumor can also be the result of a constitutional chromosomal deletion specific to each. Numerous retinoblastoma patients with deletions implicating a specific segment of the long arm of chromosome 13 (q14) have now been well documented (4,18). Two Wilms' patients with a deletion of part of the short arm of chromosome 11 were described by Riccardi et al. (13), and seven additional examples of Wilms'-aniridia patients with deletions involving 11p were recently reported (1). Thus in each of these neoplasms a sporadically occurring specific deletion acts as the equivalent of a dominant gene.

With these many similarities between retinoblastoma and neuroblastoma in mind, it seemed likely that the application of banding procedures might reveal a chromosomal aberration characteristically associated with neuroblastoma. Thus a prospective study of the G-banded karyotypes of children with neuroblastoma was initiated more than 3 years ago and this paper describes our findings.

METHODOLOGY

Whole blood cultures of phytohemagglutinin-stimulated lymphocytes were used to obtain metaphase cells for cytogenetic studies by standard techniques. Although repeated samplings were made for several neuroblastoma patients and parents, failure of cell proliferation recurred in a few.

A series of 37 patients with neuroblastoma, 7 with retinoblastoma and 6 with other neoplastic conditions, was successfully investigated (Table 1). Neuroblastoma was of primary interest but in the initial phase of this study patients with other childhood neoplastic conditions were also included. Thereafter no further samples from patients with leukemia, nor from non-neuroblastoma cancer patients, were included. Growth failures were common in blood cultures from patients with leukemia, and further samples from retinoblastoma patients became unavailable to this study because of a prior commitment of the material.

Among the 37 neuroblastoma patients there were 6 with ganglioneuroblastoma, 1 with stage I disease, 3 with stage II, 2 with stage III, 9 with stage IV, 7 with stage IV-S, and 9 who were indeterminate. One patient among those with stage II is considered a long-term survivor and is a member of the family first reported by Chatten and Voorhess (3) in which 4 out of 5 siblings were affected. Although it was obvious that chromosomal deletions related to

TABLE 1. *Cytogenetic study of children with neuroblastoma and other neoplasms*

Neoplasm	No. of patients in study	No. of patients successfully G-banded for karyotype
Neuroblastoma	44	36
Neuroblastoma plus Wilms'	1	1
Wilms', failure to thrive	1	1
Aniridia[a]	1	1
Retinoblastoma	9	7
Leukemia	7	3
Ovarian dysgeminoma	1	1
Other	3	0
Total	67	50

[a] Suspected tumor proved negative.

the occurrence of neuroblastoma might also produce dysgenesis, with the result that such patients might present first to our Clinical Genetics Service, all patients studied to date were in fact ascertained through the Oncology Division of the Cancer Center.

Where feasible, G-banded karyotypes of the parents of affected children and of certain siblings were investigated. Sixty-one parents were successfully karyotyped together with 12 siblings and other relatives. This study is thus prospective with regard to all disease-affected patients, but some of the parents and relatives were first included for study subsequent to examination of chromosomes of the relevant patient. Samples of venous blood were normally obtained from patients prior to therapy, but in four cases it was determined that therapy [cyclophosphamide (Cytoxan®) or radiation] had been administered prior to the taking of blood for chromosomal studies. In any case, acquired chromosomal abnormalities did not interfere with determinations of basic karyotypes. For differential G-band staining of metaphase chromosomes, a modification involving exposure of air-dried slides to high concentrations of trypsin was used (15).

RESULTS

Although no characteristic deletion or other specific abnormality of karyotype was identified, four different constitutional chromosomal anomalies were found in this series of 37 neuroblastoma and 13 other tumor patients. Evidence for the existence of any small deletion was actively sought, especially in relation to the region beyond 1p31 which was reported deleted in two primary neuroblastoma tumors examined by Brodeur et al. (2; see also p. 73, *this volume*). Our finding of abnormalities of karyotype of 4 children within a total population of 50 patients with childhood neoplasia appears to be significant considering the limited size of this selected pathological population. These karyotypic abnormalities were three autosomal translocations and one pericentric inversion (Table 2).

The pericentric inversion, involving chromosome 9, was detected by G-banding and was confirmed by C-banding. The inversion was demonstrable in virtually all cells examined from this child with Wilms' tumor and from the mother.

A whole-arm translocation between acrocentric chromosomes 21 and 22 was found in a child with a retinoblastoma of the unilateral type (Fig. 1). The smaller centric product presumably formed by this translocation was absent. No rearrangement was present in the mother, and because the father was unavailable it could not be determined whether this 21q;22q fusion translocation arose *de novo* or was transmitted.

Two entirely different autosomal translocations were found among 37 neuroblastoma patients studied, and in each case the translocation was reciprocal and transmitted (Figs. 2 and 3). For the translocation involving chromosomes 4 and 7, four unaffected members of the family were found to carry both chromosomal products of the initial event. Carriers in this family appeared to be at

TABLE 2. *Major abnormalities of constitutional karyotype observed in children with neoplasms and in near relatives*

Karyotype	Subject	Neoplasm involved	Origin of abnormality
46XY, inv (9) (p11 q12), 16qh+	[C0017] propositus	Wilms'	Maternal
46XX, inv (9) (p11 q12)	[C0019] mother		transmission
45XX, t(21q;22q)	[C0088] propositus	Retinobl., unilateral	?
46XX, t(4p;7p)	[C0003] propositus	Neurobl. II	Paternal
46XY, t(4p;7p)	[C0037] father		transmission
46XY, t(4p;7p)	[C0020] sibling		
46XX, t(4p;7p)	[C0022] grandmother		
46XY, t(4p;7p)	[C0023] grand uncle		
46XX, t(11q;16q)	[C0149] propositus	Ganglioneuro-blastoma	Maternal
46XX, t(11q;16q)	[C0151] mother		transmission

Abbreviations: Retinobl., retinoblastoma; Neurobl., Neuroblastoma.

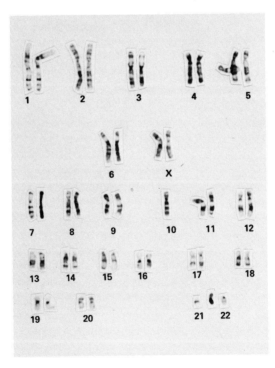

FIG. 1. Karyotype of patient C0088 with retinoblastoma. Whole-arm translocation between chromosomes 21 and 22.

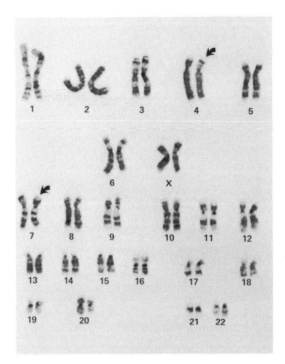

FIG. 2. Karyotype of patient C0003 with neuroblastoma, stage III. Reciprocal translocation between the short arms of chromosomes 4 and 7 *(arrows)*.

no selective disadvantage for conception or dysgenesis, implicating the balanced nature of this translocation throughout transmission involving four generations (Fig. 4). Such a segregation pattern is somewhat unusual and no histories suggestive of malignancies could be elicited within this kinship.

The second neuroblastoma-associated translocation involved exchange of parts of chromosomes 11 and 16, with break points at (q23;q24) (Fig. 3). Cytological interpretation and its occurrence in the unaffected mother of the propositus indicate that this was reciprocal.

Acquired chromosomal abnormalities observed among all cells karyotyped from children with neuroblastoma constituted 0.9% of the total (Table 3). Data from cells of the 4 patients receiving therapeutic treatment prior to sampling were of course excluded. A similarly increased value (1.0%) was observed in all cells from parents and relatives. No normal or control value for acquired abnormalities observed is available within this study; however, the incidence reported by Hecht et al. (5), which was based on a large series of subjects, is in agreement with our laboratory experience for short-term blood cultures from various subjects. Both the increases observed were statistically significant ($p \leq 0.05$).

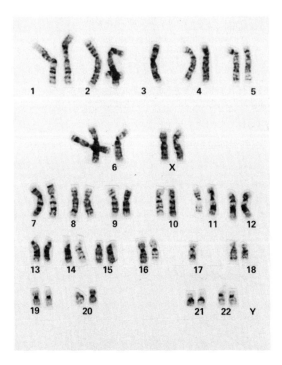

FIG. 3. Karyotype of patient C0149 with ganglioneuroblastoma. Presumably reciprocal translocation between the long arms of chromosomes 11 and 16 (left-hand member of each pair).

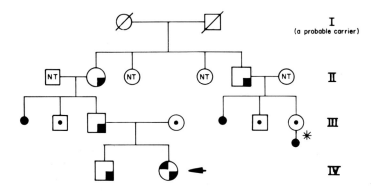

FIG. 4. Pedigree of family of patient C0003 with neuroblastoma showing segregation of the balanced translocation t(4p;7p) *(arrow denotes propositus).* NT, Not tested; dot ın center, Normal Karyotype; lower right quadrant filled in, Balanced Translocation; upper left quadrant filled in, Neuroblastoma; line through symbol, Deceased; * Not an unbalanced translocation.

TABLE 3. *Acquired abnormalities of the chromosomes observed in cells from patients with neuroblastoma and near relatives*

Subject	Neoplasm involved[a]	Deletions	Transloca- tions, re- arrangements	Aneuploidy	Incidence in sample
[C0075], propositus	Nbl.	—	—	+6	1/7
[C0146], propositus	Nbl. IV S	—	t(? → 5p)	—	1/11
[C0123], propositus	Ganglionbl.	—	t(11q;20p)	—	1/7
All propositi					3/331 cells
					0.9% [a]
[C0148], mother of [C0123]	Ganglionbl.	—	t(6q;20p)	—	1/12
[C0115], mother	Ganglionbl.	−9q	t(7q22;11q24)	—	2/20
[C0110], father	Nbl. II	−1q	—	—	1/8
[C0168], mother	Nbl.	−1q	—	—	1/7
All parents and near relatives					5/489 cells
					1.0% [a]
Various patients[b] (1,400 in number; from ref. 5)	Control				55/32,300 cells
					0.170 ± 0.021

Abbreviations: Nbl, neuroblastoma; Ganglionbl., ganglioneuroblastoma.
[a] Significantly different from control value, $p = 0.05$.
[b] Including no patients with malignancies or with instability syndromes.

DISCUSSION

Although inversions are often considered to be major chromosomal abnormalities, it seems more appropriate to regard these separately from other structural and numerical abnormalities of karyotype. The true incidence of inversion may be approximately 1% and published reports vary widely (10). Detection of inversions by G-banding is perhaps more dependent on the technical quality of the material than is detection of other types of abnormalities. Therefore, discounting the single instance of an inversion encountered, which was Wilms'-associated, we have observed three autosomal translocations among 50 patients with childhood tumors (Table 4). This provides an incidence of 6%, a value differing quite significantly ($p \leq 0.01$) from that of a normal, unselected human population (17). The incidence of major structural and numerical abnormalities found by Patil et al. (11) in a large population of children studied prospectively using G-banding techniques was 0.415%. The reliability of this as an estimate for normal human populations would seem to be confirmed by the similar incidence for such abnormalities found by Lin et al. (9) in a series of 930 newborns karyotyped by Q-banding, 0.43%.

The occurrence of two structural chromosomal rearrangements of karyotype in our series of only 37 neuroblastoma patients is in itself a significant enrichment ($p \leq 0.05$) over the values cited for major structural and numerical abnormalities of karyotype considered representative of normal human populations (Table

TABLE 4. *Incidence of major structural and numerical abnormalities of karyotype*

Population studied	Incidence[a]	Technique	Source
Children with neuroblastoma	2/37 (5.4%)[b]	G-banding	This study
Children with neoplasm	3/50 (6.0%)[c]	G-banding	This study
Consecutive newborns	4/930 (0.43%)	Q-banding	Lin et al. (9)
7–8-year-old children	18/4,342 (0.415%)	G-banding	Patil et al. (11)

[a] Values adjusted for exclusion of 0, 1, 1, and 3 inversions from these populations, respectively.
[b] Significantly different from value for 7–8-year-old children, $p = 0.05$.
[c] Significantly different from value for 7–8-year-old children, $p = 0.01$.

4). The nonspecific nature of these two translocations associated with neuroblastoma might be considered as evidence of some generally increased risk of neoplasia in persons bearing an abnormality of karyotype. However, except for sporadic case reports, evidence of such an association for abnormalities of karyotype is restricted to those involving gross genetic imbalance, such as trisomy 21 or trisomy 17. This generalization is more often stated as if it were a proved causal proposition, a predisposition to cancer deriving from the presence of the karyotypic abnormality. This may eventually prove to be the case for gross aneuploidy, but its extension to balanced forms of rearranged karyotypes is not warranted. Our observations of nonspecific rearrangements in association with neuroblastoma may well be the consequence of the presence of a genetic factor predisposing both to chromosomal rearrangement and to development of neuroblastoma tumor. The enrichment for karyotypic rearrangements in this small patient population could possibly be a secondary result of the presence of the dominant gene postulated to be the basis for disease in those afflicted children that comprise the hereditary fraction.

If such a predisposition to chromosomal exchange or rearrangement is characteristic of the cells from that fraction of our population which bears a gene factor, this may still be reflected in the general or overall frequency of acquired abnormalities observed. In fact, the incidence of such sporadic abnormalities seen was elevated both in all cells karyotyped from neuroblastoma patients and also in all cells from their parents and relatives ($p \leq 0.05$; Table 3). However, the absolute numbers observed were small.

Asking the same general question for retinoblastoma, we are aware of three prospective studies of karyotype in children with retinoblastoma. Wilson et al. (18) discovered two abnormalities of karyotype in 50 children with retinoblastoma, an XXY and a 13q⁻. Nichols *(personal communication)* found a single 13q⁻ among 31 such patients and none were found in another series of 12 retinoblastoma patients studied by Ladda et al. (8). If to this is added our finding of one autosomal translocation in 7 such patients, there occurred two

13q deletions, one case of aneuploidy, and one robertsonian translocation in a combined total of 100 children with retinoblastoma. This suggests that for both retinoblastoma and neuroblastoma, nonspecific chromosome abnormalities may be a secondary consequence of each of these dominant genes that predispose to embryonal tumor development. The possibility is raised that these 13q deletions themselves might be the result of the mutant gene's presence at that same site, a gene predisposing both to chromosomal rearrangement and to retinoblastoma. Relevant to this, a child with retinoblastoma was recently found to have a 13q deletion and her mother was heterozygous for a paracentric inversion of 13q. Most interesting is the fact that the centromeric region of the deleted 13q in the daughter was derived from the mother's normal chromosome 13 (16).

In a consideration of our original objective, the identification of a chromosomal site which may be characteristically associated with neuroblastoma, specific regions of the human idiogram which deserve special attention certainly include 1p—as discussed by Brodeur, p. 73, *this volume*—but also perhaps 11q. Although the evidence is fragmentary, certain correspondences as to particular chromosomes or chromosome arms involved were seen in the neuroblastoma families

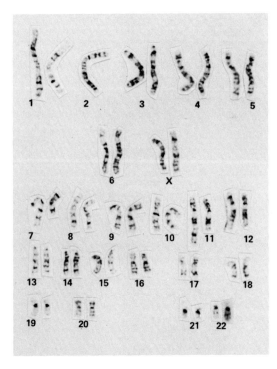

FIG. 5. Cell karyotype showing sporadic translocation between long arms of chromosomes 7 and 11 observed in 1 out of 20 cells examined from subject C0115, mother of patient C0113 with ganglioneuroblastoma.

reported here. This was true for both constitutional and acquired abnormalities noted. Chromosome arms 20p and 11q were each involved in two independent sporadic rearrangements (Table 3; Fig. 5), and the long arm of chromosome 11 was the site of one break point of the inherited reciprocal translocation, t(11q23;16q24) (Fig. 3). Also involving chromosome 11, the segment 11q23 was considered to be "abnormally thin" in all cells from the father in the unusual case of familial neuroblastoma reported by Pegelow et al. (12).

ACKNOWLEDGMENTS

The authors acknowledge the excellent technical assistance of C. Soffer, S. Amsbaugh, M. Makadon, and M. Clark. The authors wish to thank Dr. Elaine Zackai and D. Eupnu for obtaining family histories. This research was supported by PHS Grant CA 14489.

REFERENCES

1. Bader, J. L., Li, F. P., Gerald, P. S., Leiken, S. L., and Randolph, J. G. (1979): 11p chromosome deletions in four patients with aniridia and Wilms' tumor. *Cancer Res.,* 20:210 (abst. 850).
2. Brodeur, G. M., Sekhon, G. S., and Goldstein, M. N. (1978): Chromosomal aberrations in human neuroblastoma. *Cancer,* 40:2256–2263.
3. Chatten, J., and Voorhess, M. L. (1967): Familial neuroblastoma. *N. Engl. J. Med.,* 227:1230–1236.
4. Francke, U. (1976): Retinoblastoma and chromosome 13. *Cytogenet. Cell Genet.,* 14:131–134.
5. Hecht, F., McCaw, B. K., Peakman, D., and Robinson, A. (1975): Non-random occurrence of 7–14 translocations in human lymphocyte cultures. *Nature,* 255:243–244.
6. Hethcote, H. W., and Knudson, A. G. (1978): A model for the incidence of embryonal cancers: Application to retinoblastoma. *Proc. Natl. Acad. Sci. U.S.A.,* 75:2453–2457.
7. Knudson, A. G., Strong, L. C., and Anderson, D. E. (1973): Hereditary factors and cancer in man. *Prog. Med. Genet.,* 9:113–158.
8. Ladda, R., Atkins, L., Littlefield, J., and Pruett, R. (1973): Retinoblastoma: Chromosome banding in patients with heritable tumor. *Lancet,* 2:506.
9. Lin, C. C., Gedeon, M. M., Griffith, P., Smink, W. K., Newton, D. R., Wilkie, L., and Sewell, L. M. (1976): Chromosomal analysis in 930 consecutive newborns using quinacrine fluorescent banding technique. *Hum. Genet.,* 31:315–328.
10. Moorhead, P. S. (1976): A closer look at inversions. *Am. J. Hum. Genet.,* 28:294–296.
11. Patil, S. R., Lubs, H. A., Brown, J., Cohen, M., Gerald, P., Hecht, F., Kimberling, W., Myrianthopoulos, N., and Summitt, R. L. (1977): Incidence of major chromosome abnormalities in children. *Cytogenet. Cell Genet.,* 18:302–306.
12. Pegelow, C. H., Ebbin, A. J., Powars, D., and Towner, J. W. (1975): Familial neuroblastoma. *J. Pediatr.,* 87:736–765.
13. Riccardi, V. M., Sujansky, E., Smith, A. C., and Francke, U. (1978): Chromosomal imbalance in the aniridia-Wilms' tumor association: 11p interstitial deletion. *Pediatrics,* 61:604–610.
14. Schimke, R. N. (1977): Tumors of the neural crest system. In: *Progress in Cancer Research and Therapy, Vol. 3: Genetics of Human Cancer,* edited by J. J. Mulvihill, R. W. Miller, and J. R. Fraumeni, Jr., pp. 179–198.
15. Seabright, M. (1971): A rapid banding technique for human chromosomes. *Lancet,* 2:971–972.
16. Sparkes, R. S., Muller, H., and Klisak, I. (1979): Retinoblastoma with 13q- chromosomal deletion associated with maternal paracentric inversion of 13q. *Science,* 203:1027–1029.
17. Stevens, W. L. (1942): Accuracy of mutation rates. *J. Genet.,* 43:301–307.
18. Wilson, M. G., Ebbin, A. J., Towner, J. W., and Spencer, W. H. (1977): Chromosomal anomalies in patients with retinoblastoma. *Clin. Genet.,* 12(1):1–8.

Advances in Neuroblastoma Research,
edited by Audrey E. Evans.
Raven Press, New York © 1980.

Discussion: Genetics

Dr. Rajewsky (Essen) asked Dr. Gilbert if double minute and HSRs had been detected directly in material from primary tumors or only in cell lines. Dr. Gilbert replied that both long marker chromosomes and double minutes had been seen in direct preparations. *Dr. LaBrosse (Baltimore)* asked if nude mice bearing human neuroblastomas excrete elevated levels of catecholamines, and Dr. Gilbert replied that he had not tested for such metabolites. Dr. Knudson (Philadelphia) questioned whether the human chromosomes retained in a hybrid are necessary to supply the genes that make a neuroblast, and if the crucial chromosomes that are lost are the ones that would regulate this differentiation. If so, the hybrids, to be tumorigenic, must have one or more chromosomes involved in differentiation up to a certain point and must be missing chromosomes necessary for differentiation beyond that point.

Dr. Gilbert (Philadelphia) replied that this is not necessarily so. When one loses the suppressive chromosomes contributed by the mouse, one may uncover the malignant potential of the mouse, so that in fact this is a tumor not because of the positive contribution from the neuroblast but because of the loss of the negative contribution from the mouse. He postulates that the presence of HSRs or DMs might enhance tumorigenicity and allow for overgrowth of a specific cell population.

Dr. Prasad (Denver) asked if there is any change in the basal level of differentiated function or response to differentiating agents in the hybrids that were not tumorigenic. Dr. Gilbert stated that he had not studied the hybrids in terms of differentiated phenotype.

Dr. Green (Memphis) was concerned that the system requiring growth on agarose would be selective for certain clones or a membrane defect in the hybrid rather than some characteristic of human neuroblastoma. Dr. Gilbert reported that not all of the hybrids injected into the nude mouse had been passed through agarose. Although there is evidence in favor of segregation and selection, the line 4A yielded a small number of cells capable of forming a tumor when directly isolated.

There was a brisk discussion between Dr. Benedict (Los Angeles) and Dr. Brodeur on the question of his finding a normal karyotype in some of the direct preparations. Dr. Benedict stated that he had never seen "completely diploid" cells in the many direct preparations of human sarcomas, carcinomas, and in situ carcinomas that he had studied. He believed such cells might arise from normal fibroblasts or other normal cells, and it is important to characterize further those cells with a normal karyotype to prove that they are malignant. Dr. Brodeur reported that two of their nine cases had normal karyotypes; one was obtained from a primary tumor processed directly with no short-term culture, and the second was from bone marrow reportedly 100% replaced in tumor and which was studied after 2 days in culture. Although it is possible they were normal dividing cells, he believed they were indeed proliferating tumor cells and they were subsequently passaged for a period of time. In his review of the literature, 10 of 39 cases had normal diploid karyotypes, and 9 of the 10 were from primary tumors of untreated patients, processed directly.

Dr. Prasad (Denver) then asked if the extent of chromosome abnormalities was a function of age or the tumor or treatment, and Dr. Brodeur responded that he had studied only one patient under 6 months of age and that patient had a normal karyotype, Dr. Knudson (Philadelphia) asked if the infant under 6 months of age would fit the classification of stage IV-S, and the normal karyotypic finding might be evidence that the cells were not really tumor cells as ordinarily understood. Dr. Brodeur replied that the infant would be called IV-S, and he had studied only one such patient. It is not possible to assume that the normal karyotype represented a nonmalignant cell, but he believed it would be important to study tumor specimens from more than one site in such patients to determine whether IV-S tumors are really multiple primaries. If one found hyperdiploid or other abnormal modes, it would be suggested these are indeed malignant tumors.

Dr. Biedler (New York), congratulating Dr. Brodeur, suggested he had done a considerable service to focus attention on chromosome 1. She asked him what he believed was the mechanism and what the deletion might represent. Was the important event the loss from the cell or part of the chromosome, a rearrangement or a translation, and did he believe that the lesion site was important? Dr. Brodeur responded that the finding may be comparable to data on retinoblastoma and the deletion of chromosome 13. He believed the loss might be a first hit that makes the cell more susceptible to malignant transformation. He reported that he had found a lesion in the short arm of the number 1 chromosome in other tumors such as malignant melanoma and brain tumors. Perhaps there is a malignant potential at this site shared by other cells derived from neural crest.

Dr. Knudson asked Dr. Balaban-Malenbaum how the DMs arise in fresh tumors if she believes the HSRs give rise to the DMs and HSRs are not seen in fresh tumor preparations. Dr. Balaban-Malenbaum responded that she is not sure it is possible to say that there are no HSRs in fresh tumors. IMR showed them in the eighth passage, which is very early. She believed that this is a cyclic phenomenon and that when DMs are seen, the tumor has already left the HSR stage. Dr. Biedler stated that although there is a trend, going from DMs to HSRs, the evidence does not indicate that HSRs go to DMs or vice versa in a direct manner. If one accepts the view that amplification can occur extra-chromosomally, one can envision also that the DMs are groups of new amplification units that have never gone through HSR stage and never will.

Dr. Freed (Philadelphia) posed the question, "Why are double minutes double?" Most speakers had agreed that they have no centromeres, yet when the chromotids of the genome as a whole have separated, the double minutes remain double. Dr. Balaban-Malenbaum said that Barr postulates that interloops hold chromosomes together. You sometimes do see separation of DMs in anaphase preparations, but they are definitely out of phase. There are two recent cases in which DMs show this hitchhiking. Dr. Biedler added that it is not necessary to have a centromere if there is an alternative mechanism. It is known that there is a spectrum of centromeres, some having a stronger action than others, and DMs may lie at the end of the spectrum. Dr. Rajewsky (Essen) asked whether the regions of the HSRs would exchange in one piece or in several pieces if cells containing HSRs were exposed to some kind of mutagenic agent that would provide the formation of sister chromatid exchanges. Dr. Balaban-Malenbaum said that in two experiments where cells were exposed to x-ray or to mitomycin C, the HSRs were preferentially underinvolved even when the exchanges were increased 10-fold. She believed this was another piece of evidence that HSRs behave as cytologic units or single bands. Dr. Biedler had done similar experiments with HSR-containing Chinese hamster cells using mitomycin C, vincristine, and other agents known to break chromosomes and induce sister chromatid exchange and also had observed underinvolvement of the HSR region.

Dr. Knudson remarked that Dr. Moorhead's suggestion of a common agent producing both the chromosomal abnormality and the tumor reminded him of the days when people posed that Down's syndrome predisposed to leukemia. It was then noticed that sibs of Down's syndrome patients were also at increased risk for leukemia, and he asked Dr. Moorhead if he believed there was a parallel in neuroblastoma patients. Dr. Moorhead responded that although in the literature there are many sporadic cases and nearly always the conclusion is that there is a predisposition to cancer in persons bearing chromosome abnormalities, he tends to disagree and suggests that the translocation is one sign of a cellular abnormality that can lead to tumor formation.

Cell Differentiation

Advances in Neuroblastoma Research,
edited by Audrey E. Evans.
Raven Press, New York © 1980.

Section Introduction

Uriel Z. Littauer

The appearance of a variety of forms of neuroblastoma tumors has been discussed in this volume. These range from rapidly dividing neuroblast-like cells that have a high rate of spontaneous regression to more malignant cells, some of which express a variety of differentiated functions. Evidence has also accumulated to show that in some cases the tumor matures *in vivo* to a more benign form of ganglioneuroma.

Thus one would like to understand in detail the maturation process of neurons and compare it to that of neuroblastoma cells by revealing the various factors that determine the stage-by-stage development of these cells.

In general, we know that a variety of hormones and growth factors are required for cell proliferation or for its maturation. The balance between these factors, we believe, will determine the course of the cell's development. Some factors such as NGF seem to have a dual function, being required for viability and growth on one hand, as well as for cell differentiation. Similarly, many other cellular products will determine the course of cell development. A cell may, therefore, show extensive proliferation *in vivo* if the body fails to provide these factors in their correct proportion. Alternatively, the cell itself may have changed and have lost, for example, a specific receptor.

All these factors first interact with the surface membrane and in that respect glycoproteins undoubtedly play a major role. Another possible target for controlling cell maturation is the cascade reactions that take place upon induction of differentiation including the control of cyclic AMP levels and cyclic AMP dependent protein kinases.

It has been suggested that the ability of many of the malignant cells to undergo maturation has not been completely lost. Thus a number of agents have been examined for their ability to induce differentiation. These include DMSO, HMBA, dibutyryl-cAMP, phosphodiesterase inhibitors, cytotoxic drugs, or a combination of agents such as prostaglandin E_1 together with theophylline. Many mouse neuroblastoma clones have been shown to express neuronal properties when exposed to these agents. They seem to represent proliferating neuroblasts that can be induced to differentiate. However, upon withdrawal of the inducing agent, proliferation will start again. This could mean either that terminal differentiation has not been achieved or that a fraction of these cells have escaped the effect of the inducing agent altogether.

The great variability of the human neuroblastoma cell lines and the difficulty of establishing *in vitro* cultures from primary tumors has already been mentioned. Some of the human cell lines express several differentiated functions even in the absence of an inducing agent. In that respect these cell lines may represent differentiated end cells that have acquired the ability to proliferate. Other cell lines have lost several biochemical markers, that are expressed in other cases in the presence of an inducing agent. One would hope that analysis of the expression of differentiated markers may aid in classifying the various human neuroblastoma tumors and thus initiate a more logical approach to chemotherapy.

Advances in Neuroblastoma Research,
edited by Audrey E. Evans.
Raven Press, New York © 1980.

Molecular and Cellular Aspects of Chemical Neuro-Oncogenesis

Manfred F. Rajewsky

Institut für Zellbiologie (Tumorforschung), Universität Essen (GH), Federal Republic of Germany

Present experimental evidence suggests that neoplastic transformation of neural cells can be caused by carcinogenic chemicals, oncogenic viruses, and ionizing radiation (15). A number of chemical carcinogens (e.g., alkyl-nitrosoureas; azo, azoxy, and hydrazo compounds; acyl-triazenes; but also 7, 12-dimethylbenz(a)anthracene) have been shown to be neuro-oncogenic in laboratory animals, mainly in the rat (13). Analyses with various carcinogens indicate that application during the prenatal and early postnatal age period has generally a more pronounced neuro-oncogenic effect than carcinogen exposure at adult age. This is particularly evident in the case of N-ethyl-N-nitrosourea (EtNU), which has become one of the favorite model carcinogens not only for the study of neuro-oncogenesis but also for analysis of the process of chemical carcinogenesis in general (32). A single pulse of EtNU applied to fetal or newborn rats specifically results in a very high incidence of neuro-ectodermal neoplasms in the brain and peripheral nervous system. The neuro-oncogenic effect in adult rats is far less pronounced (3,10,32). The particular sensitivity of the developing neural cell system suggests that the probability of neoplastic transformation of neural (precursor) cells may be related to their proliferative and differentiated state at the time of carcinogen exposure.

PULSE CARCINOGENESIS BY EtNU IN THE RAT NERVOUS SYSTEM

Molecular Mechanisms

The neural tissue specificity of the oncogenic effect of EtNU cannot be explained by tissue differences regarding the formation of the "ultimate" electrophilic reactant of this carcinogen. The respective ethyl-cation is produced indiscriminately in all tissues, via rapid (half-life of EtNU *in vivo,* ≤ 8 min; 4) nonenzymatic decomposition. A similar molar content of ethylated bases is thus initially (i.e., at 1 hr after the EtNU pulse) found in the DNA of "high-risk" (fetal/newborn brain) and "low-risk" rat tissues (e.g., adult brain, liver; 4,32), and after EtNU application at different pre- and postnatal developmental stages (33).

Most of the ethylation products ($\sim 80\%$) initially detected in DNA after exposure to EtNU result from ethylation at exocyclic oxygen atoms (38). These products are O^6-ethyldeoxyguanosine (O^6-EtdGuo; $\sim 7\%$), O^2-ethylthymidine, O^4-ethylthymidine, O^2-ethyldeoxycytidine, and ethylphosphotriesters ($\sim 60\%$). The products formed by ethylation at ring nitrogens include 7-ethyldeoxyguanosine (7-EtdGuo; $\sim 11\%$), 3-ethyldeoxyguanosine, 1-ethyldeoxyadenosine, 3-ethyldeoxyadenosine, 7-ethyldeoxyadenosine, 3-ethyldeoxycytidine, and 3-ethylthymidine. In the case of O^6-EtdGuo, O^2-ethyldeoxycytidine, O^4-ethylthymidine, 3-ethylthymidine, 3-ethyldeoxycytidine, and 1-ethyldeoxyadenosine, the ethyl groups are thus positioned at atoms normally involved in hydrogen bonding between complementary base pairs. However, with the exception of 1-ethyldeoxyadenosine and 3-ethyldeoxycytidine, which appear to be much less frequently formed in double-stranded DNA, all products are formed at about equal relative frequencies in double-stranded and single-stranded DNA (37). Furthermore, their relative initial molar frequencies in DNA are the same, regardless of whether exposure to EtNU occurs *in vivo*, in cell culture, or in isolated DNA incubated with EtNU *in vitro*, and probably regardless of the concentration of EtNU over an extended dose range (38).

A comparison between different alkylating carcinogens shows a positive correlation of the carcinogenic effect with the relative extent of oxygen alkylation in target cell DNA in general, and with the extent of guanine-O^6 alkylation (expressed, e.g., by the molar ratio of O^6-alkyldeoxyguanosine/7-alkyldeoxyguanosine) in particular (5). Thus the initial O^6-EtdGuo/7-EtdGuo ratio in DNA for the very weakly carcinogenic diethylsulfate is 0.003 (41), whereas the corresponding value for the highly potent carcinogen EtNU is 0.63 (5,6). O^6-alkylation is generally considered to be a potentially mutagenic structural modification of deoxyguanosine (25) which can, for example, lead to transcriptional errors, or to GC $\rightarrow$ AT transition mutations in proliferating target cells.

With respect to the detection and quantitation of alkylation products in DNA, recent methodological developments have opened new possibilities. "Conventional" radiochromatographic techniques applied after target cell exposure to alkylating carcinogens labeled in the alkyl group with ^{14}C or ^{3}H permit the detection of one alkylated nucleotide in about 10^6 molecules of the same nucleotide in DNA hydrolysates (number of nucleotides/ diploid mammalian genome, $\sim 1.3 \times 10^{10}$). We have recently been able to lower this detection limit in the case of O^6-EtdGuo by developing high-affinity antibodies, specifically directed against this ethylation product, and by establishing the respective radioimmunoassay (RIA), enzyme immuno-assay (EIA), and radioimmunosorbent assay (RIST) (27,28). At present, the best antiserum (antibody affinity constant, 1–2×10^{10} 1/mol) detects ~ 50 fmol (~ 15 pg) O^6-EtdGuo in a competitive RIA (using O^6-Et[8,5'-^{3}H]deoxyguanosine as a tracer). In combination with prefractionation by high-pressure liquid chromatography (HPLC), molar concentrations of O^6-EtdGuo/deoxyguanosine of $< 10^{-7}$ can thus be determined by RIA in hydrolysates of a limited amount of DNA (e.g., DNA from two adult rat livers to determine a molar content of O^6-EtdGuo/deoxyguanosine of $\cong 10^8$). Further work now concentrates on expanding the panel of antibodies specifically directed against different carcinogen-modified constituents of DNA, particularly by the production of monoclonal antibodies (1), and on extending the immunological techniques to the detection of these products in individual cells.

As described above, the neural tissue specific, oncogenic effect of EtNU in the rat is not due to higher amounts of potentially mutagenic ethylation products formed in the DNA of neural cells as compared to the cells of other tissues. It was, therefore, interesting to find that early postnatal brain (10th day postnatally)—in contrast to other rat tissues at this developmental stage—exhibits a strongly reduced (if not entirely lacking) capability for the (enzymatic) elimination of O^6-ethyldeoxyguanosine from DNA (6,32). A similar difference is not found for any of the other ethylation products thus far studied. This selective persistence of a potentially mutagenic ethylation product in the DNA of the "high-risk" neural cells versus the "low-risk" cells of liver and other tissues, in concert with the high rate of DNA replication (required for the genetic fixation of premutational DNA lesions) during brain development, could account for an increased frequency of neoplastic transformation which would find its expression in the pronounced neuro-oncogenic effect of EtNU in rats at the perinatal age.

The nature of the enzyme(s) responsible for the recognition and elimination from DNA of O^6-alkylguanine has not yet been clarified. In principle, either a specific DNA-N-glycosylase, an endonuclease, a de- or trans-alkylase, or possibly enzymes of an entirely different nature could be involved. Current efforts by a number of research groups may soon lead to interesting results regarding this problem (12,23,24,30). Furthermore, it appears from recent observations in several laboratories that the activity of this enzyme system may be induced (stimulated) by pretreatment with very low doses (26,36), but is reduced by high concentrations of the carcinogen (14,29). Although these observations need further experimental confirmation, it seems evident that investigations are urgently required into the behavior of DNA repair-associated enzyme systems at low and very low levels of DNA modification, i.e., after exposure of target cells to carcinogen concentrations more realistic in terms of human environmental conditions. Clearly, high-sensitivity detection methods are of particular importance in this context.

Cellular Mechanisms

Thus far, the processes operating in target cells and cell populations during the time interval between their initial interaction with a carcinogen and the onset of clonal tumor growth remain unclarified. This phase, which can be best studied in pulse carcinogenesis models such as the EtNU-rat system, may involve a sequence of characteristic phenotypic and functional alterations of the presumptive cancer cells. Clearly, biochemical analyses of whole neural tissues cannot provide information on the particular types of neural (precursor) cells that undergo neoplastic conversion after exposure to EtNU. Investigations at the level of individual cells are difficult under *in vivo* conditions, although morphological and certain biochemical parameters have to some extent been studied in rat brain, as a function of time after an EtNU pulse at the 15th day of gestation or later (11,21,22,31,40,42). Appropriate cell culture systems are, therefore, required as well as phenotypic and functional "markers" for particular target cell types and stages of differentiation, and techniques for cell separation. Presently available experimental systems and parameters for these analyses are still crude and will need considerable refinement.

Recently, Laerum and Rajewsky (18) have established an *"in vivo-in vitro"* system, where a pulse of EtNU is first transplacentally administered to fetal rats of the inbred BDIX strain. The target cell population at risk, fetal rat brain cells (FBCs), are then transferred to long-term monolayer culture, thus permitting the monitoring of sequential cellular alterations during malignant transformation (see 16,19,32, and 34). In FBCs transferred to cell culture after a pulse of 75 µg of EtNU/g body weight on the 18th day of gestation, tumorigenicity (as assayed by subcutaneous reimplantation of 1 to 4×10^6 cells into baby BDIX rats) was first observed after about 200 days of culture. This time interval is similar to the median time until death with neuro-ectodermal neoplasms in the offspring of BDIX rats exposed to the same dose of EtNU at the same gestational stage. During the period of cell culture, a sequence of changes is seen which has permitted an operational subdivision into "stages" (I through V). In early primary culture (stage I), EtNU and control cultures (derived from saline-treated animals) are morphologically indistinguishable. They contain stationary glia-like cells on a growing layer of flat, epithelioid cells (probably glial precursors). The proportion of glia-like cells then gradually decreases in the control cultures (stage II; ∼ 10th day to 40th day). The control cultures are later composed almost exclusively of flat cells, and could in a number of cases be kept for up to 300 days before they finally deteriorated. "Spontaneous" transformation was thus not observed during this time period in control cultures derived from 18th day FBCs. Information regarding this point, however, is not yet available for cultures derived from FBC of earlier or later developmental stages. Other authors have in the meantime reported cases of "spontaneous" transformation in FBC cultures either after very extended culture periods (35) or under special culture conditions (2).

In contrast to the control cultures, the proportion of glia-like cells in the EtNU cultures increases slightly (or at least remains constant) during stage II. During stage III (∼ 40th to 100th day), slowly proliferating glia-like cells in the EtNU cultures gradually begin to form characteristic piled-up "nodules" which consist of tightly and irregularly arranged cells with many cytoplasmic processes. These cells exhibit a reduced substrate adherence and, after subcultivation, often show an astrocyte-like appearance.

The transition to stage IV (~ 100th to 200th day) is marked by "morphological transformation" of these cells, concomitantly with the onset of more rapid proliferation. The resulting "established" cell lines contain enlarged cells with a reduced length and number of cytoplasmic processes. At subsequent subcultures higher cell densities are reached, and the cells display a more disordered array with multiple piled-up areas (foci) of tightly packed spheroid cells. At this stage (average number of culture passages, 6 ± 2, SE), the cells have acquired the capacity to form colonies in semi-solid agar medium, with an initial average cloning efficiency of ~ 1%. After several further culture passages, the cells become tumorigenic (stage V).

The ultrastructural characteristics of both the surface and internal architecture of FBCs during the process of EtNU carcinogenesis in culture have been studied by Haugen and Laerum (7,8). Ultrastructural surface characteristics often seen on proliferative (and) neoplastic cells (e.g., high frequency of microvilli, ruffles, filopodia, zeiotic blebs, and ruffling membranes) are observed from the end of stage III onwards. Similarly, alterations of the internal cellular ultrastructure (e.g., atypically shaped nuclei with dense clumping of heterochromatin, mainly along the nuclear envelope; large nucleoli; a loss of cytoplasmic microfilament bundles; and reduced numbers of microtubules) reminiscent of tumor cells are seen from this stage onwards, i.e., before the cultures acquire tumorigenic potential.

Solid tumors developed in baby BDIX rats upon subcutaneous reimplantation of the pluriclonal neoplastic cell lines (BT lines) developed in this system appear histologically as neurinoma-, glioma-, or glioblastoma-like, and often as pleiomorphic neoplasms (20). In general, these tumors resemble the various types of neuroectodermal rat neoplasms induced by EtNU *in vivo*.

The BT lines are usually composed of multipolar glia-like cells, but also contain flatter cells with shorter and fewer cytoplasmic processes, and frequently giant cells (20). They exhibit different degrees of aneuploidy and contain, before subcloning, multiple subpopulations of cells (as reflected by plurimodal DNA distributions recorded by pulse cytophotometry; 20). Serologic analyses of selected BT-lines gave no evidence for the presence of group-specific interspecies oncornaviral antigens (20). All BT lines contain, to a varying degree and in differing proportions of the cells, the predominantly glia-specific S-100 protein (20). The amount of S-100 protein in rat brain is minimal at birth, reaching the level of adult brain only at about 25 days postnatally. In the cultured FBCs, differentiation for the expression of S-100 protein, therefore, appears to be unaffected by the process of neoplastic transformation. No indication of more than borderline neurotransmitter activity has been found in the BT lines, nor has electrical membrane excitability been detected in randomly selected BT cells (17).

From the observations mentioned above, it appears that neoplastic neurogenic cells derived from FBCs exposed to EtNU on the 18th day of gestation predominantly express phenotypic traits of glial rather than of neuronal cells. This may reflect the fact that at this particular developmental stage, the proliferative neural precursor cell compartments at risk contain a numerical excess of cells committed for the glial differentiation pathways; and the neuronal precursor cells are already close (in terms of the number of cell divisions ahead) to the stage of differentiation where their proliferation is irreversibly blocked, whereas glial cells retain their proliferative capacity. There is also the trivial explanation, that the rare occurrence of neoplastic cells with neuronal phenotypic traits is simply due to unfavorable culture conditions for neuronal precursor FBCs (so that glial phenotypes are selected for). Although the latter possibility cannot be ruled out, it seems less likely in view of the fact that the neuroectodermal neoplasms which arise *in vivo* after perinatal exposure of rats to EtNU, too, predominantly exhibit phenotypic traits normally associated with the various types of glial cells (13).

Using a similar *in vivo-in vitro* approach, other authors (35) have transferred rat brain cells into cell culture after time intervals of up to several months after the administration of EtNU *in vivo* (but before the onset of detectable tumor growth *in vivo*). Essentially confirming the findings described above, they observed the development of malignant cell lines in these cultures derived from "preneoplastic" brain. The same group has also reported an increased fibrinolytic activity at stages prior to the acquisition of the capacity to form colonies in semi-solid agar medium (9).

Regarding the search for phenotypic markers of FBCs destined to undergo neoplastic transformation, it should be noted that definite changes (e.g., morphological alterations, loss of anchorage dependence) in the cultured cells have thus far been detected only at rather advanced stages (III through V) after prenatal pulse exposure to EtNU. It must also not be overlooked that the observed phenotypic alterations (like other so-called indicators of neoplastic conversion, except for the proof of tumorigenicity *in vivo*), although apparently often associated with the transformation of cells for "permanent" proliferation ("established cell lines"), are not necessarily under the same genetic control as the "tumorigenic phenotype(s)" (39). Further work must, therefore, aim at (a) improving, standardizing, and quantifying cell culture systems; (b) obtaining more information on early (and hopefully obligatory) cellular changes connected with the process of neurocarcinogenesis; and (c) defining subpopulations of (precursor) cells, and stages of brain development and differentiation, that may be characterized by an elevated risk of neoplastic conversion by neurocarcinogens.

ACKNOWLEDGMENTS

Work in the author's laboratory is supported by the Deutsche Forschungsgemeinschaft (Ra 119/5–7), the Bundesministerium für Forschung und Technologie (CMT 04), and the U.S. National Cancer Institute, DHEW (1R01 CA20017).

REFERENCES

1. Adamkiewicz, J., and Rajewsky, M. F. In preparation.
2. Bulloch, K., Stallcup, W. B., and Cohn, M. (1977): The derivation and characterization of neuronal cell lines from rat and mouse brain. *Brain Res., 135*:25–36.
3. Druckrey, H., Landschütz, Ch., and Ivankovic, S. (1970): Transplacentare Erzeugung maligner Tumoren des Nervensystems. II. Äthyl-nitrosoharnstoff an 10 genetisch definierten Rattenstämmen. *Z. Krebsforsch., 73*:371–386.
4. Goth, R., and Rajewsky, M. F. (1972): Ethylation of nucleic acids by ethylnitrosourea-1-^{14}C in the fetal and adult rat. *Cancer Res., 32*:1501–1505.
5. Goth, R., and Rajewsky, M. F. (1974): Molecular and cellular mechanisms associated with pulse-carcinogenesis in the rat nervous system by ethylnitrosourea: Ethylation of nucleic acids and elimination rates of ethylated bases from the DNA of different tissues. *Z. Krebsforsch., 82*:37–64.
6. Goth, R., and Rajewsky, M. F. (1974): Persistence of O^6-ethylguanine in rat brain DNA: Correlation with nervous system specific carcinogenesis by ethylnitrosourea. *Proc. Natl. Acad. Sci. U.S.A., 71*:639–643.
7. Haugen, Å., and Laerum, O. D. (1978): Surface structure of fetal rat brain cells during neoplastic transformation in cell culture. *J. Natl. Cancer Inst., 61*:1415–1422.
8. Haugen, Å., and Laerum, O. D. (1979): Transmission electron microscopy of fetal rat brain cells during neoplastic transformation in cell culture. *J. Natl. Cancer Inst., 63*:455–464.
9. Hince, T. A., and Roscoe, J. P. (1978): Fibrinolytic activity of cultured cells derived during ethylnitrosourea-induced carcinogenesis of rat brain. *Br. J. Cancer, 37*:424–433.
10. Ivankovic, S., and Druckrey, H. (1968): Transplacentare Erzeugung maligner Tumoren des Nervensystems. I. Äthyl-nitrosoharnstoff (ÄNH) an BDIX-Ratten. *Z. Krebsforsch., 71*:320–360.
11. Jaenisch, W., Schreiber, D., Warzok, R., and Osske, G. (1970): Frühstadien von Geschwülsten des Zentralnervensystems. Experimentell-morphologische Untersuchungen. *Exp. Pathol. (Jena), 4*:60–68.
12. Karran, P., Lindahl, T., and Griffin, B. (1979): Adaptive response to alkylating agents involves alteration *in situ* of O^6-methylguanine residues in DNA. *Nature, 280*:76–77.
13. Kleihues, P., Lantos, P. L., and Magee, P. N. (1976): Chemical carcinogenesis in the nervous system. *Int. Rev. Exp. Pathol., 15*:153–232.
14. Kleihues, P., and Margison, G. P. (1976): Exhaustion and recovery of repair excision of O^6-methylguanine from rat liver DNA. *Nature, 259*:153–155.
15. Laerum, O. D., Bigner, D. D., and Rajewsky, M. F. (Eds.) (1978): *Biology of Brain Tumors,* UICC Technical Report Series, Vol. 30. International Union Against Cancer, Geneva.
16. Laerum, O. D., Haugen, Å., and Rajewsky, M. F. (1979): Neoplastic transformation of foetal rat brain cells in culture after exposure to ethylnitrosourea *in vivo.* In: *Neoplastic Transformation in Differentiated Epithelial Cell Systems in Vitro,* edited by L. M. Franks and C. Wigley, pp. 189–201. Academic Press, London, New York.
17. Laerum, O. D., Hülser, D. F., and Rajewsky, M. F. (1976): Electrophysiological properties of ethylnitrosourea-induced, neoplastic neurogenic rat cell lines *in vivo* and *in vitro. Cancer Res., 36*:2153–2161.
18. Laerum, O. D., and Rajewsky, M. F. (1975): Neoplastic transformation of fetal rat brain cells in culture following exposure to ethylnitrosourea *in vivo. J. Natl. Cancer Inst., 55*:1177–1187.
19. Laerum, O. D., and Rajewsky, M. F. (1978): Chemical carcinogenesis in the nervous system: Sequential phenotypic changes in neural target cell populations. In: *Biology of Brain Tumors,* edited by O. D. Laerum, D. Bigner, and M. F. Rajewsky, pp. 129–141. UICC Technical Report Series, Vol. 30. International Union Against Cancer, Geneva.
20. Laerum, O. D., Rajewsky, M. F., Schachner, M., Stavrou, D., Haglid, D., and Haugen, Å. (1977): Phenotypic properties of neoplastic cell lines developed from fetal rat brain cells in culture after exposure to ethylnitrosourea *in vivo. Z. Krebsforsch., 89*:273–295.
21. Lagemann, A., and Dietz, W. (1972): Zur Feinstruktur früher Veränderungen an Rattengehirngewebe nach Injektion von Methylnitrosoharnstoff. *Experientia, 28*:1344–1345.
22. Lantos, P. L., and Pilkington, G. J. (1979): The development of experimental brain tumours.

A sequential light and electron microscope study of the subependymal plate. I. Early lesions (abnormal cell clusters). *Acta Neuropathol. (Berl.)*, 45:167–175.

23. Laval, J. (1978): Recent progress in excision repair of DNA. *Biochimie*, 60:1123–1134.
24. Lindahl, T. (1979): DNA glycosylases, endonucleases for apurinic/apyrimidinic sites, and base excision-repair. *Prog. Nucleic Acid Res. Mol. Biol.*, 22:135–192.
25. Loveless, A. (1969): Possible relevance of O^6-alkylation of deoxyguanosine to the mutagenicity and carcinogenicity of nitrosamines and nitrosamides. *Nature*, 223:206–207.
26. Montesano, R., Brésil, H., and Margison, G. (1979): Increased excision of O^6-methylguanine from rat liver DNA after chronic administration of dimethylnitrosamine. *Cancer Res.*, 39:1798–1802.
27. Müller, R., and Rajewsky, M. F. (1978): Sensitive radioimmunoassay for detection of O^6-ethyldeoxyguanosine in DNA exposed to the carcinogen ethylnitrosourea *in vivo* or *in vitro*. *Z. Naturforsch.*, 33c:897–901.
28. Müller, R., and Rajewsky, M. F. (1979): Immunological detection of ethylation products in DNA exposed to ethylnitrosourea *in vivo* or *in vitro*. In: *Short Term Tests for Prescreening of Potential Carcinogens*, edited by L. Santi and S. Parodi, pp. 70–75. Istituto Scientifico per lo Studio e la Cura dei Tumori, Genova.
29. Nicoll, J. W., Swann, P. F., and Pegg, A. E. (1975): Effect of dimethylnitrosamine on persistence of methylated guanines in rat liver and kidney DNA. *Nature*, 254:261–262.
30. Pegg, A. E. (1978): Enzymatic removal of O^6-methylguanine from DNA by mammalian cell extracts. *Biochem. Biophys. Commun.*, 84:166–173.
31. Pilkington, G. J., and Lantos, P. L. (1979): The development of experimental brain tumours. A sequential light and electron microscope study of the subependymal plate. II. Microtumours. *Acta Neuropathol. (Berl.)*, 45:177–185.
32. Rajewsky, M. F., Augenlicht, L. H., Biessmann, H., Goth, R., Hülser, D. F., Laerum, O. D., and Lomakina, L. Ya. (1977): Nervous system-specific carcinogenesis by ethylnitrosourea in the rat: Molecular and cellular mechanisms. In: *Origins of Human Cancer*, edited by H. H. Hiatt, J. D. Watson, and J. A. Winsten, pp. 709–726. Cold Spring Harbor Conferences on Cell Proliferation, Vol. 4. Cold Spring Harbor Laboratory, Cold Spring Harbor, N.Y.
33. Rajewsky et al. In preparation.
34. Rajewsky, M. F., and Laerum, O. D. (1978): Neoplastic transformation of rat neural cells by N-ethyl-N-nitrosourea. In: *Methods for Carcinogenesis Tests at the Cellular Level and their Evaluation for the Assessment of Occupational Cancer Hazards*, pp. 48–52. Fondazione Carlo Erba—Occupational and Environmental Health Section, Milano.
35. Roscoe, J. P., and Claisse, P. J. (1978): Analysis of N-ethyl-N-nitrosourea-induced brain carcinogenesis by sequential culturing during the latent period. I. Morphology and tumourigenicity of the cultured cells and their growth in agar. *J. Natl. Cancer Inst.*, 61:381–390.
36. Samson, L., and Cairns, J. (1977): A new pathway for DNA repair in *Escherichia coli. Nature*, 267:281–283.
37. Singer, B. (1979): N-nitroso alkylating agents: Formation and persistence of alkyl derivatives in mammalian nucleic acids as contributing factors in carcinogenesis. *J. Natl. Cancer Inst.*, 62:1329–1339.
38. Singer, B., Bodell, W. J., Cleaver, J. E., Thomas, G. H., Rajewsky, M. F., and Thon, W. (1978): Oxygens in DNA are main targets for ethylnitrosourea in normal and xeroderma pigmentosum fibroblasts and fetal rat brain cells. *Nature*, 276:85–88.
39. Stanbridge, E. J., and Wilkinson, J. (1978): Analysis of malignancy in human cells: Malignant and transformed phenotypes are under separate genetic control. *Proc. Natl. Acad. Sci. U.S.A.*, 75:1466–1469.
40. Stavrou, D., and Haglid, K. G. (1973): Morphologische und immunologische Untersuchungen zur Histogenese experimenteller Hirntumoren. *J. Neurol. Sci.*, 20:39–50.
41. Sun, L., and Singer, B. (1975): The specificity of different classes of ethylating agents towards various sites of HeLa cell DNA *in vitro* and *in vivo*. *Biochemistry*, 14:1795–1802.
42. Swenberg, J. A., Clendenon, N., Denlinger, R., and Gordon, W. A. (1975): Sequential development of ethylnitrosourea-induced neurinomas: Morphology, biochemistry, and transplantability. *J. Natl. Cancer Inst.*, 55:147–152.

Advances in Neuroblastoma Research,
edited by Audrey E. Evans.
Raven Press, New York © 1980.

Control Mechanisms of Malignancy and Differentiation in Cultures of Nerve Cells

K. N. Prasad

*Department of Radiology, University of Colorado Medical Center,
Denver, Colorado 80262*

The relationship between the regulation of malignancy (capacity of cells to form tumor in syngeneic host) and differentiation is not well understood. The expression of abnormal differentiation may be the result of malignant transformation of normal cells. The spontaneous transformation of normal cells to cancer cells probably results from exposure to ionizing radiation, viruses, chemical carcinogens, or any combination of these or other agents. However, these transformed malignant cells do not always establish themselves as a cancer in the host. This may be because the cellular repair mechanism of the host may correct the defect and/or the host's immune system may kill the transformed cells. Thus the environment of the host's body exerts considerable selection pressure on the first or first few transformed cells. Some of the transformed cells may respond to this pressure by undergoing additional mutations, thus creating additional independent loci for control of malignancy. Such tumor cells may then escape the host's cellular repair system as well as the host's immune surveillance mechanism. These transformed cells would continue to grow in the host and eventually develop into clinical cancer. The number of additional mutations during tumor growth may continue to accumulate in cancer cells. Since many of the tumor therapeutic agents are carcinogenic, the surviving tumor cells after therapy may contain more complex mechanisms of regulation of malignancy than those found before the treatment.

In order to stop the progression of the neoplasms in a highly selective manner, identification of all sites for control of malignancy is important. It appears equally important to identify those physiological substances which exhibit antitumor activity. Since tumor cells escape the host's selection pressure, physiological substances that exhibit anticancer property may theoretically be found. Indeed, using clonal lines of neuroblastoma (NB) cells, we have identified one locus for control of malignancy, namely, the adenosine 3',5'-cyclic monophosphate (cyclic AMP) system. In addition, we have found three physiological substances (butyric acid, ascorbic acid, and vitamin E) which exhibit antitumor activity *in vitro.* The antitumor activity of these substances has been measured by the criteria of induction of differentiation, growth inhibition (due to cell death and reduction in cell division), and potentiation of the cytotoxicity of currently useful antitumor agents.

ROLE OF CYCLIC AMP IN DIFFERENTIATION AND MALIGNANCY OF NEUROBLASTOMA CELLS

In Vitro Studies

An elevation of the intracellular level of cyclic AMP by prostaglandin E_1 (PGE$_1$), inhibitors of cyclic nucleotide phosphodiesterase, or analogues of cyclic AMP in certain clones of NB cells increases the expression of several differentiation functions which are associated with mature neurons (13,18). These include formation of long neurites which exhibit action potential; increase in sizes of soma and nucleus; increase in total RNA and protein contents; blockade of cells in the G_1 phase of the cell cycle; increase in activities of tyrosine hydroxylase, dopamine β-hydroxylase, choline acetyltransferase, acetylcholinesterase, glutamate decarboxylase, cyclic AMP phosphodiesterase, and cyclic AMP-dependent phosphorylation; increase in levels of cAMP binding proteins and Poly A-containing messenger RNA; decrease in synthesis of histones and phosphorylation of H_1 histone; increase in sensitivity of adenylate cyclase to dopamine and norepinephrine; and abolition or decrease in malignancy. However, the activity of lactic acid dehydrogenase (LDH), a rate-limiting enzyme in anaerobic glycolysis, increases in cyclic AMP-induced differentiated cells (K. Prasad, R. Prasad, and N. Prasad, *unpublished observation*).

It is well known that a shift from anaerobic glycolysis to aerobic glycolysis occurs during differentiation of normal nervous tissue. However, this shift did not occur in differentiated NB cells. Cells which are resistant to PGE$_1$, inhibitors of cyclic nucleotide phosphodiesterase, or both exist in the tumor mass. Cyclic GMP appears to have no role in regulating the expression of differentiation in NB cells. In addition to cyclic AMP, other agents such as X-irradiation, 5-bromodeoxyuridine, 6-thioguanine, sodium butyrate, glial factor, nerve growth factor, dexamethasone, and heat-inactivated and dialyzed calf serum increase one or more differentiated functions in NB cells. Many of these agents do not increase the intracellular level of cyclic AMP (13,17,18,20).

In vitro studies have provided the following concepts: (a) Cyclic AMP is one of the important factors in the regulation of several differentiated functions and of malignancy in NB cells. Most of the differentiated functions are regulated by more than one mode, and cyclic AMP represents one of them. (b) An increase in cyclic AMP phosphodiesterase activity in dividing neuroblasts may be one of the early lesions of malignancy because the effects of dopamine, norepinephrine, PGE$_1$, and adenosine (in some clones) on the cyclic AMP level can not be measured until cyclic AMP phosphodiesterase activity is inhibited. Other lesions in the steps of cyclic AMP metabolism and in the mechanisms of cyclic AMP effect may exist in NB cells, but they have not been identified as yet. In addition, the control of malignancy may reside in loci which are independent of cyclic AMP. (c) The expressions of morphological and biochemical differentiation are independently regulated in the sense that the level of one can be increased without any change in the level of other. For example, the neurites can be formed in the absence of any change in the activity of tyrosine hydroxylase, and vice versa. (d) No individual differentiated function is linked with malignancy; however, when the levels of several differentiated functions are increased in a coordinate manner, the malignancy is decreased or abolished. (e) The expressions of malignancy and low activity of neural-specific enzyme may be only casually related. A mutant clone of NB cell isolated in a tyrosine-free medium contains tyrosine hydroxylase activity that is similar to that observed in the mature brain (3). (f) Of the mice that failed to develop tumors after subcutaneous injection of cyclic AMP-induced differentiated NB cells, 30% rejected the malignant NB cells administered subcutaneously (18). This suggested that the tumor-specific antigens may become unmasked in differentiated cells which then may evoke immune response against certain malignant NB cells. Human NB cells in culture possess tumor-specific transplantation antigens against which an immune reaction can be demonstrated by using colony inhibition assay (8).

HYPOTHESIS FOR THE MALIGNANCY OF NERVE CELLS

Figure 1 shows a diagrammatic model to explain the malignancy of nerve cells. This model suggests that a mutation in the regulatory gene for cyclic AMP phosphodiesterase within a single and/or a group of dividing neuroblasts may result from exposure to viruses, chemical carcinogens, ionizing radiation, or any combination of these and other agents; and this mutational change may increase phosphodiesterase activity in mutated cells. The high cyclic AMP phosphodiesterase activity prevents any further increase in the intracellular level of cyclic AMP, after stimulation by dopamine, norepinephrine, PGE_1, and adenosine. This also prevents any rise in the level of cyclic AMP binding proteins, because cyclic AMP appears to regulate the levels of cAMP binding protein (18). These changes might then prevent the expression of neuronal differentiated functions in the mutated nerve cell, causing it to become a cancer cell.

The regulatory genes for other differentiated functions in the daughter cancer cells may consequently become more susceptible to mutagenic changes, which then may produce further molecular lesions. This may account for the fact that the NB cells obtained from a tumor differ quantitatively and qualitatively from one another with respect to expression of cellular properties and to sensitivity to different drugs. The mutated nerve cell appears to maintain the capacity to differentiate into various forms of nerve cells. This is supported by the fact that the NB tumor contains four major types of nerve cells (1,10,13): (a) adrenergic cells, (b) cholinergic cells, (c) sensory-like cells, and (d) serotonergic

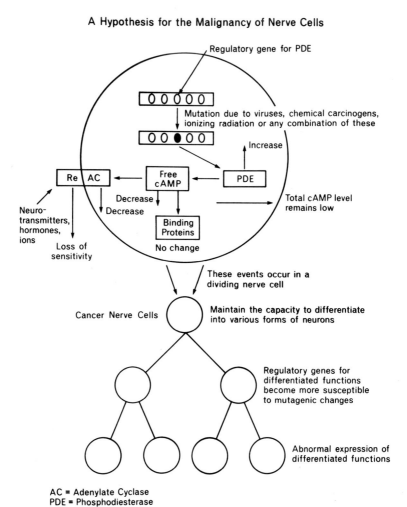

A Hypothesis for the Malignancy of Nerve Cells

AC = Adenylate Cyclase
PDE = Phosphodiesterase
Re = Receptor

FIG. 1. A diagrammatic model to explain the postulated mechanism for the development of cancer of nerve cells. cAMP, adenosine 3′,5′-cyclic monophosphate; PDE, cAMP phosphodiesterase; AC, adenylate cyclase; Re, receptor; DA, dopamine; NE, norepinephrine. From Prasad (18).

cells. However, the differentiated functions of these nerve cells are not adequately expressed, and therefore they continue to divide. Whether or not the first cancer nerve cell will lead to the formation of a detectable neoplasm depends on the host's repair system and immunological environment. If the host's repair mechanism and immunological response are normal, the mutated nerve cell may be repaired or rejected, and no malignant lesion will ever appear. On the other hand, if the host has an unresponsive immune system or poor repair mechanisms, the malignant neoplasm may become detectable in a few months or years after the appearance of the first cancer cells.

In Vivo Studies

Based on *in vitro* studies, we suggested that the addition of differentiating agents in the currently used therapeutic models may improve their effectiveness. The combination of dibutyryl cyclic AMP, papaverine, and theophylline reduces the growth of mouse NB cells for a transient period (5). Papaverine treatment of nude mice carrying human NB cells reduces the growth of tumor (7); however, papaverine does not reduce the growth of C-1300 NB tumor in A/J mice, but the treatment of mice bearing NB tumor with papaverine completely prevents all detectable metastases (22). The exact mechanism of this phenomenon is unknown. A partial explanation of this suppression of metastases may be due to the fact that the tumor-specific antigens in papaverine-induced differentiated NB cells may become unmasked and thereby may evoke immune response with destruction of micrometastases (18). Helson (6) has added papaverine and trifluoromethyl-2-deoxyuridine to his treatment protocol containing vincristine and cyclophosphamide. A marked regression of tumor was observed in all patients over 2 years of age with stage IV neuroblastoma and the conversion from neuroblastoma to ganglioneuroma was observed (6). These studies failed to show whether papaverine-induced differentiation *in vivo* is mediated by cyclic AMP. However, a study by Imashuku et al. (9) shows that the spontaneously occurring ganglioneuroma and sympathetic ganglia have eight times more cyclic AMP than immature round cell NB. One patient with immature NB who had been treated with papaverine showed a threefold higher cyclic AMP level than that observed in untreated patients. Thus cyclic AMP is one of the important factors in regulating the expression of differentiation *in vitro* as well as *in vivo*. However, additional sites for control of malignancy must exist in the same or different NB cells *in vivo*.

ANTITUMOR ACTIVITY OF PHYSIOLOGICAL SUBSTANCES

Sodium Butyrate

Butyric acid, a 4-carbon fatty acid, occurs naturally in the body; sodium butyrate (0.5 to 1.0 mM) either appears to be innocuous or produces reversible growth inhibition and morphological and biochemical alterations in several mammalian cells in culture (17). However, it causes cell death and reversible growth inhibition and elevates levels of differentiation in NB cells. Sodium butyrate also enhances (14) the growth inhibitory effect (due to cell death and inhibition of cell division) of ionizing radiation (Fig. 2) and chemotherapeutic agents on mouse NB cells. Sodium butyrate also increases the growth inhibitory effects of cyclic AMP stimulating agents on human amelanotic melanoma cells in culture (16).

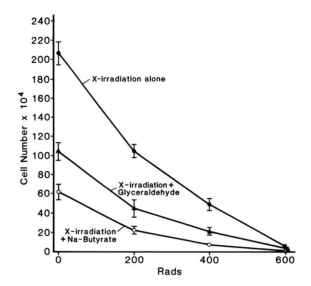

FIG. 2. Neuroblastoma cells (50,000) were plated in Falcon plastic culture dishes (60 mm). Sodium butyrate (0.5 mM) and DL-glyceraldehyde (0.25 mM) were added immediately after various doses of X-irradiation. Each value represents an average of at least 6 samples. The bar at each point is SD. The vertical bars of the points not shown in the figure were too small to be located on the graph.

Because sodium butyrate inhibits anaerobic glycolysis by reducing lactic acid dehydrogenase activity (Prasad et al., *unpublished observation*), and because NB cells are more sensitive to the inhibition of anaerobic glycolysis than other cell types (21), sodium butyrate-induced cell death in NB cells in part may be due to inhibition of anaerobic glycolysis. The fact that DL-glyceraldehyde, an inhibitor of anaerobic glycolysis, also inhibits growth and increases the radiation response of neuroblastoma cells in culture (Fig. 2) supports the above view. The number of cells depending on the anaerobic glycolysis for survival may vary from one tumor type to another, and from one individual to another for the same tumor type. Sodium butyrate also increases the cellular cyclic AMP, but this effect is not apparent until 3 days after treatment. Therefore sodium butyrate-induced increase in differentiated functions of NB cells may be related to a rise in the cellular cyclic AMP level (17).

Although the clinical value of sodium butyrate cannot be elevated at this time, high doses (7 to 10 g/day) of sodium butyrate produce no clinically detectable toxic effect in patients with NB (Voute and Furman, *personal communication*). Voute indicated that sodium butyrate produces a bad odor and therefore is not well suited for clinical study. However, DL-glyceraldehyde, a natural metabolite, also inhibits growth and increases the growth inhibitory effect of ionizing radiation. Therefore, DL-glyceraldehyde may be more suitable for clinical use than sodium butyrate.

Sodium Ascorbate

The beneficial effects of high doses of ascorbate in advanced human neoplasms has been reported (4). Sodium L-ascorbate at nonlethal concentrations potentiated the growth inhibitory effect of 5-fluorouracil (5-FU) (12-fold), X-irradiation (14-fold), bleomycin (3-fold), R020–1724 (75-fold), PGE$_1$ (3-fold), and sodium butyrate (3-fold) on NB cells, but did not produce such an effect on glioma cells (19). Sodium L ascorbate did not enhance the cytotoxic effect of vincristine, 6-thioguanine, adriamycin, or CCNU on NB cells, except at higher drug doses (18). Sodium D-ascorbate was equally effective. Although glutathione was more cytotoxic than ascorbate, it did not potentiate the effect of 5-FU. Thus the potentiating effect of sodium L-ascorbate may not be due entirely to its reducing or vitamin C property. Sodium ascorbate completely prevented the cytotoxic effects of DTIC and partially (about 50%) prevented the effect of methotrexate on NB cells (19). If such a phenomenon is also observed *in vivo,* a reduction in the vitamin C level in blood prior to the administration of methotrexate and DTIC may increase their effectiveness or may reduce the drug requirements for the same effect on tumor cells. Thus it is important that sodium ascorbate is combined with only those drugs with which the potentiating effects are observed.

Some of the mechanisms of the sodium ascorbate effect include low catalase levels in tumor cells (2); either formation of H$_2$O$_2$ intracellularly and excreted in the medium or formation of H$_2$O$_2$ at the cell surface (12); formation of dehydroascorbate exogenously, intracellularly, or both (19); and inhibition of superoxide dismutase by ascorbate leading to an intracellular accumulation of free radicals (19). The fact that the addition of catalase to the medium prevents the cytotoxic effect supports the involvement of H$_2$O$_2$ in the mechanism of high doses of sodium ascorbate effect on cultured cells. Because sodium ascorbate inhibits catalase activity *in vitro* (11), we suggest that this mechanism could become important in those tumor cells that have predominantly catalase activity with little or no peroxidase because of a mutational event. The inhibition of catalase activity would lead to an accumulation of H$_2$O$_2$ in such cells and thereby would cause cell death. Normal cells or other tumor cells that do not have this particular biochemical lesion would not die under a similar experimental condition, because they can get rid of cellular H$_2$O$_2$ by peroxidase in spite of inhibition of catalase activity. The number of cells having predominantly catalase activity with little or no peroxidase activity may differ from one tumor type to another, and from one individual to another for the same tumor type.

Vitamin E

Vitamin E caused dramatic increase in morphological differentiation of NB cells, but not of glioma cells in culture (15). This is not related to a rise in the cyclic AMP level. A significant increase in morphological differentiation

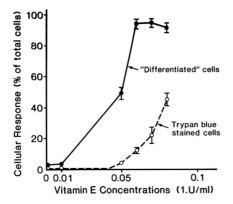

FIG. 3. Neuroblastoma cells (10⁴) were plated in Lux tissue culture dishes (60 mm), and vitamin E was added 24 hr later. Drug and medium were changed at 2 days after treatment, and the number of morphologically differentiated cells was counted 3 days after treatment. The number of trypan blue stained cells among attached cell population was also determined. Each value represents an average of at least 6 samples. The bar at each point is SD. The bars not shown in figure were equal to sizes of symbols. From Prasad et al. (15).

of NB cells was observed at a concentration of 0.05 IU/ml (Fig. 3), and as early as 1 day after treatment. The concentration range which caused a maximal increase in the formation of neurites was very narrow (0.06 to 0.08 IU/ml). The cell death was marked after treatment of the cultures with higher concentrations (0.07 to 0.08 IU/ml) of vitamin E, and on the frequency of change of growth medium and vitamin E. The cultures of higher cell density (5 × 10⁴/dish) required higher concentrations (0.07 to 0.08 IU/ml) of vitamin E to produce an effect similar to that produced in cultures of lower cell density (1 × 10⁴) by lower concentrations of vitamin E (0.05 to 0.06 IU/ml). The daily change of growth medium and vitamin E (0.06 IU/ml) produced more differentiated cells than those in which medium and drug were changed only once during a 3-day period (15). Cells resistant to vitamin E exist in NB cell culture even

TABLE 1. *Effect of vitamin E in combination with ionizing radiation and certain pharmacological agents*

Treatment	% Morphologically differentiated cells
Control	3 ± 1[a]
Vitamin E (0.05 IU/ml)	46 ± 4
Prostaglandin E_1 (10 µg/ml)	47 ± 3
Vitamin E + prostaglandin E_1	89 ± 3
Bleomycin (0.004 U/ml)	2 ± 1
Bleomycin + vitamin E	90 ± 3
X-irradiation (400 rads)	20 ± 2
Vitamin E + 400 rads	72 ± 4

[a] Standard deviation.
Neuroblastoma cells (NBP₂, 50,000) were plated in Lux culture dishes (60 mm). Drugs were added 24 hr after plating. The drug and medium were changed 2 days after treatment, and the percent morphologically differentiated cells was determined 3 days after treatment. Each value represents an average of 6 samples.

after treatment with high concentrations of vitamin E, because a few surviving cells eventually reach confluency.

The combination of ionizing radiation (15), sodium butyrate, or papaverine with vitamin E produced an additive effect on NB cells for the criterion of growth inhibition *(unpublished observation)*. The combination of vincristine, 5-fluorouracil, bleomycin, prostaglandin E_1, or R020–1724 with vitamin E produced a synergistic effect on NB cells for the same criterion. X-irradiation and cyclic AMP stimulating agents cause morphological differentiation of NB cell culture (13). The combination of ionizing radiation (400 rads), PGE_1 (10 μg/ml), or bleomycin (0.004 U/ml) with vitamin E (0.05 IU/ml) produced an additive effect on morphological differentiation of NB cells (Table 1).

CONCLUSIONS

In vitro and *in vivo* data support the hypothesis that cyclic AMP may be one of the important factors in regulating the expression of malignancy and differentiation of NB cells. *In vitro* data suggest that the addition of differentiating agents, vitamin C, vitamin E, and butyric acid to the currently used tumor therapeutic modalities may improve their effectiveness by enhancing the levels of differentiation, by increasing the lethality of tumor cells, by reducing the exposure to ionizing radiation, by decreasing the doses of chemotherapeutic agents, or by maintaining the integrity of the host's immune system.

REFERENCES

1. Amano, T., Richelson, E., and Nirenberg, M. (1972): Neurotransmitter synthesis by neuroblastoma clones. *Proc. Natl. Acad. Sci. U.S.A.,* 69:259–263.
2. Benade, L., Howard, T., and Burk, D. (1969): Synergistic killing of Ehrlich ascites carcinoma cells by ascorbate and 3-amino-1, 2, 4-triazole. *Oncology,* 23:33–43.
3. Breakefield, X. O., and Nirenberg, M. W. (1974): Selection for neuroblastoma cells that synthesize certain transmitters. *Proc. Natl. Acad. Sci. U.S.A.,* 71:2530–2533.
4. Cameron, E., and Pauling, L. (1976): Supplemental ascorbate in the supportive treatment of cancer. *Proc. Natl. Acad. Sci. U.S.A.,* 73:3685–3689.
5. Chang, J. H. T., and Prasad, K. N. (1976): Differentiation of mouse neuroblastoma cells in vitro and in vivo induced by cyclic adenosine monophosphate (cAMP). *J. Pediatr. Surg.,* 11:847–858.
6. Helson, L. (1975): Management of disseminated neuroblastoma. *CA,* 25:264–277.
7. Helson, L., Helson, C., Peterson, R. F., and Das, S. K. (1976): A rationale for the treatment of metastatic neuroblastoma. *J. Natl. Cancer Inst.,* 57:727–729.
8. Helstrom, J. G., Helstrom, K. E., Pierce, G. E., and Bill, A. H. (1968): Demonstration of cell bound and humoral immunity against neuroblastoma cells. *Proc. Natl. Acad. Sci. U.S.A.,* 60:1231–1238.
9. Imashuku, S., Todo, S., Amano, T., Mizukawa, K., Sugimoto, T., and Kusunoki, T. (1977): Cyclic AMP in neuroblastoma, ganglioneuromas and sympathetic ganglia. *Experientia,* 33:1507.
10. Knapp, S., and Mandell, A. J. (1974): Serotonin biosynthetic capacity of mouse C-1300 neuroblastoma cells in culture. *Brain Res.,* 66:547–551.
11. Orr, E. W. M. (1962): Studies on ascorbic acid. Factors influencing the ascorbate. *Biochemistry,* 6:2995–2999.
12. Peterkofsky, B., and Prather, W. (1977): Cytotoxicity of ascorbate and other reducing agents

towards cultured fibroblasts as a result of hydrogen peroxide formation. *J. Cell. Physiol.,* 90: 61–70.

13. Prasad, K. N. (1975): Differentiation of neuroblastoma cells in culture. *Biol. Rev.,* 50:129–165.

14. Prasad, K. N. (1979): Effect of sodium butyrate in combination with X-irradiation, chemotherapeutic and cyclic AMP stimulating agents on neuroblastoma cells in culture. *Experientia,* 35:906–907.

15. Prasad, K. N., Ramanujam, S., and Gaudreau, D. (1979): Vitamin E induces morphological differentiation and increases the effect of ionizing radiation on neuroblastoma cells. *Proc. Soc. Exp. Biol. Med.,* 161:570–573.

16. Prasad, K. N., and Sakamoto, A. (1978): Effect of sodium butyrate in combination with prostaglandin E_1 and inhibitors of cyclic nucleotide phosphodiesterase on human amelanotic melanoma cells in culture. *Experientia,* 34:1575–1576.

17. Prasad, K. N., and Sinha, P. K. (1976): Effect of sodium butyrate on mammalian cells in culture: A review. *In Vitro,* 12:125–132.

18. Prasad, K. N., and Sinha, P. K. (1978): Regulation of differentiated functions and malignancy in neuroblastoma cells in culture. *Cell Differentiation and Neoplasia,* edited by G. F. Sauders, pp. 111–141. Raven Press, New York.

19. Prasad, K. N., Sinha, P. K., Ramanujam, M., and Sakamoto, A. (1979): Sodium ascorbate potentiates the growth inhibitory effect of certain agents on neuroblastoma cells in culture. *Proc. Natl. Acad. Sci. U.S.A.,* 76:829–832.

20. Prasad, K. N., Spuhler, K., Arnold, E. B., and Vernadakis, A. (1979): Modification of response of mouse neuroblastoma cells in culture by serum type. *In Vitro,* 15:807–812.

21. Sakamoto, A., and Prasad, K. N. (1972): Effect of DL-glyceraldehyde on mouse neuroblastoma cell culture. *Cancer Res.,* 32:532–534.

22. Wajsman, Z., Williams, P., and Murphy, G. P. (1978): A study of the effect of papaverine in neuroblastoma using the experimental C-1300 murine system. *Oncology,* 35:1–4.

Advances in Neuroblastoma Research,
edited by Audrey E. Evans.
Raven Press, New York © 1980.

Adenosine 3′:5′-Monophosphate (cAMP) Levels and Characteristics of cAMP-Dependent Protein Kinases in Human Neuroblastoma

*Shinsaku Imashuku, Milligan C. Fossett, III, Alexander A. Green, and F. Ann Hayes

Division of Hematology-Oncology, St. Jude Children's Research Hospital, Memphis, Tennessee 38101

Over the past decade, studies of mouse neuroblastoma have provided valuable information concerning the basic mechanism of maturation of this tumor. Most data indicate that adenosine 3′:5′-monophosphate (cAMP) plays a key role in this process, probably through activation of cAMP-dependent protein kinases (1,12–14). Binding of intracellular cAMP to the regulatory (R) subunit of protein kinases dissociates the catalytic subunit, which phosphorylates a number of proteins and therefore could be responsible for the control of tumor growth and differentiation (14).

Since cAMP will induce many functions in neuroblasts characteristic of mature neurons, some investigators have attempted to stimulate morphologic differentiation of the tumor with chemotherapy that increases intracellular levels of the cyclic nucleotide (5,6,12). Despite these efforts toward a more effective clinical treatment, little is known about the mechanism by which human neuroblastoma differentiates into ganglioneuroma *in vivo*. More recently, studies with experimental cell lines and animal tumors have identified an abnormal response to cAMP due to altered binding by the R subunit of cAMP-dependent protein kinases (2,4,10,15,16). These findings have raised the question of whether human neuroblastoma has an intact cAMP-dependent protein kinase system.

Presented in this report are studies in which we assessed the tissue content of cAMP as well as the properties of cAMP-dependent protein kinases in human neuroblastoma and ganglioneuroma.

MATERIALS AND METHODS

Tumor specimens were obtained during surgery from 15 patients with neuroblastoma and from 8 with ganglioneuroma; adrenal glands were obtained from

---

*On leave of absence from the Department of Pediatrics, Kyoto Prefectural University of Medicine, Kyoto, Japan.

3 patients at autopsy. All tissues were quickly frozen in liquid nitrogen and stored at −70°C. Cultured cells, either human neuroblastoma (SK-N-SH, EW, and HW lines) or mouse C-1300 neuroblastoma (N-18), were maintained in RPMI 1640 medium containing 10% fetal calf serum and harvested at confluency.

Preparation of Tissue Extract

Tissues and cultured cells were homogenized with 3 to 5 volumes of 10 mM Tris-HCl (ph 7.5), 2 mM ethylenediaminetetraacetic acid, and 20 mM benzamidine buffer. A clear supernatant fluid (cytosol) was obtained by centrifuging the homogenate at 105,000 × g for 60 min, dialyzed overnight, and used for protein kinase determination. For assay of tissue cAMP content, tumor specimens were homogenized with 6% trichloroacetic acid.

Assay Procedures

Tissue concentrations of cAMP were determined by the method of Gilman (3), and [³H]cAMP-binding activity and histone kinase activity were measured as described previously (7). DEAE-cellulose column chromatography was performed as reported earlier (7). Photoaffinity labeling and autoradiographic analysis were done by the procedure of Walter et al. (17), as follows: the standard reaction mixture contained 50 mM morpholinoethanesulfonate (pH 6.2), 10 mM MgCl$_2$, 0.3 to 0.6 μM 8-N$_3$-[³²P]cAMP (obtained from ICN, Irvine, California), with or without 20 μM cAMP, and 40 μl of tissue extract (200 to 300 μg of protein) in a final volume of 100 μl. The mixture was irradiated for 10 min with ultraviolet light (254 nm) from a Mineralite UVSL-25 hand lamp at a distance of 10 cm. Samples were mixed with sodium dodecyl sulfate (SDS) containing stop solution (11) and heated at 100°C for 30 sec. A 100-μl portion of the mixture was then subjected to SDS-polyacrylamide slab gel electrophoresis with 7.5% acrylamide, as described by Laemmli (11). The gels were stained with 0.025% Coomassie blue, destained, and dried. Autoradiographs were developed by exposing the dried gels to 3M XD Trimax Medical X-ray films for 5 days at room temperature, and were scanned with an Ortec 4310 Densitometer. Peak densitometric readings were used to measure ³²P incorporation into individual protein bands.

RESULTS AND DISCUSSION

Tissue Levels of cAMP

Findings for 11 neuroblastomas and 8 ganglioneuromas were compared. Neuroblastoma specimens had a median cAMP content of 8.1 pmol/mg protein (range 1.5 to 15.6), whereas that of ganglioneuroma was 39.1 (range 19.3 to

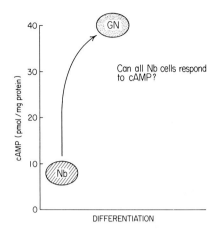

FIG. 1. Schematic representation of correlation between cAMP tissue content and degree of tumor differentiation. Neuroblastoma (Nb) contains a median cAMP concentration of 8.1 pmol/mg protein, whereas ganglioneuroma (GN) contains a median of 39.1.

61.8) ($p < 0.002$). Comparison of cAMP concentrations as pmol per mg DNA disclosed a similar difference: median cAMP content of 161 pmol/mg DNA (range 42.5 to 239) for neuroblastoma versus a median of 2,286 (range 677 to 3,842) for ganglioneuroma. Since the cAMP content of ganglioneuroma is the same as that of human sympathetic ganglia (9), these results could indicate a cAMP deficiency in neuroblastoma. If so, maturation of the tumor may depend on increasing levels of the cyclic nucleotide, as depicted schematically in Fig. 1. Such an association would support the therapeutic concept that increased intracellular cAMP induces differentiation of human neuroblastoma. This model, although attractive, does not take into account the dependency of cAMP action on an intact cAMP-dependent protein kinase system.

Characterization of cAMP-Dependent Protein Kinases in Human Neuroblastoma

cAMP-dependent protein kinases are distinguished by their order of elution with salt from a DEAE-cellulose column. By this procedure, cytosol of both human neuroblastoma and ganglioneuroma yields type I and type II enzymes (7,8). Because the abnormal cAMP-dependent protein kinases identified in experimental tumors were associated with *altered* cAMP-binding proteins (R subunits), we characterized the R subunits of protein kinases in human neuroblastoma and ganglioneuroma, using photoaffinity labeling to resolve the cAMP-binding proteins. As shown in Fig. 2, we identified multiple cAMP-binding proteins in cytosol fractions of human neuroblastoma as well as adrenal gland. Similar results were obtained for ganglioneuroma. Characterization of protein kinases and their binding proteins in tumor cytosol disclosed that type I enzyme has a single R subunit with an apparent molecular weight (MW) of 47,000, and type II enzyme has two species of R subunits with MW 55,000 and 51,000 (7,8). Figure 2 also demonstrates a difference in the cAMP-binding proteins

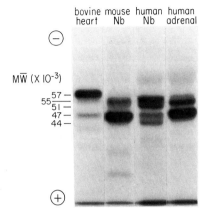

FIG. 2. Autoradiographic comparison of cAMP-binding proteins in cytosol from mouse and human neuroblastoma (Nb). Cytosol fractions from bovine heart (a tissue containing mainly type II protein kinase) and human adrenal gland were examined on the same gel. Molecular weights were determined as described previously (7). An MW 44,000 protein identified in human neuroblastoma is a proteolytic product of the MW 51,000 protein.

of mouse versus human neuroblastoma. Whereas human tissues contain two proteins with MW 55,000 and 51,000, mouse neuroblastoma contains a single protein only, with MW of 53,000 to 54,000. By contrast, the R subunit of type I enzyme, MW 47,000, is found in all tissue extracts. These findings appear to indicate a species difference in molecular size of the R subunit of type II cAMP-dependent protein kinase.

Several biochemical properties of the cAMP-binding proteins of human neuroblastoma are summarized in Table 1. Similar properties were found for these proteins in ganglioneuroma and adrenal gland, suggesting that the multiple R subunits in malignant neuroblastoma are capable of normal function.

Heterogeneity of cAMP-Dependent Protein Kinases in Human Neuroblastoma

As shown in Table 2, we have identified at least three different distribution patterns of these binding proteins. Six of seven ganglioneuromas had pattern

TABLE 1. *Characteristics of heterogenous R subunits of human neuroblastoma protein kinases[a]*

	Molecular weight class of subunits		
	47,000	51,000	55,000
Protein kinase type	I	II	II
cAMP binding			
Affinity (M)	5×10^{-9}	6×10^{-8}	6×10^{-8}
pH optimum	6.2	4	4
Heat stability	−	+	−
Autophosphorylation	−	+	+
Affinity for cGMP	+	−	−
cIMP	+	−	−

[a] Temperature sensitivity was tested after preincubation of cytosol at 50°C for 15 min. The incorporation of 8-N_3-[^{32}P]cAMP into the MW 47,000 protein was decreased in the presence of guanosine 3′,5′-monophosphate (cGMP) and inosine 3′,5′-monophosphate (cIMP). Procedures for autophosphorylation were described previously (7).

TABLE 2. *Distribution of cAMP-binding proteins in cytosol fractions of human neuroblastoma and ganglioneuroma*

	No. of specimens with pattern[a]		
	1	2	3
Neuroblastoma ($N = 15$)	2	10	3
Ganglioneuroma ($N - 7$)	1	6	0
Adrenal gland ($N = 3$)	1	2	0

[a] Based on relative incorporation of 8-N_3-[^{32}P]cAMP, as follows:

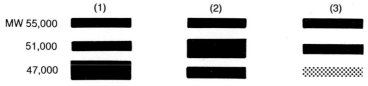

2, whereas a third pattern, characterized by a minimal amount of MW 47,000 protein, was found in rapidly growing tissues from 3 patients with recurrent neuroblastoma. The variation in distribution patterns obtained with the photoaffinity labeling technique has consistently matched the protein kinase profiles obtained by DEAE-cellulose column chromatography. The significance of heterogeneous cAMP-dependent protein kinase patterns is still uncertain and most likely will not be known until tumor protein kinase profiles, morphologic features of tumor specimens, and clinical data from each patient are correlated. Further clarification of the functional roles of type I and type II protein kinases and their R subunits is likewise needed.

ACKNOWLEDGMENTS

The authors wish to gratefully acknowledge the technical assistance of Ms. Sharon Nooner for her preparation of tissue culture material and Mr. John Gilbert's assistance in preparation of this manuscript. This work was supported by CORE Grant CA 21765 and Program Grant CA 23099 from the National Cancer Institute, by the Ruby Levi Research Fund, and by ALSAC.

REFERENCES

1. Chang, J. H. T., and Prasad, K. N. (1976): Differentiation of mouse neuroblastoma cells *in vitro* and *in vivo* induced by cyclic adenosine monophosphate (cAMP). *J. Pediatr. Surg.,* 11:847–858.
2. Cho-Chung, Y. S., Clair, T., Yi, P. N., and Parkison, C. (1977): Comparative studies on cyclic AMP binding and protein kinase in cyclic AMP-responsive and -unresponsive Walker 256 mammary carcinomas. *J. Biol. Chem.,* 252:6335–6341.
3. Gilman, A. G. (1970): A protein binding assay for adenosine 3′,5′-cyclic monophospate. *Proc. Natl. Acad. Sci. U.S.A.,* 67:305–312.

4. Granner, D. K. (1974): Absence of high-affinity adenosine 3',5'-monophosphate binding sites from the cytosol of three hepatic-derived cell lines. *Arch. Biochem. Biophys.*, 165:359–368.
5. Helson, L. (1975): Management of disseminated neuroblastoma. *CA*, 25:264–277.
6. Helson, L., Helson, C., Peterson, R., and Das, S. K. (1976): A rationale of the treatment of metastatic neuroblastoma. *J. Natl. Cancer Inst.*, 57:727–729.
7. Imashuku, S., Fossett, M. C., III, and Green, A. A. (1979): Characterization of adenosine 3',5'-monophosphate binding proteins in human neuroblastoma. *Cancer Res. (in press)*.
8. Imashuku, S., Fossett, M., Green, A., and Hayes, A. (1979): Heterogeneity of adenosine 3',5'-monophosphate (cAMP)-dependent protein kinases in human neuroblastoma (Nb) and ganglioneuroma (GN). *Proc. Am. Assoc. Cancer Res.*, 20:195 (abst.).
9. Imashuku, S., Todo, S., Amano, T., Mizukawa, T., Sugimoto, T., and Kusunoki, T. (1977): Cyclic AMP in neuroblastoma, ganglioneuroma and sympathetic ganglia. *Experientia*, 33:1507.
10. Insel, P. A., Bourne, H. R., Coffino, P., and Tomkins, G. M. (1975): Cyclic AMP-dependent protein kinase, pivotal role in regulation of enzyme induction and growth. *Science*, 190:896–898.
11. Laemmli, U. K. (1970): Cleavage of structural proteins during the assembly of the head of bacteriophage T4. *Nature*, 227:680–685.
12. Prasad, K. N., and Kumar, S. (1975): Role of cyclic AMP in differentiation of human neuroblastoma cells in culture. *Cancer*, 36:1338–1343.
13. Prasad, K. N., Sahu, S. K., and Sinha, P. K. (1976): Cyclic nucleotides in the regulation of expression of differentiated functions in neuroblastoma cells. *J. Natl. Cancer Inst.*, 57:619–631.
14. Ryan, W. L., and Heidrick, M. L. (1974): Role of cyclic nucleotides in cancer. *Adv. Cyclic Nucleotide Res.*, 4:81–116.
15. Schimmer, B. P., Tsao, J., and Knapp, M. (1977): Isolation of mutant adrenocortical tumor cells resistant to cyclic nucleotides. *Mol. Cell Endocrinol.*, 8:135–145.
16. Simantov, R., and Sachs, L. (1975): Temperature sensitivity of cyclic adenosine 3',5'-monophosphate-binding proteins and the regulation of growth and differentiation in neuroblastoma cells. *J. Biol. Chem.*, 250:3236–3242.
17. Walter, U., Uno, I., Liu, A.Y.-C., and Greengard, P. (1977): Identification, characterization and quantitative measurement of cyclic AMP receptor proteins in cytosol of various tissues using a photoaffinity ligand. *J. Biol. Chem.*, 244:4406–4412.

Advances in Neuroblastoma Research,
edited by Audrey E. Evans.
Raven Press, New York © 1980.

Neurotransmitter-Synthesizing Enzymes in Human Neuroblastoma Cells: Relationship to Morphological Diversity

*Robert A. Ross, *Tong Hyub Joh, *Donald J. Reis,
**Barbara A. Spengler, and **June L. Biedler

*Laboratory of Neurobiology, Department of Neurology, Cornell University Medical College, New York, New York 10021; and **Laboratory of Cellular and Biochemical Genetics, Memorial Sloan-Kettering Cancer Center, Walker Laboratory, Rye, New York 10580

The establishment *in vitro* of continuous cell lines of human neuroblastoma permits a variety of studies relevant to clinical control of this tumor, to genetic correlates of normal and malignant cell growth, and to study of the development and expression of a neuronal phenotype. Recently, a number of human neuroblastomas have been adapted to cell culture and partially examined with respect to some of their morphological and biochemical characteristics (2,14,16).

One of the interesting characteristics of neuroblastoma cells is their ability to synthesize proteins unique to a neuronal phenotype. One class of these marker proteins is the enzymes required for the biosynthesis of neurotransmitter substances. Although many of the currently available human neuroblastoma cell lines have been analyzed for some of the neurotransmitter-biosynthetic enzymes, none have been systematically analyzed for the presence of a large number of these specific marker proteins. Thus, for example, little is known about the expression of all four of the enzymes required for the biosynthesis of catecholamines (tyrosine hydroxylase, TH; aromatic L-amino acid decarboxylase, AADC; dopamine-β-hydroxylase, DBH; and phenylethanolamine-N-methyl transferase, PNMT) or of the presence of activity for either tryptophan hydroxylase or glutamic acid decarboxylase in human neuroblastoma cells (2,14,16).

In addition, human neuroblastoma cells are heterogenous with respect to morphological phenotypes. Tumors and cell lines consist of cells with epithelial, neuroblast, or intermediate phenotypes. However, it is not known whether these divergent cell types differ with respect to their ability to express activities of the neurotransmitter-synthesizing enzymes, whether there is any relationship between morphological cell type and level of enzyme activity, and, finally, whether these different cell types are immutable or capable of interconversion.

METHODS

Cell Lines and Culture Techniques

The human neuroblastoma parental cell lines included in this study are listed in Table 1. The origin of each cell line and the culture conditions under which it was established and maintained, as well as the methods used to establish clones from several cell lines, are discussed in the accompanying chapter (Biedler et al., *this volume*, p. 81).

Enzyme Assays

Cells in stationary growth phase were collected and centrifuged, as previously described (2), and cell pellets were stored at −70°C. At the time of enzyme assay, cells were homogenized in 5 mM potassium phosphate buffer (pH 7.4) containing 0.2% Triton X-100 and protein measured (11). The homogenate was then centrifuged and enzyme activity analyzed in the supernatant.

Enzymes involved in catecholamine biosynthesis were assayed as follows: tyrosine hydroxylase by a modification (8) of the method of Coyle (5), aromatic L-amino acid decarboxylase by the method of Lamprecht and Coyle (10), dopamine-β-hydroxylase using the double-enzyme procedure of Molinoff et al. (12), and phenylethanolamine-N-methyl transferase by the method of Axelrod (1). Choline acetyltransferase (CAT) was assayed according to the method of Fonnum (6). Glutamic acid decarboxylase activity was assayed by the method of Chalmers et al. (4), and tryptophan hydroxylase was assayed by a modification of the method of Ichiyama (9).

TABLE 1. *Neurotransmitter biosynthetic enzymes in human neuroblastoma cell lines*

Line	CAT	TH	AADC	DBH	PNMT
A. Adrenergic					
SK-N-BE(1)	0	42.8 ± 2.8	6.5 ± 0.7	10.54 ± 0.64	0
SK-N-BE(2)	0	54.1 ± 1.9	22.9 ± 1.6	5.79 ± 0.45	0
SK-N-SH	0	0.017 ± 0.002	5.7 ± 0.5	14.66 ± 0.42	0
IMR-32	0	1.47 ± 0.32	1.26 ± 0.07	0	0
LA-N-1	0	3.05 ± 0.53	0	0	0
B. Cholinergic					
SK-N-MC	3.52 ± 0.28	0	0	0	0
C. Mixed					
LA-N-2	9.40 ± 1.04	0.23 ± 0.002	0.16 ± 0.05	3.69 ± 0.12	0
NAP	1.72 ± 0.20	0.76 ± 0.003	0	4.97 ± 0.24	0

A "0" denotes activity that was less than 2 times the blank value. Enzyme activity is expressed as nmoles of product formed/hr/mg protein, and each value represents the mean ± SEM of 4–15 individual cultures.

RESULTS

Enzyme Activities in Human Neuroblastoma Parental Cell Lines

We have examined eight of the currently available human neuroblastoma cell lines with respect to the neurotransmitter-synthesizing enzymes characteristic of catecholaminergic (TH, AADC, DBH, and PNMT), cholinergic (CAT), serotonergic (tryptophan hydroxylase), and GABAergic (glutamic acid decarboxylase) neurons. As shown in Table 1, all of the parental cell lines contained the enzymes required for the synthesis of adrenergic and/or cholinergic transmitters; none were inactive (16).

Adrenergic

Five neuroblastoma lines were defined as adrenergic since they contained activity for TH, the presumed rate-limiting enzyme in catecholamine biosynthesis. TH activity varied in these lines over a 3,000-fold range: the lowest activity was found in SK-N-SH cells and the highest in cells of the SK-N-BE(2) line. The TH activity in each line was comparable in magnitude to that found in primary tumors of human neuroblastoma as well as in human adrenal glands (7). In addition, the wide range of activities expressed in the different human neuroblastoma cell lines is also seen in normal human adrenal glands (7).

In four of the five adrenergic lines AADC activity was detected. The presence of this enzyme in human neuroblastoma cells stands in contrast to its apparent absence in mouse neuroblastoma cells (15).

In three of the adrenergic lines DBH activity, in addition to TH and AADC, was detected; thus these cells contained all of the enzymes required for the synthesis of norepinephrine. PNMT activity was not detectable in any of the cell lines nor could its activity be induced by addition of dexamethasone to the culture media.

Cholinergic

In only one cell line, SK-N-MC, was CAT activity present exclusive of other neurotransmitter-synthesizing enzymes. Thus this line is defined as purely cholinergic. This finding confirms a previous study with these cells which showed not only the presence of this enzyme but also the capacity of these cells to synthesize acetylcholine (2).

Mixed (Adrenergic/Cholinergic)

Two of the eight cell lines contained activities of both adrenergic and cholinergic enzymes. LA-N-2 contained all of the enzymes necessary for the synthesis of norepinephrine and acetylcholine. NAP contained all of these enzymes except AADC.

The cause of these findings is unknown. Since LA-N-2 contains a polyploid number of chromosomes (15; Biedler et al., *this volume*), the presence of multiple neurotransmitter-biosynthetic enzymes could be due to the fusion of cells with different neurotransmitter phenotypes. The NAP cell line, however, is near diploid (Biedler et al., *this volume*), and thus another mechanism must account for these findings. Although it is possible that cells with different neurotransmitter-synthesizing enzymes could exist within the parental cell line, we have recently discovered that a clonal line derived from NAP (NAP-22) expresses activities of enzymes for both adrenergic and cholinergic biosynthesis.

Clonal Cell Lines of Neuroblastoma Cells

To determine the degree of heterogeneity in parental cell lines with respect to the expression of the activities of the neurotransmitter-synthesizing enzymes, clones from three human neuroblastoma cell lines were isolated and assayed.

SK-N-BE(2)

Eight clones were isolated and characterized for TH and DBH activities (Table 2, A). Of interest was the finding that not all clones expressed the parental phenotype; whereas one clone [BE(2)-C] expressed activities for these enzymes near to that found in the parental line, another clone [BE(2)-K2] contained activity for only TH. The remaining clones expressed intermediate activity values for both enzymes. There was no correlation between the size or chromosomal location of the homogeneously staining region (Biedler et al., *this volume*) found in these clones and the activity levels of the neurotransmitter-synthesizing enzymes.

SK-N-MC

Twice-cloned isolates of SK-N-MC, designated MC-IXC and MC-IIE, were analyzed biochemically for CAT activity (Table 2, B). Both clones contained enzyme activity with one line (MC-IXC) having 10-fold greater CAT activity than the other line (MC-IIE).

SK-N-SH

Two cell lines were cloned from SK-N-SH (Table 2, C). One line (SH-SY5Y) expressed a neuroblast-like morphology and contained TH and DBH activities. Another clone (SH-EP) had an epithelial morphology and TH and DBH activities

TABLE 2. *Enzyme activity of clonal populations derived from SK-N-BE(2), SK-N-SH, and SK-N-MC*

A. SK-N-BE(2)

	Enzyme activity	
Clone	TH (nmol/hr/mg)	DBH (nmol/hr/mg)
BE(2)-B	3.5 ± 0.6	4.2 ± 0.5
BE(2)-C	46.7 ± 5.2	9.6 ± 1.0
BE(2)-H	6.3 ± 0.2	3.2 ± 0.5
BE(2)-J	4.5 ± 0.3	1.4 ± 0.1
BE(2)-K2	1.5 ± 0.3	0
BE(2)-M17	14.3 ± 1.8	1.6 ± 0.2
BE(2)-N	2.6 ± 0.2	2.7 ± 0.5
BE(2)-Q32	34.6 ± 1.1	0

B. SK-N-MC

Clone	Cat activity (nmol/hr/mg)
MC-IIE	1.82 ± 0.02
MC-IXC	23.75 ± 2.0

C. SK-N-SH

	Enzyme activity	
Clone	TH (nmol/hr/mg)	DBH (nmol/hr/mg)
SH-SY5Y	0.007 ± 0.001	11.5 ± 0.4
SH-IN	0.056 ± 0.003	8.1 ± 0.4
SH-EP	0	0

Enzyme activity is expressed as mean ± SEM of 4–10 individual cultures.

were not detectable within cultures of these cells. A third clone (SH-IN) also expressed enzyme activities for TH and DBH.

Stability of Enzyme Activity over Time

To determine whether the level of enzyme activity within these clones was stable with time in continuous culture, assays were performed over a 16-month period in several of these clones. In the majority of clones examined [e.g., SH-SY5Y and BE(2)-C], neurotransmitter enzyme activity was stable and unchanged over this period. However, in one clone [BE(2)-Q32] enzyme activity decreased with time in culture (Fig. 1).

Coordinate Morphological and Biochemical Interconversion

The SK-N-SH cell line consists primarily of two morphologically distinct cell types. One is a neuroblast-like cell type with a small, rounded cell body, large nucleoli, and often long and delicate neurite-like processes. A clonal cell

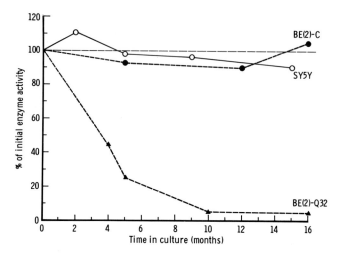

FIG. 1. Stability of enzyme activity in human neuroblastoma clones with time in culture. Each point represents the mean of enzyme activity for at least 2 individual cultures. Enzyme activities are TH in BE(2)-C (●) and BE(2)-Q32 (▲), and DBH activity in SH-SY5Y (○).

line of this morphological phenotype, SH-SY5Y, has been isolated (Fig. 2a). The second cell type is characterized by a flattened, epithelial-like morphology. A clonal cell type with these characteristics has also been isolated (Fig. 2b).

Morphological Interconversion

Since earlier observation had led us to speculate that neuroblast-like cells and epithelial cells of the SK-N-SH line are morphological extremes in a spectrum of phenotypic expression (3), we devised experiments to obtain evidence of morphological interconversion.

Neuroblast to epithelial cell. To determine the morphological purity of the SH-SY5Y line with time in culture, cells of this clone were seeded into tissue culture plates and, after varying periods of time, the morphological phenotypes of colonies were assessed. After 2 to 3 weeks of growth, all of the stained colonies were comprised of neuroblast-like cells. However, after 20 weeks of cultivation and subsequent plating, 3 colonies out of 1,000 consisted entirely of epithelial-like cells. Finally, after 32 and 44 weeks of growth, 5% of the colonies consisted, in whole or in part, of epithelioid cells. Thus cells with a neuroblast-like morphology can convert to cells resembling the epithelial-like components of the SK-N-SH line.

Epithelial to neuroblast cell. To determine whether morphological interconversion between the two cell types was bidirectional, similar experiments were conducted with the epithelial-like SH-EP clone. Karyotype analysis revealed the presence of a unique, structurally abnormal chromosome (isochromosome 1q) that was contained in 35% of SH-EP cells examined and was not seen

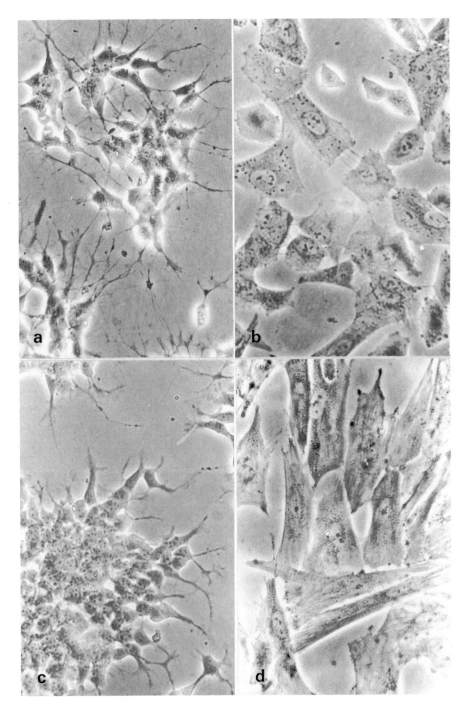

FIG. 2. Phase contrast photomicrographs of human neuroblastoma SK-N-SH clones and SH-EP subclones (×100). **a:** SH-SY5Y, thrice-cloned neuroblast-like cell line. **b:** SH-EP, epithelial-like clone. **c:** SH-EP15, neuroblast-like clone of SH-EP. **d:** SH-EP12 epithelial-like cell.

TABLE 3. *Coordinate changes in cell morphology and DBH activity in SH-EP subclones*

Subclone	Morphology	DBH activity (nmoles/hr/mg)
SH-EP1	Epithelial	0
SH-EP12	"	0
SH-EP7	Intermediate	4.26 ± 0.05
SH-EP13	"	3.48 ± 0.36
SH-EP16	"	3.99 ± 0.40
SH-EP17	"	2.95 ± 0.45
SH-EP2	Neuroblast	5.20 ± 0.02
SH-EP5	"	5.83 ± 0.05
SH-EP15	"	6.29 ± 0.73

Enzyme activity is expressed as mean ± SEM of 4–6 individual cultures.

in SH-SY5Y. This unique marker chromosome could thus serve to identify neuroblast-like cells, should they arise, as being derived solely from SH-EP cells.

After about 4 months of serial cultivation, cultures began to show foci of dense, multilayering cells if allowed to remain in the same culture flask for 3 to 4 weeks. By this culturing schedule, we were able to select for cells which mounded and were morphologically different from the flattened, monolayering cells characteristic of the SH-EP clone. A mounding culture of SH-EP cells was used to seed plates with microwells and several subclones were isolated (Table 3).

Morphologically, two subclones (SH-EP1 and SH-EP12) were epithelial-like (Fig. 2d), while three subclones (SH-EP2, SH-EP5, and SH-EP15) were neuroblast-like (Fig. 2c). Karyotype analysis of these subclones revealed that all contained the marker chromosome unique to SH-EP cells. Since all of the subcloned cells observed possessed the isochromosome 1q marker, we conclude that the subclones with a neuroblast-like morphology were derived from epithelial-like SH-EP cells by some process of morphological transformation.

Biochemical Interconversion

Since we had previously shown that the epithelial-like SH-EP clone did not contain detectable activities for the neurotransmitter-synthesizing enzymes, we sought to determine if the morphological transformation observed within SH-EP subclones to a neuroblast-like cell type would also produce a change in the biochemical expression of these enzymes as well. Initially, cells with either an epithelial, intermediate, or neuroblast-like morphological phenotype were assayed for DBH activity (Table 3). Surprisingly, subclones transformed to a neuroblast-like morphology expressed DBH activity while subclones which had

TABLE 4. *Coordinate biochemical changes in neurotransmitter enzymes in SH-EP subclones*

Subclone	Morphology	TH activity (pmoles/hr/mg)	AADC activity (nmoles/hr/mg)	DBH activity (nmoles/hr/mg)
SH-EP1 SH-EP12	Epithelial	0	0	0
SH-EP7 SH-EP17	Intermediate	0.63 ± 0.13	8.43 ± 0.48	3.71 ± 0.16
SH-EP5 SH-EP15	Neuroblast	1.17 ± 0.28	11.28 ± 1.14	5.86 ± 0.35

Enzyme activity is expressed as mean $\pm$ SEM of 4 individual cultures.

retained the epithelial phenotype were still inactive for this enzyme. Cells which appeared intermediate in morphology were also intermediate in DBH activity. Further biochemical analysis (Table 4) showed that all of the neurotransmitter-synthesizing enzymes characteristic of adrenergic cells were expressed in the neuroblast-like subclones of SH-EP and not in the epithelial-like ones.

SUMMARY AND CONCLUSIONS

Using the neurotransmitter-synthesizing enzymes as specific markers of a neuronal phenotype, we have systematically studied the expression of these proteins in human neuroblastoma parental cell lines and clones. Three basic conclusions can be drawn.

Firstly, all of the parental cell lines had characteristics of cells of neural crest origin; the lines contained enzymes for catecholamine and/or acetylcholine biosynthesis. The magnitude and wide range of enzyme activities expressed in neuroblastoma cells in culture are similar to that for TH activity in primary neuroblastoma tumors as well as in normal human adrenal glands (7), suggesting that there is a natural heterogeneity in the phenotypic expression of these marker proteins.

Secondly, our finding of the presence of enzymes for more than one neurotransmitter in some of the neuroblastoma cell lines confirms previous studies (2). These findings are strengthened by the appearance of enzymes for more than one neurotransmitter in a near diploid clone (NAP-22) and support the hypothesis that this condition is representative of a natural phenotypic variation within cells of neural crest origin.

Finally, clones derived from some of the human neuroblastoma cell lines show varying but, in most cases, stable levels of enzyme activity. Comparison of these results with each cell's morphology suggests that there is a relationship between the morphology and biochemical phenotypes, such that cells with a neuronal morphology express enzymes specifically required for neurotransmitter biosynthesis, whereas cells with a flattened, epithelial-like morphology are inactive for these marker proteins. Of interest is the finding that these two cell types, under selective conditions, can show bidirectional interconversion. Whether such interconversion occurs *in vivo* and represents different naturally occurring phenotypic variations of cells of neural crest origin remains to be elucidated. Moreover, the ability to predict and control the interconversion between the different cell types of human neuroblastoma may enable more effective treatment and provide for a better prognosis in patients with this disease.

ACKNOWLEDGMENTS

This research was supported by Grants NS06911, HL18974, CA08748, and CA18856 from the National Institutes of Health.

REFERENCES

1. Axelrod, J. (1962): Purification and properties of phenylethanolamine-N-methyl transferase. *J. Biol. Chem.*, 237:1657–1660.
2. Biedler, J. L., Roffler-Tarlov, S., Schachner, M., and Freedman, L. S. (1978): Multiple neurotransmitter synthesis by human neuroblastoma cell lines and clones. *Cancer Res.*, 38:3751–3757.
3. Biedler, J. L., Spengler, B. A., and Lyser, K. M. (1975): Morphological interconversion of human neuroblastoma cells. *In Vitro*, 10:380.
4. Chalmers, A., McGeer, E. G., Wickson, V., and McGeer, P. L. (1970): Distribution of glutamic acid decarboxylase in the brains of various mammalian species. *Comp. Gen. Pharmacol.*, 1:385–390.
5. Coyle, J. T. (1972): Tyrosine hydroxylase in rat brain-cofactor requirements, regional and subcellular distribution. *Biochem. Pharmacol.*, 21:1935–1944.
6. Fonnum, F. (1969): Radiochemical micro-assays for the determination of choline acetyltransferase and acetylcholinesterase activities. *Biochem. J.*, 115:465–472.
7. Imashuku, S., Takada, H., Sawadad, T., Nakamura, T., and LaBrosse, E. H. (1975): Studies on tyrosine hydroxylase in neuroblastoma, in relation to urinary levels of catecholamine metabolites. *Cancer*, 36:450–457.
8. Joh, T. H., Geghman, C., and Reis, D. J. (1973): Immunochemical demonstration of increased accumulation of tyrosine hydroxylase protein in sympathetic ganglia and adrenal medulla elicited by reserpine. *Proc. Natl. Acad. Sci. U.S.A.*, 70:2767–2771.
9. Joh, T. H., Shikimi, T., Pickel, V. M., and Reis, D. J. (1975): Brain tryptophan hydroxylase: Purification of, production of antibodies to, and cellular and ultrastructural localization in serotonergic neurons of rat midbrain. *Proc. Natl. Acad. Sci. U.S.A.*, 72:3575–3579.
10. Lamprecht, F., and Coyle, J. T. (1972): DOPA decarboxylase in the developing rat brain. *Brain Res.*, 41:503–506.
11. Lowry, O. H., Rosebrough, N. J., Farr, A. L., and Randall, R. J. (1951): Protein measurement with the folin phenol reagent. *J. Biol. Chem.*, 193:265–275.
12. Molinoff, P. B., Weinshilboum, R. W., and Axelrod, J. (1971): A sensitive enzymatic assay for dopamine-β-hydroxylase. *J. Pharmacol. Exp. Ther.*, 178:425–431.
13. Patterson, P. H., and Chun, L. L. Y. (1977): The induction of acetylcholine synthesis in primary cultures of dissociated rat sympathetic neurons. Effect of conditioned medium. *Dev. Biol.*, 56:263–280.
14. Schlesinger, H. R., Gerson, J. M., Moorhead, P. S., Maguire, H., and Hummeler, K. (1976): Establishment and characterization of human neuroblastoma cell lines. *Cancer Res.*, 36:3094–3100.
15. Waymire, J. C., and Waymire, K. (1978): Adrenergic enzymes in cultured mouse neuroblastoma: Absence of detectable aromatic L-amino acid decarboxylase. *J. Neurochem.*, 31:693–698.
16. West, G. J., Uki, J., Hershman, H. R., and Seeger, R. C. (1977): Adrenergic, cholinergic, and inactive human neuroblastoma cell lines with the action-potential Na$^+$ ionophore. *Cancer Res.*, 37:1372–1376.

Advances in Neuroblastoma Research,
edited by Audrey E. Evans.
Raven Press, New York © 1980.

Serum-Free Culture of Neuroblastoma Cells

Jane E. Bottenstein

Department of Pediatrics, University of California, Los Angeles, California 90024

The addition of serum to synthetic medium has been a *sine qua non* for proliferation or survival in culture of all but highly selected cell lines. Homologous serum is not always easily obtainable, so that fetal calf or horse sera have been most widely used for mammalian cells. The well-known variability of serum lots, as well as the complex and undefined nature of this medium supplement, have been a major source of variability and irreproducibility of experimental results. The ideal culture medium would contain only optimal concentrations of defined components essential for the growth and/or differentiation of a specific cell type or tissue.

In order to obtain more defined media, serum requirements for growth have recently been replaced by complexes of hormones and other factors for a wide variety of normal and tumorigenic cell lines in a series of publications from Sato's laboratory (2–4,9,10,12,18). There are apparently unique sets of growth requirements for specific cell types, which permit selection for these cell types from a mixed population of cells, i.e., primary cultures (6,13,25,26). In particular, the problem of fibroblast overgrowth can be eliminated with the appropriate medium.

The benefits of a more defined medium for studying the regulation of growth and differentiation of neuronal cells are obvious (see review, 27). This chapter will describe the formulation of such a defined medium and its specificity. These studies were begun with a rat neuroblastoma, a clonal cell line of central nervous system origin (21,22). The strategy for finding this growth medium was to begin with commercially available synthetic media with insulin and transferrin added, since these substances have been common requirements of all the various cell types in Sato's laboratory thus far. To this basic mixture a large number of substances were added, singly and in combinations: steroid and peptide hormones, growth factors, neurotransmitters, neuropeptides, trace elements, vitamins, fatty acids, prostaglandins, and other known serum constituents. Commercially available or easily obtainable substances were used at all times to ensure wide applicability of the final medium.

EFFECT OF N2 MEDIUM ON GROWTH OF RAT
NEUROBLASTOMA CELLS

The resulting N2 medium has recently been described (3,4) and is shown in Table 1. In these initial experiments it was found that B104 cells could not be plated directly into N2 medium; for proliferation to occur, B104 cells required a serum preincubation period, followed by washing, and then switching to N2 medium. Table 2 shows that B104 cells grown in N2 medium have a growth rate 72% of that in serum-containing medium, whereas cells without any supplementation of the basal medium are unable to proliferate. The responses of B104 cells to deletions of the individual supplements of N2 medium are shown in Table 3. The most stringent growth requirement appears to be transferrin, since its deletion results in the greatest loss in cell number; only 8% of the number of cells found in the presence of fully supplemented N2 medium are obtained. Insulin is also a stringent requirement, whereas progesterone, selenium, and putrescine are required to a lesser though significant extent. Only insulin and transferrin show any growth stimulatory effect when added singly to the basal medium, and fully supplemented N2 medium results in a synergistic increase in the number of cells (4). The effects of other steroids on the growth of B104 cells were also reported (4). The only other trace element added was cadmium, which could not replace selenium at an equimolar concentration *(unpublished results)*.

In order to evaluate the specificity of N2 medium, a number of other neuronal and non-neuronal cell lines were grown in this medium. Several subclones of the C1300 mouse neuroblastoma (1), of peripheral nervous system origin, were capable of rapid proliferation in N2 medium (4). Table 4 indicates the growth response of two non-neuronal cell lines in N2 medium. The C62B cell line is

TABLE 1. *Supplements added to serum-free medium for growth of B104 cells (N2 medium)*

Supplement	Concentration
Insulin	5 μg/ml
Transferrin	100 μg/ml
Progesterone	20 nM
Selenium	30 nM
Putrescine	100 μM

Supplements were added at optimal concentrations to a basal medium, which consisted of a 1:1 mixture of Ham's F12 medium and Dulbecco-Vogt's modification of Eagle's medium containing: 1.2 g/l $NaHCO_3$; 15 mM HEPES buffer; 40 mg/l penicillin, 8 mg/l ampicillin, and 90 mg/l streptomycin. Triple-distilled water was used to prepare the medium.

TABLE 2. *Growth of B104 neuroblastoma cells in various media*

Medium	Cells/dish $\times 10^{-4}$		Doubling time (hr)
	Day 3	Day 5	
Basal[a]	10.7 ± 0.6	11.2 ± 0.6	—
N2[a]	38.1 ± 2.0	106.0 ± 2.8	32
Basal + 10% FCS	126.4	530.0 ± 8.5	23

100,000 cells/60-mm dish were plated in 3 ml of basal medium supplemented with 10% fetal calf serum (FCS). After 19 hr, medium was aspirated, cultures were washed twice with basal medium, and 3 ml of experimental medium was added as indicated. After trypsinization, cell number was determined with a Coulter counter. Values are expressed as the mean of duplicate or triplicate ($\pm$SD) cultures.

[a] See Table 1.

TABLE 3. *Effect of single deletions of N2 supplements on B104 neuroblastoma cells*

Medium	Cells/dish $\times 10^{-4}$	% N2
Basal[a]	6.4 ± 0.2	4
N2–Insulin	26.3 ± 1.6	16
N2–Transferrin	12.7 ± 0.1	8
N2–Progesterone	68.3 ± 6.4	42
N2–Selenium	56.6 ± 3.7	35
N2–Putrescine	64.1 ± 6.6	39
N2[a]	163.6 ± 0.9	100

Inoculum was 75,000 cells/60 mm dish. Experimental conditions were as in Table 2. Cells were counted on day 5; values are expressed as the mean ($\pm$SD) of triplicate cultures.

[a] See Table 1.

TABLE 4. *Growth of non-neuronal cell lines in various media*

Cell line	Medium	Cells/dish $\times 10^{-4}$	Doubling time (days)
C62B	Basal[a]	7.1 ± 0.7	9.0
	N2[a]	7.8 ± 0.7	5.2
	Basal + 6% FCS	18.0	1.2
Balb/c 3T3	Basal	1.6 ± 0.4	—
	N2	3.3 ± 0.2	4.2
	Basal + 10% FCS	11.1 ± 0.8	1.2

C62B: 50,000 cells/60 mm dish were plated in 3 ml of basal medium supplemented with 6% fetal calf serum (FCS); after 18 hr, medium was aspirated, cultures were washed 3 times with basal medium, and 3 ml of experimental medium was added as indicated. *Balb/c 3T3:* 19,000 cells/35 mm dish were plated in 2 ml of basal medium supplemented with 10% FCS; after 17 hr, medium was aspirated, cultures were washed twice with basal medium, and 2 ml of experimental medium was added as indicated. Cells were counted on day 3 for both cell lines; values are expressed as the mean of duplicate or triplicate ($\pm$SD) cultures.

[a] See Table 1.

a rat glioma from the central nervous system and it grows very poorly in this medium, with a doubling time five times greater than in the optimal 6% serum-containing medium. The Balb/c 3T3 mouse fibroblast cell line also grows poorly in N2 medium, with a much slower doubling time as compared to 10% serum-containing medium. On the basis of these data, N2 medium appears to be more specific for neuronal growth. The extremely slow growth of the non-neuronal cell lines is probably due to their common media supplements: insulin and transferrin (2).

SUBSTANCES INHIBITORY TO GROWTH OF RAT NEUROBLASTOMA CELLS

Although the original objective of these studies was to find agents which would stimulate the growth of B104 cells, many inhibitory or cytotoxic substances were also revealed in these serum-free cultures. Table 5 lists some of these agents and the concentration(s) at which they were effective.

The most cytotoxic agents were adenosine, epinephrine, oleic acid, and the prostaglandins PGE_2 and PGD_2 (7). It was previously reported that 1×10^{-3} M adenosine in the presence of serum inhibits the growth of B104 cells (20); proliferation of many other cell types has also been inhibited by adenosine (8). Other investigators have found an inhibitory effect of β-estradiol or testosterone (40 μM) on the growth of C1300 mouse neuroblastoma cells (19), as is found with B104 cells. This is the first report of an inhibitory effect of PGD_2 on neuroblastoma growth, although PGE_1 and PGE_2 have both been reported as growth inhibitory to mouse neuroblastoma cells (17) and WI38 human fibro-

TABLE 5. *Inhibitors of the growth of B104 neuroblastoma cells in serum-free media*

Substance	Concentration
Adenosine	$\geq 10\ \mu$M
Epinephrine	$\geq 10\ \mu$M
β-Estradiol	≥ 20 nM
Glucagon	$\geq 0.1\ \mu$g/ml
Norepinephrine	$100\ \mu$M
Oleic acid	$10\ \mu$M
PGD_2	$\geq 5\ \mu$M
PGE_2	$\geq 10\ \mu$M
Selenium	$\geq 0.3\ \mu$M
Testosterone	≥ 20 nM
Triiodothyronine	$\geq 0.1\ \mu$M

Summary of the results of 8 different experiments in serum-free supplemented media. The criterion for inhibition was a 50% decrease in cell number relative to the control, in which the substance was absent.

blasts (16). Although selenium at 3×10^{-8} M is required for growth of B104 cells, concentrations above this are cytotoxic. More extensive studies are now in progress on the effect of these inhibitory substances on neuroblastoma growth.

ELIMINATION OF THE SERUM PREINCUBATION

Still remaining was the problem of having to plate B104 cells into serum-containing medium before switching to N2 medium. Unknown residual serum factors could be contributing to the growth response seen, and indefinite subculture under serum-free conditions was not possible. When B104 cells were plated directly into N2 medium, although the cells were attached there was no proliferation (5). It was hypothesized that perhaps an impairment of the cell-substrate interaction prevented cell division. Accordingly, two substances known to affect cell-substrate adhesion were tried: polylysine (14,30) and fibronectin (11,15,29). It was found that a poly-D-lysine precoating of the tissue culture dish and addition of 5 to 10 $\mu g/ml$ fibronectin, isolated from human plasma, would replace the serum preincubation (5). Now B104 cells could be serially subcultured indefinitely in N2 medium, using soybean trypsin inhibitor to inactivate the trypsin after removal of the cells from the plate, and their growth rate was now the same as in N2 medium with a serum preincubation. It was also reported that under these conditions N2 medium permitted colony formation when cells were inoculated at very low densities (5).

GROWTH RESPONSE OF HUMAN NEUROBLASTOMA CELLS TO N2 MEDIUM

Recently, N2 medium has been tested on the LA-N-1 human neuroblastoma cell line (24,28), derived from bone marrow metastases. Since the B104 rat neuroblastoma required modification of the surface of the tissue culture dish for growth in N2 medium (5), a similar evaluation of this requirement was made for LA-N-1 cells. In Table 6 it is evident that the same modification is most permissive for growth of LA-N-1 cells as for B104 cells, i.e., precoating with polylysine and adding fibronectin to N2 medium. There is no significant increase in cell number in basal medium regardless of any other modification. Also, no proliferation of LA-N-1 cells occurs in N2 medium alone, whereas a polylysine precoating of the dish results in an increase in cell numbers in N2 medium. When fibronectin is added to culture dishes in the absence or presence of N2 supplementation, it appears to interfere with adhesion of LA-N-1 cells to the substrate, unlike B104 cells (5), and this results in large numbers of floating cells. However, when fibronectin is added to a polylysine-precoated dish, there is a further increase in the number of LA-N-1 cells in N2 medium as compared to polylysine precoating without fibronectin.

After the best substrate conditions were established, the growth response of LA-N-1 cells as a function of time was determined (Table 7). Basal medium

TABLE 6. *Effect of substrate modification on the growth of LA-N-1 neuroblastoma cells*

Modification	Medium	Cells/dish $\times$ 10^{-4}
None	Basal[a]	6.4 $\pm$ 0.4
Polylysine coated (Lys)	Basal	5.5 $\pm$ 0.3
Fibronectin, 5 μg/ml	Basal	3.4 $\pm$ 0.3
Lys + fibronectin	Basal	7.9 $\pm$ 0.4
None	N2[a]	4.8 $\pm$ 0.5
Lys	N2	12.3 $\pm$ 0.6
Fibronectin	N2	3.0 $\pm$ 0.1
Lys + fibronectin	N2	16.0 $\pm$ 0.8

Falcon plastic tissue culture dishes (35 mm) were utilized. Poly-D-lysine (Lys) precoating: just before medium was added, dishes were precoated for 5 min at room temperature with 0.5 ml of a sterile 0.1 mg/ml Lys solution in triple-distilled water, followed by a 2 ml water wash. Fibronectin was added separately to dishes containing the indicated medium. See ref. 5 for further details of substrate modification and plating conditions.

50,000 cells/dish were plated in 2 ml of the indicated medium. Cells were counted on day 5; values are expressed as the mean ($\pm$SD) of triplicate cultures.

[a] See Table 1.

TABLE 7. *Growth of LA-N-1 neuroblastoma cells in various media*

Medium	Cells/dish $\times$ 10^{-4}		
	Day 1	Day 4	Day 6
Basal[a]	14.7 $\pm$ 2.0	14.5 $\pm$ 0.6	13.2 $\pm$ 0.5
N2[a] (Lys + Fibronectin[b])	20.9 $\pm$ 0.6	34.9 $\pm$ 1.5	54.5 $\pm$ 3.2
Basal + 30% FCS	17.6 $\pm$ 1.4	28.3 $\pm$ 2.4	50.3 $\pm$ 1.5

200,000 cells/35 mm dish were plated in 2 ml of the indicated medium. Cultures containing basal medium $\pm$ serum had unmodified substrates. Values are expressed as the mean ($\pm$SD) of triplicate cultures.

[a] See Table 1.
[b] See Table 6.

does not sustain LA-N-1 cell division, whereas cells in N2 medium grow as well as or better than in serum-containing medium. To date LA-N-1 cells have been growing in N2 medium in the total absence of serum for 50 days with five subcultures. The medium is changed at 5 days initially and every 2 days thereafter until subculture. Fibronectin is added only at the time of subculture.

There is a difference in the morphology of LA-N-1 cells in the respective media. When a single cell suspension of LA-N-1 cells is plated, the cells tend to cluster together in the presence of serum (Fig. 1A) and to remain more dispersed in N2 medium (Fig. 1C). Figure 2A shows these cells in N2 medium at a higher density. In comparison, if one plates clusters of LA-N-1 cells rather than single cells into N2 medium, profuse neurite extension occurs, presumably

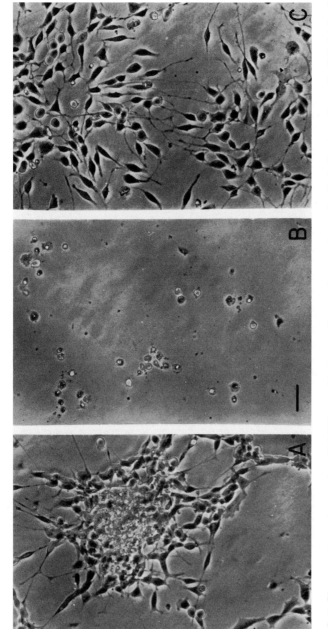

FIG. 1. Phase contrast micrographs of LA-N-1 neuroblastoma cells in various media on day 6. **A:** Basal medium with 30% fetal calf serum. **B:** Basal medium alone. **C:** N2 medium with 5 µg/ml fibronectin added and a polylysine-precoated dish. See Table 1 for media constituents and Table 6 for details of substrate modification. Scale bar, 50 µm.

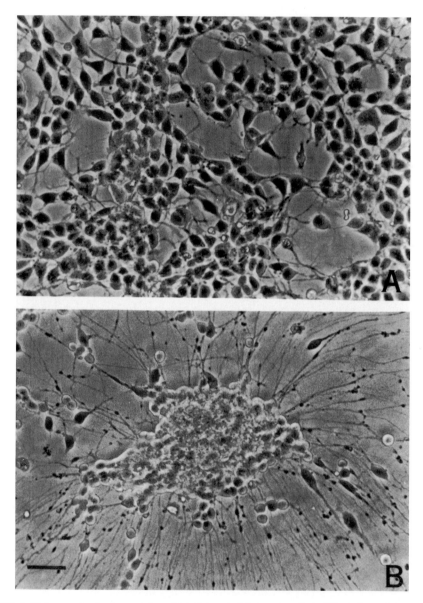

FIG. 2. Phase contrast micrographs of LA-N-1 neuroblastoma cells in N2 medium with 5 μg/ml fibronectin added. Culture dishes were precoated with polylysine just prior to medium addition. **A:** Plating of single cells after 6 days in culture. **B:** Plating of clusters of cells after 5 days in culture. See Table 1 for medium constituents and Table 6 for details of substrate modification. Scale bar, 50 μm.

enhanced by cell-cell interactions (Fig. 2B). The pattern of neurite formation seen in N2 medium is much more elaborate than any observed in serum-containing medium, suggesting that a serum factor modulates neurite extension. Consistent with this idea is the report that α_1-, α_4-, and β-globulin fractions from fetal calf serum inhibit neurite formation in C1300 mouse neuroblastoma cells (23).

CONCLUSIONS

Serum-free N2 medium should prove extremely useful in studying growth regulation and differentiation of neuroblastoma cells. If inhibition of the maturation of normal neuroblasts results in neuroblastoma, a serum-free culture system should be ideal for identifying and elucidating the mechanism(s) of action of physiological and pharmacological effectors which restrict or promote expression of differentiation. In addition, the investigation of cell-substrate or cell-cell adhesion under more defined conditions may further elucidate the phenomenon of metastasis.

ACKNOWLEDGMENTS

The author wishes to thank Gordon H. Sato for his inspiration and encouragement of these studies. This research was supported by a National Institutes of Health Postdoctoral Individual Research Award 5F32NS05482-02.

REFERENCES

1. Augusti-Tocco, G., and Sato, G. (1969): Establishment of functional clonal lines of neurons from mouse neuroblastoma. *Proc. Natl. Acad. Sci. U.S.A.,* 64:311–315.
2. Bottenstein, J., Hayashi, I., Hutchings, S., Masui, H., Mather, J., McClure, D., Ohasa, S., Rizzino, A., Sato, G., Serrero, G., Wolfe, R., and Wu, R. (1979): The growth of cells in serum-free hormone-supplemented media. *Meth. Enzymol.,* 58:94–109.
3. Bottenstein, J. E., Mather, J. P., and Sato, G. H. (1979): Growth of neuroepithelial derived cell lines in serum-free hormone supplemented media. In: *Hormones and Cell Culture,* edited by G. Sato and R. Ross, pp. 531–544. Cold Spring Harbor Laboratories, Cold Spring Harbor, New York.
4. Bottenstein, J. E., and Sato, G. H. (1979): Growth of a rat neuroblastoma cell line in serum-free supplemented medium. *Proc. Natl. Acad. Sci. U.S.A.,* 76:514–517.
5. Bottenstein, J. E., and Sato, G. H. (1979): Fibronectin and polylysine requirement for growth of neuroblastoma cells in serum-free medium. Submitted for publication.
6. Bottenstein, J. E., Skaper, S. D., Varon, S. S., and Sato, G. H. (1979): Selective survival of neurons in chick embryo sensory ganglionic cultures utilizing serum-free supplemented medium. *Exp. Cell Res. (in press).*
7. Dray, F., Sato, G., and Bottenstein, J. (1979): Effect of primary prostaglandins on neuroblastoma cells cultured in a defined medium. *International Prostaglandin Conference* (abstract in press).
8. Fox, I. H., and Kelley, W. N. (1978): The role of adenosine and 2'-deoxyadenosine in mammalian cells. *Annu. Rev. Biochem.,* 47:655–686.
9. Hayashi, I., and Sato, G. (1976): Replacement of serum by hormones permits growth of cells in a defined medium. *Nature,* 259:132–134.
10. Hutchings, S., and Sato, G. (1978): Growth and maintenance of HeLa cells in serum-free medium supplemented with hormones. *Proc. Natl. Acad. Sci. U.S.A.,* 75:901–904.

11. Letourneau, P. C., Ray, P. N., and Bernfield, M. R. (1979): The regulation of cell behavior by cell adhesion. In: *Biological Regulation and Development,* edited by R. Goldberger. Plenum Press, New York *(in press).*

12. Mather, J., and Sato, G. (1979): The growth of mouse melanoma cells in hormone-supplemented serum-free medium. *Exp. Cell Res.,* 120:191–200.

13. Mather, J. P., and Sato, G. H. (1979): The use of hormone-supplemented serum-free media in primary cultures. *Exp. Cell Res.,* 124:215–221.

14. McKeehan, W. L., and Ham, R. G. (1976): Stimulation of clonal growth of normal fibroblasts with substrata coated with basic polymers. *J. Cell Biol.,* 71:727–734.

15. Orly, J., and Sato, G. (1979): Fibronectin mediates cytokinesis and growth of rat follicular cells in serum-free medium. *Cell,* 17:295–305.

16. Polgar, P., and Taylor, L. (1977): Effects of prostaglandin on substrate uptake and cell division in human diploid fibroblasts. *Biochem. J.,* 162:1–8.

17. Prasad, K. N. (1972): Morphological differentiation induced by prostaglandin in mouse neuroblastoma cells in culture. *Nature [New Biol.],* 236:49–52.

18. Rizzino, A., and Sato, G. (1978): Growth of embryonal carcinoma cells in serum-free medium. *Proc. Natl. Acad. Sci. U.S.A.,* 75:1844–1848.

19. Sandquist, D., Williams, T. H., Sahu, S. K., and Kataoka, S. (1978): Morphological differentiation of a murine neuroblastoma clone in monolayer culture induced by dexamethasone. *Exp. Cell Res.,* 113:375–381.

20. Schubert, D. (1974): Induced differentiation of clonal rat nerve and glial cells. *Neurobiology,* 4:376–387.

21. Schubert, D., Carlisle, W., and Look, C. (1975): Putative neurotransmitters in clonal cell lines. *Nature,* 254:341–343.

22. Schubert, D., Heinemann, S., Carlisle, W., Tarikas, H., Kimes, B., Patrick, J., Steinbach, J., Culp, W., and Brandt, B. (1974): Clonal cell lines from the rat central nervous system. *Nature,* 249:224–227.

23. Seeds, N. W., Gilman, A. G., Amano, T., and Nirenberg, M. W. (1970): Regulation of axon formation by clonal lines of a neural tumor. *Proc. Natl. Acad. Sci. U.S.A.,* 66:160–167.

24. Seeger, R. C., Rayner, S. A., Banerjee, A., Chung, H., Lang, W. E., Neustein, H. B., and Benedict, W. F. (1977): Morphology, growth, chromosomal pattern, and fibrinolytic activity of two new human neuroblastoma cell lines. *Cancer Res.,* 37:1364–1371.

25. Shoemaker, W. J., Bottenstein, J. E., Milner, R. J., Clark, B. R., and Bloom, F. E. (1979): Serum-free culture medium maintains differentiated properties of neurons in fetal rat brain explants. *Society for Neuroscience Meeting (abstract in press).*

26. Varon, S., Skaper, S. D., Adler, R., Bottenstein, J., and Sato, G. (1979): Purified neuronal cultures from ganglionic and central nervous system tissues of several species by use of a defined, serum-free medium. *Society for Neuroscience Meeting (abstract in press).*

27. Waymouth, C. (1977): Nutritional requirements of cells in culture, with special reference to neural cells. In: *Cell, Tissue, and Organ Cultures in Neurobiology,* edited by S. Fedoroff and L. Hertz, pp. 631–648. Academic Press, New York.

28. West, G., Uki, J., Herschman, H. R., and Seeger, R. C. (1977): Adrenergic, cholinergic, and inactive human neuroblastoma cell lines with the action-potential Na$^+$ ionophore. *Cancer Res.,* 37:1372–1376.

29. Yamada, K. M., and Olden, K. (1978): Fibronectins-adhesive glycoproteins of cell surface and blood. *Nature,* 275:179–184.

30. Yavin, E., and Yavin, Z. (1974): Attachment and culture dissociated cells from rat embryo cerebral hemispheres on polylysine-coated surface. *J. Cell Biol.,* 62:540–546.

Advances in Neuroblastoma Research,
edited by Audrey E. Evans.
Raven Press, New York © 1980.

Glycoproteins Associated with Differentiating Neuroblastoma Cells in Culture

Mary Catherine Glick, Maria Y. Giovanni, and *Uriel Z. Littauer

Department of Pediatrics, University of Pennsylvania Medical School, and The Children's Hospital of Philadelphia, Philadelphia, Pennsylvania 19104

Human neuroblastoma cells in culture possess differentiated neuronal properties such as neurotransmitter synthesizing enzymes and active Na$^+$ channels (5). Because of the near diploid chromosomal number and the human derivation, they represent an excellent system for the study of the biochemical properties associated with the maturation of neuronal cells. In contrast to the clones of mouse neuroblastoma C-1300 (10) which are derived from a single tumor, the human neuroblastoma cell lines originate from different tumors. Moreover, these tumors probably arise at various stages of nerve cell maturation so that among the cell lines there may be a variety of differentiated properties.

As with mouse neuroblastoma, the human neuroblastoma cells can be differentiated with dimethyl sulfoxide (DMSO) (4,5), but unlike the former cells several highly differentiated functions are already displayed in cells growing logarithmically in the absence of an inducing agent. Figure 1 illustrates this point. The growth curve of human neuroblastoma cells, CHP-134, is compared to choline acetyltransferase (CAT) activity. In these experiments the cells are rapidly growing between days 1 and 7 in the absence of DMSO, whereas in the presence of 2% DMSO growth is less rapid. The CAT activity (Fig. 1B) is already high on day 1 for the cells grown without DMSO and after an initial drop remains approximately the same throughout the growth period with or without DMSO. On the other hand, mouse neuroblastoma cells, NS-20, which are growing logarithmically, show low CAT activity which increases when the cells reach the confluent state of growth (10).

The establishment of active Na$^+$ channels, however, was more similar in the mouse and human cells (2,5,6). Examination of this neuronal function by ^{86}Rb efflux (8) revealed that the cells expressed this differentiated function only after time in culture and that growth in the presence of DMSO increased this activity (5,6).

The most striking finding was the presence of a glycoprotein of approximate

---

* Permanent address: Department of Neurobiology, Weizmann Institute of Science, Rehovot, Israel.

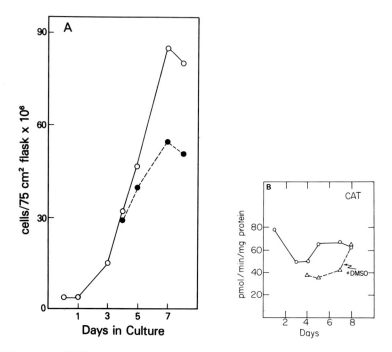

FIG. 1. Growth and CAT activity of human neuroblastoma CHP-134 in the presence or absence of DMSO as inducing agent. **A:** Growth curve of CHP-134 expressed as cell count with (●) or without (○) 2% DMSO added to complete medium at day 3 and every 48 hr thereafter in fresh medium. **B:** CAT activity (10) was measured in homogenates of the cells grown as shown in (**A**) in the presence (△) or absence (○) of 2% DMSO. The assay was performed by Ms. D. Saya, Weizmann Institute.

molecular weight 200,000 which was associated with cells displaying active Na^+ channels. Table 1 summarizes the results obtained with the human neuroblastoma cells, CHP-134 (5), and several clonal cell lines of mouse neuroblastoma, C-1300 (6). In all cases, the presence of active Na^+ ionophores correlated with the presence of the glycoprotein, 200,000 M_r. This glycoprotein was found in the neurites and membranes of the differentiated cells but not in the membranes of nondifferentiated cells. Furthermore, under some conditions when neurites were prepared from NIE-115 cells which were differentiated morphologically but did not show active ^{86}Rb efflux, lesser amounts of the glycoprotein were found associated with the neurites (see DMSO, day 0 in Table 1). A reciprocal relationship between the appearance of the high molecular weight glycoprotein in the membrane and the growth medium was observed (Table 1). That is, when active Na^+ channels were not highly developed, the high molecular weight glycoprotein was found in the growth medium, whereas in the presence of active Na^+ flux, a high molecular weight glycoprotein was associated with the cell surface (6). This relationship was dramatically demonstrated using clonal cell line NIA-103 from mouse neuroblastoma, which is unable to undergo differentiation in culture (Table 1).

TABLE 1. *Correlation of active Na$^+$ channels with a high molecular weight glycoprotein*

Cell type	Active Na$^+$ channels[a]	High molecular weight glycoprotein[b]	
		Neurites/ membranes[c]	Media[d]
CHP-134	+++	+++	−
NIE-115			
DMSO—day 3	++	+++	−
DMSO—day 0	−	−	±
Log	−	−	++
Confluent	±	±	+
NIA-103	−	−	+++

[a] Measured by the efflux of ^{86}Rb (5,6).
[b] M_r = 200,000 as defined by SDS polyacrylamide gel electrophoresis of radioactive fucose-containing glycoproteins (5,6).
[c] Prepared from radioactive cells (5,6). All cells were metabolically labeled with L-[^{3}H]fucose for 48 hr before harvest.
[d] Precipitated with heparin (6).

Table 2 summarizes the known characteristics of this glycoprotein. The glycoprotein is called "Excitoporin" because of its association with cells which possess excitable membranes. "Porin" denotes the association with the Na$^+$ channel which is conceptually referred to as a pore and is schematically depicted in Fig. 2. Excitoporin indeed fulfills at least some of the criteria of an ion channel. As a glycoprotein, it possesses a hydrophilic portion extending partially to the external surface of the cell. The carbohydrate portion is demonstrated by the metabolic labeling with radioactive L-fucose and D-glucosamine, precursors of glycoproteins. The hydrophobic portion which would attract the lipid bilayer has yet to be demonstrated. It is noteworthy that a protein, 230,000 M_r, has been reported by Agnew et al. (1) as the tetrodotoxin binding component of *Electroporus*. Whether or not Excitoporin will show these characteristics remains to be demonstrated.

In keeping with the recent theories of the sodium gating currents (3,7), one can speculate that the activated state of the sodium channel would involve the assembly of several Excitoporin molecules. Regardless of the precise role or the mechanism, the association of Excitoporin with the surface of neuroblastoma cells possessing an excitable membrane has been demonstrated.

TABLE 2. *Characteristics of Excitoporin*

Fucose and glucosamine-containing glycoprotein
~ MW 200,000
3–7% of the total neurite glycoproteins
Increases with development of excitable membranes
Enriched in neurites and surface membranes
Present in differentiated cells
Present in culture medium of nondifferentiated cells

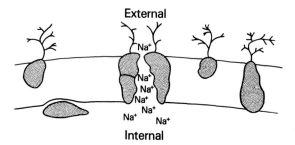

FIG. 2. Schematic representation of the Na^+ channel in a surface membrane. Glycoproteins extend as branches from the membrane, and either traverse the membrane or are found only on the external side. The Na^+ channel is depicted as a pore.

Even though many differentiated properties are well developed in some of the human neuroblastoma lines, the cells are still capable of forming tumors in nude mice (9). Therefore, we conclude that the simple concept that to increase the degree of differentiation necessitates loss of tumorigenicity does not seem to be valid. Rather, a more basic and systematic approach to the processes of the maturation of the various neuronal markers and their relationship to tumorigenicity is warranted for a complete understanding of the enigmatic neuroblastoma cell.

ACKNOWLEDGMENTS

This work was supported by NIH PO1-HD08356, PO1-CA14489, The Canuso Foundation, and the United States-Israel Binational Foundation.

REFERENCES

1. Agnew, W. S., Levinson, S. R., Brabson, J. S., and Raftery, M. A. (1978): Purification of the tetrodotoxin-binding component associated with the voltage-sensitive sodium channel from *Electrophorus electricus* electroplax membranes. *Proc. Natl. Acad. Sci. U.S.A.,* 75:2606–2610.
2. Catterall, W. A. (1977): Activation of the action potential Na^+ ionophore by neurotoxins. *J. Biol. Chem.,* 252:8669–8676.
3. Hille, B. (1978): Ionic channels in excitable membranes. *Biophys. J.,* 22:283–294.
4. Kimhi, Y., Palfrey, C., Spector, I., Barak, Y., and Littauer, U. Z. (1976): Maturation of neuroblastoma cells in the presence of dimethylsulphoxide. *Proc. Natl. Acad. Sci. U.S.A.,* 73:462–466.
5. Littauer, U. Z., Giovanni, M. Y., and Glick, M. C. (1979): Differentiation of human neuroblastoma cells in culture. *Biochem. Biophys. Res. Commun.,* 88:933–939.
6. Littauer, U. Z., Giovanni, M. Y., and Glick, M. C. (1979): A glycoprotein from neurites of neuroblastoma cells differentiated. Submitted for publication.
7. Neumann, E., and Bernhardt, J. (1977): Physical chemistry of excitable biomembranes. *Annu. Rev. Biochem.,* 46:117–141.
8. Palfrey, C., and Littauer, U. Z. (1976): Sodium dependent efflux of K^+ and Rb^+ through the activated sodium channel of neuroblastoma cells. *Biochem. Biophys. Res. Commun.,* 72:209–215.

9. Schlesinger, H. R., Gerson, J. M., Moorhead, P. S., Maguire, H., and Hummeler, K. (1976): Establishment and characterization of human neuroblastoma cell lines. *Cancer Res.*, 36:3094–3100.
10. Schrier, B. K., Wilson, S. H., and Nirenberg, M. (1974): Cultured cell systems and methods for neurobiology. *Methods Enzymol.*, 32:765–788.

Advances in Neuroblastoma Research,
edited by Audrey E. Evans.
Raven Press, New York © 1980.

A Surface Glycoprotein as a Human Neuroblastoma Antigen Detected by Monoclonal Antibodies

*Mariko Momoi, **Roger H. Kennett, and †Mary Catherine Glick

*Departments of *†Pediatrics, and **Human Genetics, University of Pennsylvania Medical School, and *†The Children's Hospital of Philadelphia, Philadelphia, Pennsylvania 19104*

Monoclonal antibodies directed toward the cell surface are powerful tools for isolating membrane components. The availability of a large amount of monoclonal antibody with appropriate specificity facilitates the purification of responsive molecules in biological systems. Ideally, in the case of neuroblastomas, the antibodies can be used to distinguish neuronal and tumor-specific components.

Using the monoclonal antibody to human neuroblastoma cells (PI153/3) we have been able to isolate a membrane glycoprotein by virtue of its antigenic activity. The specificity of the monoclonal antibody has been described (5; Kennett et al., *this volume*), and with the exception of some leukemias the antibody appears to react mainly with cells of neuronal origin.

The surface receptor for the antibody was isolated from cultured human neuroblastoma cells (3) labeled metabolically with L-[³H]fucose or D-[³H]glucosamine, either as glycoproteins or as glycopeptides (Fig. 1). For the isolation of the glycoprotein, extraction was with 0.5% Nonidet P-40, whereas the glycopeptides were isolated by treating the cells with low concentrations of trypsin (2).

The surface antigen was purified by double-antibody affinity chromatography using immobilized anti-IgM (anti-μ). The affinity purification involved three main steps as shown in Fig. 2. First, anti-μ was coupled to Sepharose-4B (6). In the second step, the coupled anti-μ was mixed with the antibody-containing ascites fluid (PI153/3), and the specific antibody was bound. In the third step, the Sepharose-immune complex was incubated with fucose- or glucosamine-labeled glycoconjugates prepared from the cells (Fig. 1). Finally, to obtain the surface antigen, the radiolabeled glycoproteins or glycopeptides which were bound to the Sepharose-immune complex were eluted with glycine buffer.

PREPARATION OF SURFACE ANTIGEN

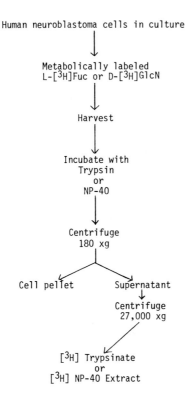

Human neuroblastoma cells in culture

↓

Metabolically labeled
L-[³H]Fuc or D-[³H]GlcN

↓

Harvest

↓

Incubate with
Trypsin
or
NP-40

↓

Centrifuge
180 xg

Cell pellet   Supernatant

↓

Centrifuge
27,000 xg

[³H] Trypsinate
or
[³H] NP-40 Extract

FIG. 1. Radioactive glycoproteins and glycopeptides were prepared from human neuroblastoma cells, CHP-134 and IMR-5. The cells were cultured for 5 days at 37°C, and labeled with L-[³H]fucose or D-[³H]glucosamine for 48 hr before harvest (3). The cells were harvested after washing with 0.16 M NaCl by a mild trypsinization (2) or extraction with 0.5% Nonidet P-40. The supernatants obtained by both procedures were centrifuged further at 27,000 × g for 20 min and were used as the source of radioactive glycoproteins, [³H]NP-40 extract, or glycopeptides [³H]trypsinate.

Figure 3 shows the elution profile from an affinity column of glucosamine-containing glycoconjugates extracted with NP-40 from IMR-5, a human neuroblastoma clonal cell line (Gilbert, *this volume*). This affinity system was specific both to antibody and to the source of the membrane antigen. The specificity to the antibody was shown by substituting for the neuroblastoma antibody a control monoclonal antibody to prepare the affinity complex. This affinity system, using a human B-cell line-derived monoclonal antibody (4), bound less than 10% of the radioactive membrane components bound by the specific antibody. The specificity of the source of the membrane receptor was shown by using radioactive glycopeptides from different cell lines such as NP5TP76B, a hybrid of human neuroblastoma × mouse fibroblast (Gilbert, *this volume*). The membrane glycoconjugates from this hybrid did not bind to the affinity complex. On the other hand, the glycoproteins from CHP-134, another human neuroblastoma cell line (3), did bind to the affinity beads. Both of these specificities were similar to those described for this monoclonal antibody using a binding assay with [¹²⁵I] anti-Fab (5).

The antigen was a glycoprotein as shown by the binding of radioactive fucose

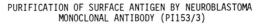

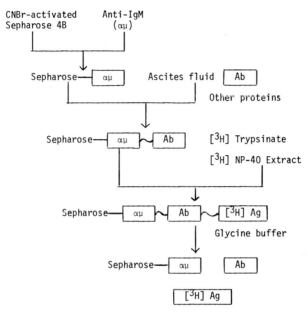

FIG. 2. Double-affinity complex to Sepharose 4B. Goat anti-mouse IgM ($\alpha\mu$) was reacted with CNBr-activated Sepharose 4B. Hybridoma-derived ascites fluid, PI153/3 (5; Kennett et al., *this volume*) was reacted with this complex and the monoclonal antibody was bound. The human neuroblastoma-derived radioactive glycopeptides, [³H]trypsinate or glycoproteins [³H]NP-40 extract, were bound to the Sepharose-$\alpha\mu$-antibody complex. Elution of the radioactive antigen, [³H]Ag, and antibody, Ab, was with 50mM glycine buffer.

or glucosamine-containing material to the affinity column, since L-fucose and D-glucosamine are glycoprotein precursors. In addition, the trypsinate (Fig. 1) retained binding activity for the affinity beads. The trypsinate represents approximately 15% of the membrane glycopeptides, possessing a spectrum of molecular weights.

In order to further define the binding specificity, the trypsinate was digested with the general protease, Pronase, to remove the amino acids from the glycopeptides. The carbohydrate portion will remain intact after this enzyme digestion. To demonstrate the binding activity, the Pronase-digested trypsinate from IMR-5 cells metabolically labeled with D-[³H]glucosamine was passed through a Sephadex G-50 column, the retained fractions were pooled and subjected to the affinity chromatography. This fraction showed a specific binding activity to the affinity column, and the bound radioactivity per 10^8 cells was comparable to that of the glucosamine-labeled Nonidet P-40 extract or trypsinate. This leads to the suggestion that the binding capacity of the surface antigen resides in the carbohydrate portion of the glycoprotein rather than in the polypeptide backbone.

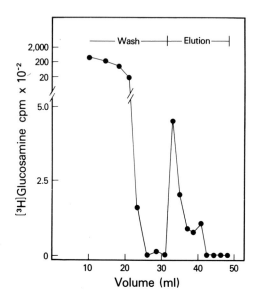

FIG. 3. Elution profile of an NP-40 extract of IMR-5 cells from the antibody affinity column. The NP-40 extract containing radioactive glycoproteins was washed from the column with 30 ml of buffer, and elution of specific glucosamine-containing antigens was with 50 mM glycine buffer. (See Figs. 1 and 2.)

We have partially purified and characterized a membrane antigen which is recognized by a monoclonal antibody to human neuroblastoma cells. The antigen is a glycoprotein derived from the surface of human neuroblastoma cells, CHP-134 and IMR-5. The isolation was by virtue of its antigenic properties which appeared to be retained in the glycopeptide. It will be interesting to see how the detailed structures of the oligosaccharides from antigens derived from other sources expressing the antigen, such as fetal brain and some leukemias (Kennett et al., *this volume*), will differ from those of the neuroblastoma cell surface. Sequential enzyme degradation will be used to elucidate the partial structure in a manner analogous to that used to define a membrane glycopeptide from virus-transformed hamster cells (7).

The use of monoclonal antibodies such as the one described gives an opportunity to define membrane components which may be unique to neuronal cells, and aids in defining the architecture of the surface membrane. Furthermore, since surface components contribute to many normal and aberrant functions of the cell, including metastasis (1), such a systematic dissection, combining immunological and chemical techniques, may eventually sort out some of the differences observed in the clinical stages of this disease (Evans, *this volume*).

ACKNOWLEDGMENTS

This work was supported by the Yoshida Foundation for Science and Technology, Japan; NIH Grants PO1 CA 14489 and CA 24263; and NSF Grant PCM76-82997.

REFERENCES

1. Glick, M. C. (1976): Cell surface changes associated with malignancy. In: *Fundamental Aspects of Metastasis,* edited by L. Weiss, pp. 9–23. North-Holland Publishing Company, Amsterdam.
2. Glick, M. C., Kimhi, Y., and Littauer, U. Z. (1973): Glycopeptides from surface membranes of neuroblastoma cells. *Proc. Natl. Acad. Sci. U.S.A.,* 70:1682–1687.
3. Glick, M. C., Schlesinger, H., and Hummeler, K. (1976): Glycopeptides from the surface of human neuroblastoma cells. *Cancer Res.,* 36:4520–4524.
4. Kennett, R. H., Denis, K. A., Tung, A. S., and Klinman, N. R. (1978): Hybrid plasmocytoma production. *Curr. Top. Microbiol. Immunol.,* 81:77–91.
5. Kennett, R. H., and Gilbert, F. (1979): Hybrid myelomas producing antibodies against a human neuroblastoma antigen present on fetal brain. *Science,* 203:1120–1121.
6. Livingston, D. M. (1974): Immunoaffinity chromatography of proteins. *Methods Enzymol.,* 34:725–726.
7. Santer, U. V., and Glick, M. C. (1979): Partial structure of a membrane glycopeptide from virus-transformed hamster cells. *Biochemistry,* 18:2533–2540.

Advances in Neuroblastoma Research,
edited by Audrey E. Evans.
Raven Press, New York © 1980.

Production of Sulfated Glycosaminoglycans by Human Neuroblastoma Cell Cultures

*J. T. Gallagher, **I. N. Hampson, and **S. Kumar

*Cancer Research Campaign Department of Medical Oncology, Manchester University, and Christie Hospital and Holt Radium Institute; and **Clinical Research, Christie Hospital and Holt Radium Institute, Manchester, England

Cell surface glycoproteins and glycosaminoglycans (GAGs) have been studied in a wide variety of cultured cells and a role for the carbohydrate portion of these molecules in cell recognition and related phenomenon is assumed from localization of the sugar residues on the external surface of the membrane. There is now extensive documentation of abnormalities in these components in tumor cells (2; M. C. Glick, *personal communication*), but the significance of such changes remains obscure. Of the sulfated GAGs associated with the cell surface, heparan sulfate (HS) is usually the major component and chondroitin sulfate (CS) the minor one. Although these macromolecules, together with hyaluronic acid, undoubtedly contribute to the elastic and compressibility properties of connective tissues, specific biological functions at the cellular level have not been elucidated despite strong evidence on the requirement for a suitable cellular microenvironment, partly formed by GAGs, in the differentiation and maturation of embryonic cells (3,5).

To help further our understanding of the biological properties of GAGs, we decided to examine the GAG composition of a human neuroblastoma cell line, CHP-100 (kindly provided by Dr. H. Schlesinger), with the initial objectives of identifying the constituent GAGs both at the cell surface and in the culture medium and with the longer term aims of studying GAG variations during *in vitro* differentiation of neuroblastoma cells. To this end, GAGs were first radiolabeled in confluent cultures to facilitate analysis. $Na_2{}^{35}SO_4$ and ^3H-glucosamine (10 $\mu Ci/ml$ and 5 $\mu Ci/ml$, respectively) were added to the cell cultures for 48 hr, the spent medium removed, and the washed monolayers trypsinized for 15 min in 0.05% w/v trypsin. The cell suspension obtained was centrifuged for 5 min at 800 g and the supernatant (the trypsin extract or "trypsinate") was considered to represent a combined cell surface/cell matrix GAG and glycopeptide population. Nondiffusible components in the trypsinate and spent culture medium were analyzed by gradient elution on DEAE-cellulose chromatography (Figs. 1 and 2).

A single, doubly labeled peak, on occasions partially resolved into two compo-

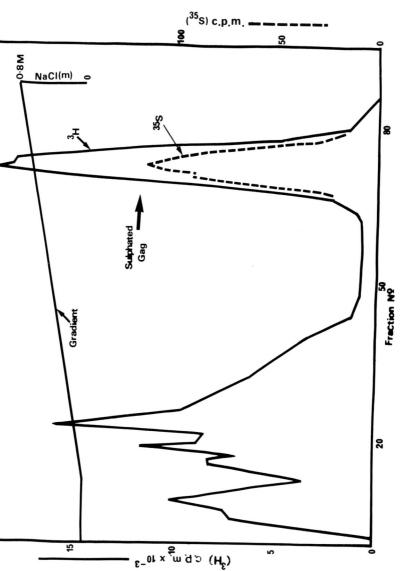

FIG. 1. DEAE-cellulose chromatography of the "trypsinate" of human neuroblastoma cell cultures. Confluent cultures were labeled with ^{3}H-glucosamine and Na$_2$^{35}SO$_4$, as described in the text. A trypsin extract of the cells was dialyzed, concentrated, and applied to a DEAE-cellulose DE-52 column (10 cm × 1 cm) equilibrated with 5 mm sodium phosphate buffer, pH 6.8. Bound components were eluted with a NaCl gradient (0 → 0.8 M) at a flow rate of 10 ml/hr. Fraction volumes were 2.4 ml

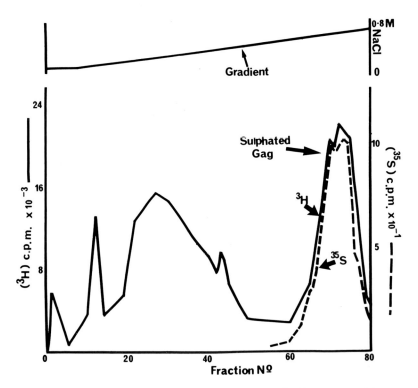

FIG. 2. DEAE-cellulose chromatography of the "spent medium" of human neuroblastoma cell cultures. Spent medium from confluent cultures described in Fig. 1 was processed and fractionated as described in the legend to Fig. 1.

nents, emerged from the column at around 0.65 M NaCl. In both media and trypsinate fractions, susceptibility to chondroitinase—"ABC" and "AC" digestion together with electrophoretic analysis indicated that HS and CS were present. CS components consisted of chondroitin sulfates A/C and dermatan sulfate. HS:CS ratio was higher in the trypsinate than in the medium. So far we have not attempted to characterize hyaluronic acid (HA) in this system, but no clearly defined peak of ^{3}H-labeled HA was found in the DEAE-chromatograms. Pronase digests of the sulfated GAGs were mainly excluded from Sephadex G-200.

The apparent enrichment of HS at the cell surface in our system is of interest as it accords with findings of other workers (4). The observation that murine neuroblastoma cells show a retention of HS during differentiation (1) emphasizes the need for corresponding studies in differentiating human neuroblastoma.

REFERENCES

1. Augusti-Tocco, G., and Chiarugi, V. P. (1976): Surface glycosaminoglycans as a differentiation cofactor in neuroblastoma cell cultures. *Cell Differ.*, 5(3):161–170.

2. Chiargu, V. P., Vannucchi, S., Cella, C., Fibbi, G., Del Rosso, M., and Cappelletti, R. (1978): Intercellular glucosaminoglycans in normal and neoplastic tissues. *Cancer Res.,* 38(12):4717–4721.
3. Hay, E. D. (1977): Interaction between the cell surface and extracellular matrix in corneal development. Cell and tissue interactions. *Soc. Gen. Physiol. Ser.,* 32:115–137.
4. Kraemer, P. M., and Tobey, R. A. (1972): Cell-cycle dependent desquamation of heparin sulfate from the cell surface. *J. Cell. Biol.,* 55:713–717.
5. Toole, B. P., and Linsenmayer, T. F. (1975): Proteoglycan collagen interaction: Possible developmental significance. In: *Extracellular Matrix Influences on Gene Expression,* edited by H. C. Slaukin and R. C. Grealich, pp. 341–346. Academic Press, New York.

Advances in Neuroblastoma Research.
edited by Audrey E. Evans.
Raven Press, New York © 1980.

Endocytosis of Ricin and Cholera Toxin by Murine Neuroblastoma

Nicholas K. Gonatas

Department of Pathology, University of Pennsylvania School of Medicine,
Philadelphia, Pennsylvania 19104

Murine neuroblastoma has certain morphologic, biochemical, and electric properties of sympathetic neurons (3,10,15,16). Neuroblastoma cells cultured in media containing dibutyryl cyclic AMP show enhanced electrical excitability and morphologic "differentiation" (3,15). Furthermore, it has been shown that nerve growth factor binds specifically on murine neuroblastoma cells (16). For these reasons murine neuroblastoma has been used as a model of cultured neurons (10).

In previous papers we have reported our observations on the receptor-mediated (adsorptive) endocytosis of ricin and cholera toxin by cultured neurons (1,6,7, 12,18,19). Many biologically important molecules—such as hormones, growth factors, neurotransmitters, lectins, toxins, and viruses—bind to specific plasma membrane receptors. The mechanism of action of these agents is not clearly understood, but it is reasonable to assume that their binding with corresponding plasma membrane receptors, the subsequent redistribution of receptor-ligand complexes, and their eventual endocytosis are linked with the initiation, propagation, and possibly termination of their specific physiologic or pathologic effects.

In our previous studies of adsorptive endocytosis of ricin or cholera toxin by cultured neurons we utilized conjugates of the ligands with the tracer enzyme horseradish peroxidase (HRP) (5–7,12). Using the cytochemical reaction for HRP of Graham and Karnovsky, we were able to detect the endocytosed ligand within the cisternae of the Golgi apparatus, and more specifically in the elements of Golgi-endoplasmic reticulum-lysosome (GERL) (14). According to Novikoff, GERL is involved in cellular secretion. The functional implications of the adsorptive endocytosis of ricin and cholera toxin into GERL is unknown; we have postulated that this special route of endocytosis of plasma membrane receptor-ligand complexes may be related to plasma membrane retrieval for recycling, or for degradation (4,6). Further studies of the mechanisms and implications of adsorptive endocytosis require the use of homogeneous cell populations and of quantifiable assays. Cultured neurons are not suitable for these studies, and for this reason we have explored the feasibility of cultured murine neuroblastoma to study adsorptive endocytosis.

In this chapter we shall review our work on the endocytosis of ricin and cholera toxin by cultured murine neuroblastoma. Our conclusions are that (a) cultured neuroblastoma cells are endowed with an acid phosphatase positive system of cisternae and tubules corresponding to GERL of sympathetic neurons, (b) conjugates of HRP with ricin and with cholera toxin undergo endocytosis into lysosomes and elements of GERL, (c) exogenous monosialoganglioside (GM_1), the natural receptor of cholera toxin, probably becomes incorporated with the plasma membranes of murine neuroblastoma so that about 96% of the cells are stained with cholera toxin-HRP after preincubation of cells with GM_1, whereas only about 9% of cells not exposed to GM_1 bind cholera toxin-HRP. Part of these findings have been published (8,13).

MATERIALS AND METHODS

Culture

In this study the neuro-2A line (CCL-131) obtained from the American Type Culture Collection was used (Rockville, Md.). Cells were grown in Falcon bottles (Falcon, Labware, Div. of Becton, Dickinson and Co., Oxnard, Calif.) in Dulbecco's Modified Eagle's Medium (Grand Island Biological Co., Grand Island, N.Y.) with 2 mM glutamine and 10% fetal calf serum (13). Cells for ultrastructural studies were grown on plastic strips (Aclar 33c, 5 mil, Allied Chemical Corp., Specialty Chemical Div., Morristown, N.J.).

Ligands

With the possible exception of the NS_3 antigen, the antigenic or chemical composition of the plasma membranes of murine neuroblastoma is virtually unknown (17). For that reason we have selected a lectin, ricin (D-galactose), and cholera toxin (GM_1 ganglioside) as probes of neuroblastoma cell surfaces (5,19). Although the specificities of these ligands are widespread, they bind with high affinity with moieties containing terminal D-galactose (ricin) or GM_1 ganglioside (cholera toxin).

Conjugation with HRP

The ligands were covalently linked with HRP with glutaraldehyde according to the method of Avrameas and Ternynck and co-workers (2,5,12,13). Conjugates with molar ratios 1:1 of ligand and HRP were obtained.

Processing of Cells for Electron Microscopy

Cells were washed at 4°C with Earle's balanced salt solution buffered with carbonate or 10 mM Hepes at 7.35 (N-2-hydroxylethylpiperazine-N'-ethanesulfonic acid; Schwarz/Mann). Ligands at concentrations of 10 to 50 μg/ml were incubated for 1 hr at 4°C; after several washes with buffered Earle's, cells were either fixed immediately for study of surface binding or incubated at 37°C for various periods of time in a medium free of ligand and then fixed (adsorptive endocytosis). Thus under the conditions of the experiment the initial binding between ligand and plasma membrane receptor occurs at 4°C, a temperature which precludes the endocytosis of the ligand; subsequently, cells are transferred at 37°C in a medium free of ligand; therefore the observed endocytosis of HRP is presumably representing the uptake of membrane-bound ligand (adsorptive endocytosis). Exogenous GM_1 was introduced according to described methods (13).

Cytochemical Demonstration of HRP

This was performed according to the method of Graham and Karnovsky (9) with diaminobenzidine tetrahydrochloride as substrate.

Cytochemical Demonstration of Acid Phosphatase

This was performed according to the method of Novikoff and Novikoff (14) with disodium salt of cytidine-5'-monophosphoric acid (Sigma, St. Louis, Mo.) as the substrate.

RESULTS

Surface staining after incubations of cells with ricin-HRP or cholera toxin-HRP at 4°C: When cells were incubated with the ligands at 4°C and fixed for electron microscopy immediately thereafter, a diffuse surface stain of oxidized diaminobenzidine (DAB) was noted. The stain was noted on perikarya, processes, and growth cones. Whereas all cells stained with ricin-HRP, only about 9% of cells stained with cholera toxin-HRP. However, if cells were incubated with 10 μg/ml of GM_1 at 4°C for 1 hr prior to their incubation with cholera toxin-HRP, 96% of cells showed a surface stain. These results indicate that: (a) receptors to ricin or GM_1 are diffusely present on cell surfaces, and (b) introduction of exogenous GM_1 increases the binding of cholera toxin-HRP.

Specificity of Binding

Incubation of ^{125}I-labeled ricin in the presence of 0.1 M of lactose abolished 88 to 92% of the binding *(unpublished observations)*. Incubation of cholera toxin-HRP with GM_1 abolished completely the binding of the toxin on cells, whereas incubation of cholera toxin-HRP with an asialo derivative of GM_1 did not affect the binding of the toxin on cells (13).

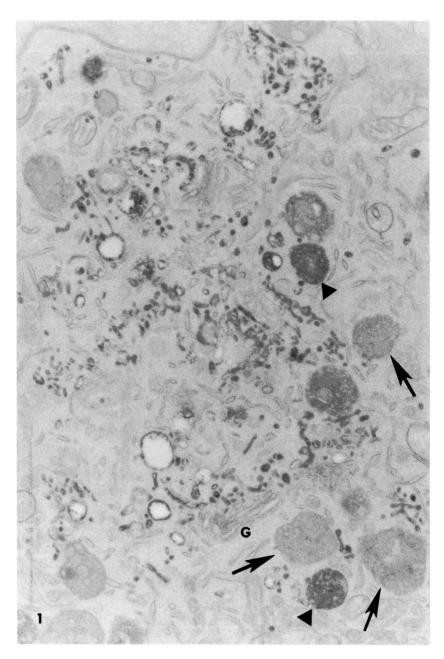

FIG. 1. Endocytosis of ricin-HRP by murine neuroblastoma. Note numerous vesicles and cisternae containing peroxidase-positive material. G, unstained cisternae of Golgi apparatus; arrows, peroxidase-negative lysosomes; arrowheads, peroxidase-positive lysosomes. × 31,000.

Surface Redistributions at 37°C

Redistribution of ricin-HRP or cholera toxin-HRP in patches or "caps" was not seen; this implies that the "receptors" or, more likely, the ligands used are monovalent.

Endocytosis

In our original studies of endocytosis of lectin-HRP or cholera toxin-HRP by cultured neurons, we identified the ligands in cisternae and vesicles of GERL (6,7,12). A similar pattern of endocytosis of cholera toxin into murine neuroblastoma has been observed (13); subunit B (the binding subunit) of cholera toxin showed a similar endocytosis into neuroblastoma GERL (13); since the binding subunit B of cholera toxin does not stimulate the adenylate cyclase, it was concluded that endocytosis of the entire toxin or of its subunit B into GERL did not require activation of the adenylate cyclase (13,19).

A similar route of endocytosis of ricin-HRP into GERL was observed in cultured neuroblastoma cells (Fig. 1). Furthermore, acid phosphatase cytochemistry confirmed that neuroblastoma cells have a system of vesicles and cisternae corresponding to GERL of neurons *(unpublished observations)*. Endocytosis of ricin-HRP or cholera toxin-HRP into neuroblastoma GERL was noted after incubations at 37°C for 30 to 60 min. After longer incubations (2 to 3 hr) peroxidase stain was seen in dense bodies probably representing lysosomes. Thus we concluded that the principal destinations of endocytosed, presumed, plasma membrane receptor-ligand complexes are the vesicles and cisternae of GERL.

The functional implications and the mechanism of this unusual endocytic pathway of plasma membrane moieties are under current study; several possibilities are being examined, such as retrieval of plasma membrane glycoproteins and glycolipids for reutilization (recycling) (4,6,11), degradation of plasma membranes, and failure of fusion of endocytosed vesicles of plasma membrane origin with lysosomes.

The role of the Golgi apparatus in secretion and glycosylations has been fairly well established, and a role of GERL in secretion has been proposed (14). Therefore the observation of the endocytosis of plasma membrane moieties in the general area of probable biosynthesis and/or assembly of certain plasma membrane moieties is intriguing and deserves further exploration.

SUMMARY

Conjugates of horseradish peroxidase with ricin (D-galactose) and cholera toxin (GM_1 ganglioside) were used for a cytochemical detection of the surface distribution and endocytosis of glycoproteins and glycolipids with terminal D-galactose or GM_1 ganglioside of murine neuroblastoma. Binding of cholera toxin-HRP by murine neuroblastoma was enhanced after the exogenous introduction of GM_1 ganglioside. Cells were labeled at 4°C with the above ligands, and the adsorptive endocytosis of presumed receptor-ligand complexes was studied after incubations of labeled cells at 37°C in a medium free of ligand. Ricin and cholera toxin underwent endocytosis in cisternae and vesicles of GERL. We suggest that GERL is the primary recipient of adsorptively endocytosed plasma membrane "receptor"-ligand complexes which may be thus degraded or possibly reutilized.

ACKNOWLEDGMENT

This work was supported by USPHS Grant NS-05572.

REFERENCES

1. Antoine, J. C., Avrameas, S., Gonatas, N. K., Stieber, A., and Gonatas, J. O. (1974): Plasma membrane and internalized immunoglobulins of lymph node cells studied with conjugates of antibody or its Fab fragments with horseradish peroxidase. *J. Cell Biol., 63*:12–23.
2. Avrameas, S., and Ternynck, T. (1971): Peroxidase labeled antibody and Fab conjugates with enhanced intracellular penetration. *Immunochemistry, 8*:1175–1179.
3. Chalazonitis, A., and Greene, A. L. (1974): Enhancement in excitability properties of mouse neuroblastoma cells cultured in the presence of dibutyryl cyclic AMP. *Brain Res., 72*:340–345.
4. Farquhar, M. (1978): Recovery of surface membrane in anterior pituitary cells. Variations in traffic detected with anionic and cationic ferritin. *J. Cell Biol., 77*:R35–R42.
5. Gonatas, N. K., and Avrameas, S. (1973): Detection of plasma membrane carbohydrates with lectin peroxidase conjugates. *J. Cell Biol., 59*:436–443.
6. Gonatas, N. K., Kim, S. U., Stieber, A., and Avrameas, S. (1977): Internalization of lectins in neuronal GERL. *J. Cell Biol., 73*:1–13.
7. Gonatas, N. K., Stieber, A., Kim, S. U., Graham, S. I., and Avrameas, S. (1975): Internalization of neuronal plasma membrane ricin receptors into the Golgi apparatus. *Exp. Cell Res., 94*:426–431.
8. Graham, D. I., Gonatas, N. K., and Charalampous, F. C. (1974): The undifferentiated and extended forms of C-1300 murine neuroblastoma. *Am. J. Pathol., 76*:285–306.
9. Graham, R. C., Jr., and Karnovsky, M. K. (1966): The early stages of absorption of injected horseradish peroxidase in the proximal tubules of mouse kidney: Ultrastructural cytochemistry by a new technique. *J. Histochem. Cytochem., 14*:291–302.
10. Haffka, S. C., and Seeds, N. (1975): Neuroblastoma: The *E. coli* of neurobiology. *Life Sci., 16*:1649–1658.
11. Herzog, I., and Farquhar, M. (1977): Luminal membrane retrieved after exocytosis reaches most Golgi cisternae in secretory cells. *Proc. Natl. Acad. Sci. U.S.A., 74*:5073–5077.
12. Joseph, K. C., Kim, S. U., Stieber, A., and Gonatas, N. K. (1978): Endocytosis of cholera toxin into neuronal GERL. *Proc. Natl. Acad. Sci. U.S.A., 75*:2815–2819.
13. Joseph, K. C., Stieber, A., and Gonatas, N. K. (1979): Endocytosis of cholera toxin in GERL-like structures of murine neuroblastoma cells pretreated with GM_1 ganglioside. *J. Cell Biol., 81*:543–554.
14. Novikoff, A. B., and Novikoff, P. M. (1977): Cytochemical contributions to differentiating GERL from the Golgi apparatus. *Histochem. J., 9*:525–551.
15. Prasad, K. N., and Hsie, A. W. (1971): Morphologic differentiation of mouse neuroblastoma cells induced in vitro by dibutyryl adenosine 3':5'-cyclic monophosphate. *Nature, 233*:141–142.
16. Revoltella, R., Bertolini, L., Pediconi, M., and Vigneti, E. (1974): Specific binding of nerve growth factor (NGF) by murine C-1300 neuroblastoma cells. *J. Exp. Med., 140*:437–451.

17. Schachner, M., and Wortham, K. A. (1975): Nervous system antigen-3 (NS-3). An antigenic cell surface component expressed on neuroblastoma C-1300. *Brain Res.,* 99:201–208.
18. Silverstein, S. C., Steinman, R. M., Cohn, Z. A. (1977): Endocytosis. *Annu. Rev. Biochem.,* 46:669–722.
19. Van Heyningen, S. (1974): Cholera toxin interactions of subunits with ganglioside GM_1. *Science,* 183:656–657.

Advances in Neuroblastoma Research,
edited by Audrey E. Evans.
Raven Press, New York © 1980.

Discussion: Cell Differentiation

Dr. Ross (Ithaca) asked Dr. Rajewsky if the mechanism of carcinogenesis which varies with the time of gestation could be due to development of a blood-brain barrier, and Dr. Rajewsky offered some data against this explanation.

Dr. Seeger (Los Angeles) asked Dr. Ross whether the discordant expression of neurotransmitter could be based on variations in a normal cell or was a reflection of tumorigenicity. Dr. Ross hypothesized several possibilities: that variations in enzymes could be natural phenotypic variations or that they could be a result of the culture techniques.

Dr. Danon (Los Angeles) asked Dr. Prasad to clarify the connections between differentiation and cell cycle. Dr. Prasad said it was possible to induce morphological differentiation without inhibiting cell division.

Dr. Danon asked Dr. Rajewsky to comment more on the specificity of the carcinogen studied and why the majority of the tumors in the rats are of brain origin. Dr. Rajewsky responded that at the time of carcinogen pulse the neuronal differentiation in the brain is a bit earlier than the glial, so that there is a numerical excess of glial precursors as compared to neuronal precursors in sensitive stages. He also speculated that the neuronal cells might be closer to differentiation than the corresponding glial precursors at the time of the pulse.

There followed a discussion among *Dr. Anderson (Denver), Dr. Imashuku (Memphis),* and *Dr. Littauer (Israel)* regarding the extent to which answers in the mouse neuroblastoma model can be extrapolated to human neuroblastoma lines. Dr. Littauer emphasized the complexity of the problem. The mouse model has been established as neuroblastoma-like cells which under certain conditions can be induced to differentiate. In the case of the human neuroblastoma, we are faced with a variety of tumors with different properties. He referred to the studies reported by Dr. Glick which showed that some human cell lines are already differentiated to start with and do not need inducing agents to express some of the biochemical properties. Other cell lines may be blocked and unable to express one or all of the differentiated functions. In such cases the rationale of attacking cells by agents that induce differentiation may fail, and it is important to bear in mind that of the variety of tumors found in man, only some will be comparable to the mouse model.

Dr. Hayes (Memphis) pointed out that human cell lines are excellent models for some studies since most of them are drug resistant and induction of differentiation can be studied in some. She noted that Dr. Anderson's findings that prostaglandin can induce differentiation *in vivo* should be emphasized. She commented on the fact that clinically neuroblastoma has been seen to differentiate into ganglioneuroma.

Dr. Benedict (Los Angeles) observed that terminology presents a problem in discussing "differentiation." It is important to determine whether people are talking about morphologic changes, specific enzyme changes, or cell membrane changes, and none of these may have any relationship to the clinical development of ganglioneuroma. He observed that the so-called differentiated cells that have been described have never reached the stage of terminal differentiation: all are still viable and able to divide. Dr. Littauer agreed that no one, to his knowledge, has found a method by which terminal (or irreversible) differentiation can be induced. He also commented that we do not have a clear picture as to which specific biochemical markers are associated with this process.

Dr. Castor (Philadelphia) asked Dr. Bottenstein if the addition of polylysine onto the culture dish and fibronectin to the medium is necessary only for a brief period at the beginning when the cells are added to synthetic medium, and she said this was so. When the medium is changed subsequently no more fibronectin is added. She commented further that the polylysine coating and fibronectin are required at every stage of subculture. Dr. Littauer asked her if she had correlated any selective responses of PC12 cells. Dr. Bottenstein replied that she had done so, but had not included them in her presentation because they are not strictly neuronal cells. They also grow in serum-free media as long as the basal medium is DME only; she added, for those not familiar with these cells, that they are derived from an adrenomedullary tumor and will proliferate in serum-containing medium in the absence of nerve growth factor (NGF). When NGF is added they stop dividing, extend the processes, and synthesize neurotransmitter enzymes. Although they will grow in the serum-free defined medium, they grow better in serum-containing medium. The addition of NGF did produce neurite extension. She responded to Dr. Prasad's question regarding the effect of prostaglandin or dopamine that PGD_2 and PGE_2 were cytotoxic in the concentrations used. These cells were much more sensitive to the prostaglandin in the absence of the serum than when in a serum-containing medium.

Dr. Rajewsky (Germany) asked Dr. Bottenstein if she could discuss the success of inducing primary explants in serum-free medium. Dr. Bottenstein replied that she plans to culture primary neuroblastomas but has not yet done so.

Dr. Schlesinger (Philadelphia) commented that he had attempted on several occasions to culture tumors from bone marrow or primary neuroblastomas in the serum-free medium, but had so far been unsuccessful.

Dr. LaBrosse (Baltimore) asked Dr. Prasad if he had studied cyclophosphamide in his cell system, and Dr. Prasad said that he had not because of its requirement for liver enzyme activation.

Dr. Reynolds (Dallas) expressed concerns regarding comparative studies of neuroblastoma and ganglioneuroma since he believed that neuroblastomas are composed mostly of tumor cells whereas ganglioneuromas and sympathetic ganglia have a degree of stroma such as glia and fibroblasts. A member of the audience commented that most of the stroma of ganglioneuroma is composed of the fibrillary nerve processes. It was agreed, however, that fresh tumor tissue, ganglioneuroma, and neuroblastoma tissue from different stages and ages had to be examined in addition to the neuroblastoma cell lines.

Immunology

Advances in Neuroblastoma Research,
edited by Audrey E. Evans.
Raven Press, New York © 1980.

Expression of Fetal Antigens by Human Neuroblastoma Cells

Robert C. Seeger, *Yehuda L. Danon, **Paul M. Zeltzer, Jack E. Maidman, and Sylvia A. Rayner

Department of Pediatrics, UCLA School of Medicine, Los Angeles, California 90024; and Department of Obstetrics and Gynecology, Charles R. Drew Postgraduate Medical School, Los Angeles, California 90059

A number of cell surface antigens (CSAs) of neuroblastomas also are expressed by cells in mature brain (1,3,9,12); however, only one has been described which is associated with cells in fetal but not adult brain (7,8). Because of their relatively restricted expression, fetal antigens potentially have advantages over antigens expressed by postnatal cells for immunodiagnosis and immunotherapy. Also, fetal antigens may provide markers for the phase of differentiation where malignant transformation occurred. Therefore, we are seeking to define neuroblastoma-associated CSAs which are expressed by fetal cells. In this chapter we report three CSAs which are expressed only in fetal tissues; one is expressed in many fetal tissues and two are limited to fetal brain. Because the latter are expressed by both neoplastic cells and fetal neural cells, they are termed fetal onconeural antigens. In addition to these CSAs, we describe a fourth new neuroblastoma-associated antigen that is associated with cells of both fetal and adult brain.

MATERIALS AND METHODS

Three CSAs were identified using a rabbit antiserum raised against human first trimester fetal brain. It was raised by three subcutaneous injections at weekly intervals of a homogenate of three first trimester fetal brains in complete Freund's adjuvant; the fetuses were 10 to 11 weeks fertilization age, 30 to 48 gm, and 8 to 9 cm crown-rump length. Fetuses were the products of abortions induced with prostaglandin for medical reasons; informed consents were obtained for use of all abortuses. The antiserum was heat inactivated and then absorbed until activity against adult brain, lung, liver, kidney, skin, and muscle tissues, lymphocytes, erythrocytes, and fetal calf serum was removed (12,16).

The fourth CSA was defined with monoclonal antibody C10.115, which was

---

* Present address: Department of Pediatrics, Beilinson Hospital, Petah Tikva, Israel.
** Present address: Department of Pediatrics, University of Texas, San Antonio, Texas.

prepared by fusing spleen cells from Balb/c mice injected with LA-N-1 human neuroblastoma cells with S194/5.XXO.BU.1 Balb/c myeloma cells. Details of fusion with polyethylene glycol and selection of antibody-producing lymphocyte hybridomas have been reported (10,15).

Binding of antibodies to CSA was determined with the 131 I-staphylococcal protein A (131 I-SpA) binding assay as previously described (16). Briefly, antiserum or antibody was incubated with 125 I-iododeoyxyuridine-labeled target cells, nonbound antibodies were removed by washing, 131 I-SpA was added, and nonbound 131 I-SpA was removed by washing. Counts per minute (cpm) of bound 131 I-SpA were determined, and the cpm bound per 5 μg of target cell protein or per 3×10^5 target cells was calculated.

Specificity of antibody reactivity was determined directly with the 131 I-SpA binding test using panels of cultured or fresh cells and indirectly by absorbing antiserum or antibody, centrifuging the absorbent and then retesting the nonabsorbed supernatant against LA-N-1 neuroblastoma cells. Details of cell lines, absorbents, and absorption procedures have been reported (12).

RESULTS

Neuroblastoma CSAs Defined by Anti-First Trimester Fetal Brain Serum

Considerable reactivity with LA-N-1 neuroblastoma cells remained after the rabbit antiserum was absorbed with normal adult tissues and cells including brain. In three 131 I-SpA binding tests, there were 4,421 ± 348, 3,937 ± 351, and 7,082 ± 287 cpm bound per 5 μg LA-N-1 protein. To determine if CSAs on LA-N-1 cells recognized by this serum were limited to fetal brain, it was further absorbed with first trimester brain, liver, lung, kidney, muscle, and intestine (Table 1). Three sequential absorptions with fetal brain (the immunogen) removed 82% and with non-neural tissues removed 43 to 47% of anti-LA-N-1 activity. This indicated that LA-N-1 cells have fetal antigens that are common to both fetal brain and non-neural tissues and others that are unique to fetal brain. For subsequent studies, antibodies directed against non-neural fetal antigens were removed by absorption with first trimester liver, muscle, and kidney. The resulting antiserum recognized antigens on LA-N-1 cells that were expressed by fetal brain alone (i.e., fetal neural antigens).

The expression of fetal neural antigens by noncultured neuroblastomas and other tumors was determined using absorptions tests (Table 2). Absorption of the antiserum and then retesting of it on LA-N-1 cells demonstrated that 10 of 12 neuroblastomas and 1 of 1 leiomyosarcoma removed more than 65% of reactivity. The neuroblastomas were obtained from patients with localized or metastatic disease, indicating that expression of antigen(s) was independent of the stage of disease. Of 29 other tumors tested, 22 removed 35 to 65% and seven removed less than 35% of antibody activity.

To determine if neuroblastomas expressed a fetal neural antigen that was

TABLE 1. *Absorption of anti-first trimester brain serum with first trimester tissues[a]*

First trimester absorbent[a]	% of anti-LA-N-1 activity removed
Brain	82
Liver	47
Lung	46
Kidney	46
Muscle	43
Intestine	46

[a] Antiserum was preabsorbed with adult non-neural and neural tissues until it was nonreactive with them. This preabsorbed antiserum (1/100 dilution) still reacted with LA-N-1 neuroblastoma cells to give $3,937 \pm 351$ CPM (mean $\pm$ SD) per 5 μg LA-N-1 protein. Data are from a representative experiment.

[b] Each absorbent (100 mg wet weight for 0.4 ml of a 1/100 dilution of the antiserum) was used 3 times, and values for all tissues except brain represent complete removal of activity against that absorbent. Adult liver and kidney homogenate (negative control) did not remove activity.

different from that expressed by the non-neuroblastoma tumors, activity against the latter was removed by absorption. Activity against LA-N-1 still remained which could be removed by absorption with noncultured neuroblastoma cells (Table 3). Thus LA-N-1 cells express one fetal neural antigen(s) which is common to neuroblastomas and some non-neuroblastoma tumors and another which is limited to neuroblastomas.

TABLE 2. *Absorption of anti-first trimester brain serum with tumor homogenates[a]*

	No. tumors removing anti-LA-N-1 activity % activity removed		
Tumor absorbent[b]	65–85	35–65	0–35
Neuroblastoma	10	2	0
Leiomyosarcoma	1	0	0
Rhabdomyosarcoma	0	2	0
Osteogenic sarcoma	0	0	3
Ewing's sarcoma	0	1	0
Wilms' tumor	0	5	1
Renal cell carcinoma	0	1	0
Melanoma	0	3	3
Oat cell carcinoma	0	2	0
Lung adenocarcinoma	0	2	0
Colon adenocarcinoma	0	3	0
Hodgkin's lymphoma	0	2	0
Teratocarcinoma	0	1	0

[a] Antiserum was preabsorbed with adult tissues and cells as in Table 1 and with first trimester liver, muscle, and kidney.

[b] With 100 mg of each tumor homogenate, 0.4 ml of a 1/100 dilution of the antiserum was absorbed once.

TABLE 3. *Sequential absorption of anti-first trimester brain serum with non-neuroblastoma and then neuroblastoma homogenates[a]*

% (cumulative) of anti-LA-N-1 activity removed by absorbent						
One	$\longrightarrow$		Two	$\longrightarrow$		Three
Wilms' tumor[b]	62[c]	Wilms' tumor	65		Neuroblastoma	85
Leiomyosarcoma	69	Leiomyosarcoma	70		Neuroblastoma	87
Colon carcinoma	66	Colon carcinoma	68		Neuroblastoma	91
Melanoma	66	Melanoma	72		Neuroblastoma	85
Rhabdomyosarcoma	70	Rhabdomyosarcoma	74		Neuroblastoma	90
Neuroblastoma	86	Neuroblastoma	90		Neuroblastoma	93

[a] Antiserum was preabsorbed as in Table 2.
[b] Preabsorbed antiserum was diluted 1/100 and then absorbed with 100 mg of homogenate for each 4 μl of undiluted serum. Homogenates of single tumors were used.
[c] Data are mean value for 3 experiments.

The antiserum also was tested against 19 different leukemias. All bound less than 25% as much antibody as LA-N-1 cells; this panel included nine non-T, non-B acute lymphocytic leukemias, seven T acute lymphocytic leukemias, two acute myelogenous leukemias, and one chronic myelogenous leukemia in blast crisis.

Neuroblastoma CSAs Defined with a Monoclonal Antibody

A monoclonal antibody was prepared by fusing S194/5.XXO.BU.1 myeloma cells with spleen cells from mice immunized with LA-N-1 neuroblastoma cells. A lymphocyte hybridoma which produced antibodies reacting with LA-N-1 cells was cloned by limiting dilution, and the antibody produced by one clone, C10.115, was studied. C10.115 antibodies reacted with LA-N-1 cells and equally well with three other human neuroblastoma cell lines (Table 4). Four other neuroblastoma cell lines also expressed the antigen recognized by this antibody but to a lesser extent since they bound 35 to 59% as much antibody as did LA-N-1 cells. Eighteen non-neuroblastoma cell lines consistently bound less antibody than all neuroblastoma cell lines except CHP-100. The average ($\pm$ 1 SD) amount of antibody bound by these 18 cell lines was 22 $\pm$ 11% of that bound by LA-N-1; three cell lines bound 36 to 42% as much antibody as LA-N-1 cells. These data suggest that the antigen defined by C10.115 antibody is expressed in greatest quantity on neuroblastoma cells but that it can be expressed to a lesser extent by a few non-neuroblastoma tumor cells.

C10.115 antibody also was tested against leukemia and lymphoma cells (Table 5). The antibody reacted significantly with T cell acute lymphocytic leukemia cells from one patient and with two of three T cell acute lymphocytic leukemia cell lines. However, it reacted minimally with T chronic lymphocytic leukemia,

TABLE 4. *Reactivity of C10.115 monoclonal antibody with tumor cell lines*

Cell	Reactivity (%)[a]	Cell	Reactivity (%)
Neuroblastoma		Osteogenic sarcoma	
LA-N-1	100	MT	15
LA-N-2	121	HT-1080	16
LA-N-4	59	Rhabdomyosarcoma	
CHP-100	35	RD	17
CHP-134	138	Leiomyosarcoma	
IMR-32	86	UCLA-SO-S1	16
SK-N-SH	51	Melanoma	
SK-N-MC	49	UCLA-SO-M7	29
Medulloblastoma		UCLA-SO-M10	15
TE-671	8	UCLA-SO-M14	24
Glioma		UCLA-SO-M20	29
U-251 MG	12	Colon carcinoma	
D-54 MG	26	SK-CO-1	36
A-172 MG	42	HT-29	11
Transitional cell			
cancer bladder		Teratoma	
T24	18	Tera 1	31
J82	42	Squamous cell carcinoma of lung	
		SK-MES-1	9

[a] Undiluted supernatant of C10.115 lymphocyte hybridoma was tested on adherent cells using the 131 I-SpA binding assay. Reactivity (%) = cpm 131 I-SpA per 5 μg target cell protein/ cpm 131 I-SpA per 5 μg LA-N-1 protein ×100. Data are means for 2–4 experiments. cpm (mean ± SD) 131 I-SpA per 5 μg LA-N-1 protein were 1,745 ± 245, 1,242 ± 441, 309 ± 40, and 3,661 ± 387 for the 4 experiments.

TABLE 5. *Reactivity of C10.115 monoclonal antibody with leukemia and lymphoma cells*

Cell[a]	Reactivity (%)[b]	Cell	Reactivity (%)
Neuroblastoma		ALL, T cell	
LA-N-1	100	Patient 1	46
ALL; non-T, non-B cell		CCRF-CEM	190
Patient 1	20	CCRF-HSB-2	145*
2	3	RPMI 8402	1*
3	17	CLL, T cell	
4	7	Patient 1	7*
5	14*	Lymphoma, T cell	
REH	29*	Patient 1	21*
AML		Patient 2	4*
Patient 1	15*		
2	18*		
3	0*		

[a] ALL, acute lymphocytic leukemia; AML, acute myelogenous leukemia; CLL, chronic lymphocytic leukemia.
[b] Undiluted C10.115 supernatant was tested on cells in suspension using the 131 I-SpA binding assay. Reactivity (%) = cpm 131 I-SpA per 3 × 105 target cells/cpm 131 I-SpA per 3 × 105 LA-N-1 cells × 100. Data are means of 2 experiments or are from a single experiment (*). 131 I-SpA bound per 3 × 105 LA-N-1 cells was 1,823 ± 462 and 2,216 cpm.

T lymphoma, non-T, non-B acute lymphocytic leukemia, and acute myelogenous leukemia cells. Studies of additional lymphoma and leukemia cells are in progress which will more completely define cell types expressing this antigen.

The C10.115 monoclonal antibody has been tested against some normal cells and tissues. It did not react with erythrocytes or normal peripheral blood lymphocytes in direct binding tests. In absorption tests, homogenates (100 mg) of first trimester and adult brain removed 98% and 94%, respectively, of anti-LA-N-1 activity. Studies are in progress which will further define the distribution of this antigen among normal cells and tissues.

DISCUSSION

This chapter describes new CSAs which are expressed by both neuroblastoma cells and first trimester fetal cells. Three CSAs were defined using an exhaustively absorbed rabbit anti-first trimester fetal brain serum. The first of these CSAs is expressed by LA-N-1 neuroblastoma cells, fetal brain, and many other non-neural fetal tissues (general fetal antigen). The expression of the second and third of these tumor-associated CSAs is limited in first trimester tissues to brain; therefore, they are termed fetal onconeural antigens (FONAs). One of these antigens (FONA-1) is expressed by neuroblastoma and other types of tumor cells, whereas the other (FONA-2) is limited to neuroblastoma cells. The fourth new CSA is defined by C10.115 monoclonal antibody and is expressed by neuroblastoma, T cell acute lymphocytic leukemia, and fetal and adult brain cells. The distribution of this CSA in fetal and adult tissues and cells has not yet been completely determined; however, it is not expressed by erythrocytes and normal peripheral blood lymphocytes.

The antigens we have described can be distinguished from two other neuroblastoma CSAs which also are expressed by fetal neural cells (Table 6). Kennett and Gilbert (7) recently defined a CSA with PI 153/3 monoclonal antibody that is expressed by neuroblastoma and retinoblastoma cells and by fetal but not adult brain cells. This antigen also is on non-T, non-B, and B acute lymphocytic leukemia and B chronic lymphocytic leukemia cells (8). The general fetal, FONA-1, FONA-2, and C10.115 CSAs we describe are not expressed by these types of leukemia cells. Casper et al. (3) defined with a rabbit antiserum a CSA termed HB that is expressed by both fetal and adult brain cells, neuroblastoma, rhabdomyosarcoma, and Wilms' tumor cells. This CSA is not on T acute lymphocytic leukemia cells. Although not formally proven, HB antigen may be the same as the onconeural antigen we have described previously (12).

The CSAs described also are distinct from other fetal antigens which have been associated with neoplastic cells. Carcinofetal ferritin is associated with cultured and non-cultured neuroblastoma cells and also with placental and fetal liver cells (4,6). The antiserum that defines FONA-1 and FONA-2 is nonreactive with fetal liver. Some patients with neuroblastoma have been reported to have moderately elevated serum carcinoembryonic antigen (CEA) (5), but recent studies have shown this to be CEA-like activity due to nonspecific cross-reacting antigen (NCA) (14). NCA is in normal adult lung, with which the antiserum defining general fetal antigen, FONA-1, and FONA-2 was nonreactive. Alpha-fetoprotein (AFP) has not been reported to be associated with neuroblastoma cells; in addition, the serum defining FONA-1 and FONA-2 did not react with fetal liver which contains AFP (13).

Our investigations and those of others have defined multiple antigens on human neuroblastoma cells which tentatively can be categorized according to their expression by normal cells (Table 6). One group of CSAs apparently is limited to fetal neural tissues and thus may be fetal specific neural differentiation antigens (FONA-1, FONA-2, and PI 153/3). This conclusion is a qualified one, however, since expression of antigens in normal tissues was defined with absorption and isotope binding tests which provide information about populations of cells but not about individual cells. Conceivably, a minor population of cells in mature brain or other tissues could express antigens which are present in relatively large quantities in fetal brain; tests of single cells are necessary to define such a population. A second set of antigens are general fetal antigens;

TABLE 6. *Human neuroblastoma cell surface antigens*

	Cells/tissue expressing antigen	
Antigen	Tumor	Normal
PI 153/3[b]	Neuroblastoma, retinoblastoma, B ALL, B CLL, non-T, non-B ALL	Fetal brain
FONA-1[a]	Neuroblastoma, rhabdomyosarcoma, Wilms' tumor, oat cell carcinoma, colon adenocarcinoma, teratocarcinoma	Fetal brain
FONA-2[a]	Neuroblastoma	Fetal brain
General fetal antigen[a]	Neuroblastoma, rhabdomyosarcoma, Wilms' tumor, oat cell carcinoma, colon adenocarcinoma, teratocarcinoma	Fetal brain, liver, lung, kidney, muscle, intestine
HB[a]	Neuroblastoma, rhabdomyosarcoma, Wilms' tumor	Adult and fetal brain
C10.115[b]	Neuroblastoma, T ALL	Adult and fetal brain
MBA-2[a,dc]	Neuroblastoma	Adult brain and kidney
INMA[a,d]	Neuroblastoma	Adult brain
ONA[a]	Neuroblastoma, oat cell carcinoma, Wilms' tumor, sarcoma	Adult brain

[a] Detected by heteroantisera.
[b] Detected by monoclonal antibodies.
[c] First trimester fetal tissue in all cases except that used to characterize PI 153/3.
[d] Interspecies antigen.

their expression is extinguished in mature tissues. The same qualification holds for these antigens as for fetal specific neural differentiation antigens. A third category of antigens are expressed by fetal neural cells and continue to be expressed by adult neural cells (HB and C10.115).

A fourth group of antigens may be expressed by adult but not fetal neural cells. Although not yet demonstrated for humans, some murine neural antigens are limited to adult brain (2,11). Highly differentiated ganglioneuroma cells may be more likely than neuroblastoma cells to express such adult specific neural antigens. MBA-2 (9), INMA (1), and ONA (12) are on adult human neural cells, but additional experiments with fetal tissues are necessary to determine if they are adult specific. A final group of antigens that has been demonstrated with heteroantisera is expressed by various adult cell types and tissues. Antibodies against these general antigens that also are on neuroblastoma cells have been demonstrated by absorption tests with lung, liver, kidney, skin, muscle, lymphocytes, and erythrocytes. These antigens may be on normal fetal and adult cells or on only adult cells.

The phenotype defined for neuroblastoma cells by CSAs may be that of appropriate counterpart normal cells. Alternatively, some CSAs may be inappropriately expressed due to derepression or increased expression of normal genes in the neoplastic cell. One approach to resolving these possibilities will be to examine the CSA phenotype of cells in the adrenal medulla, sympathetic ganglia, and brain of fetuses and adults.

Neuroblastoma CSAs which also are expressed by neural cells, whether fetal or adult, provide opportunities for immunodiagnosis and possibly immunotherapy. Monoclonal antibodies such as C10.115 and PI 153/3 allow clear serological and biochemical definition of CSAs. Potentially, these antibodies are powerful reagents for use in differential diagnostic tests, in phenotyping tumor cells for prognostication, in monitoring disease state with immunoassays for soluble antigens or for single cells, and in localizing tumors with radionuclide scanning. There may be immunotherapeutic uses for monoclonal antibodies directed against neuroblastoma CSAs. These antibodies may mediate complement or effector cell dependent cytotoxicity. They may be used to target cytotoxic agents such as isotopes, drugs, and toxins. Finally, if directed against appropriate determinants, noncytotoxic monoclonal antibodies may be able to effect the expression of neoplastic properties by tumor cells.

SUMMARY

Four new neuroblastoma CSAs are described which also are expressed by first trimester fetal cells. The first three of these CSAs were defined with exhaustively absorbed rabbit anti-first trimester fetal brain serum. One CSA is expressed by LA-N-1 neuroblastoma cells, fetal brain, and many other non-neural fetal tissues. The second and third CSAs are limited in first trimester tissues to brain and, therefore, are termed fetal onconeural antigens. One of these antigens

(FONA-1) is expressed by neuroblastoma and other types of tumor cells and the other (FONA-2) is limited to neuroblastoma cells. The fourth new CSA is defined by C10.115 monoclonal antibody and is expressed by neuroblastoma, T cell acute lymphocytic leukemia, and fetal and adult brain cells.

ACKNOWLEDGMENTS

This research was supported by Grant CA22794 awarded by the National Cancer Institute, DHEW. R.C.S. is the recipient of Research Career Development Award CA00069 from the National Cancer Institute, DHEW. Y.L.D. is the recipient of International Research Fellowship TW02565, awarded by the National Institute of Health, DHEW, and is a Fulbright Scholar. We thank Mr. F. Hoover for technical assistance.

REFERENCES

1. Akeson, R., and Seeger, R. C. (1977): Interspecies neural membrane antigens on cultured human and murine neuroblastoma cells. *J. Immunol.,* 118:1995–2003.
2. Bock, E. (1978): Nervous system specific proteins. *J. Neurochem.,* 30:7–14.
3. Casper, J. T., Borella, L., and Sen, L. (1977): Reactivity of human brain antiserum with neuroblastoma cells and nonreactivity with thymocytes and lymphoblasts. *Cancer Res.,* 37:1750–1756.
4. Drysdale, J. W., and Alpert, E. (1975): Carcinofetal human isoferritins. *Ann. N.Y. Acad. Sci.,* 259:427–434.
5. Frens, D. B., Bray, P. F., Wu, J. T., and Lahey, M. E. (1976): The carcinoembryonic antigen assay: Prognostic value in neural crest tumors. *J. Pediatr.,* 88:591–594.
6. Hann, H. L., Levy, H. M., Evans, A. E., and Drysdale, J. W. (1979): Serum ferritin and neuroblastoma. *Proc. Am. Assoc. Cancer Res.,* 20:126.
7. Kennett, R. H., and Gilbert, F. (1979): Hybrid myelomas producing antibodies against a human neuroblastoma antigen present on fetal brain. *Science,* 203:1120–1121.
8. Kennett, R. H., Jonak, Z., and Bechtel, K. B. (1979): Characterization of antigens with monoclonal antibodies. *This volume.*
9. Martin, S. E., and Martin, W. J. (1975): Expression by human neuroblastoma cells of an antigen recognized by naturally occurring mouse anti-brain autoantibody. *Cancer Res.,* 35:2609–2612.
10. Nowinski, R. C., Lostrom, M. E., Tam, M. R., Stone, M. R., and Burnette, W. N. (1979): The isolation of hybrid cell lines producing monoclonal antibodies against the P15 (E) protein of ecotropic murine leukemia viruses. *Virology,* 93:111–126.
11. Schachner, M., Wortham, K., and Kincade, P. W. (1976): Detection of nervous-system specific cell surface antigen(s) by heterologous anti-mouse brain serum. *Cell. Immunol.,* 22:369–374.
12. Seeger, R. C., Zeltzer, P. M., and Rayner, S. A. (1979): Onco-neural antigen: A new neural differentiation antigen expressed by neuroblastoma, oat cell carcinoma, Wilms' tumor, and sarcoma cells. *J. Immunol.,* 122:1548–1555.
13. Sell, S., Becker, F. F., Leffert, H. L., and Watalee, H. (1976): Expression of an oncodevelopment gene product (alpha fetoprotein) during fetal development and adult oncogenesis. *Cancer Res.,* 36:4239–4249.
14. Sugimoto, T., Sawada, T., and Kusunoki, T. (1979): Immunologic and biochemical studies on the carcinoembryonic like substance in human neuroblastoma. *Pediatr. Res.,* 13:91–95.
15. Trowbridge, I. S. (1978): Interspecies spleen-myeloma hybrid producing monoclonal antibodies against mouse lymphocyte surface glycoprotein, T 200. *J. Exp. Med.,* 148:313–323.
16. Zeltzer, P. M., and Seeger, R. C. (1977): Microassay using radioiodinated protein A from *Staphylococcus aureus* for antibodies bound to cell surface antigens of adherent tumor cells. *J. Immunol. Methods,* 17:163–175.

Advances in Neuroblastoma Research,
edited by Audrey E. Evans.
Raven Press, New York © 1980.

Characterization of Antigens with Monoclonal Antibodies

*Roger H. Kennett, **Zdenka Jonak, and **Kathleen B. Bechtol

*Department of Human Genetics, University of Pennsylvania School of Medicine; and
**Wistar Institute of Anatomy and Biology, Philadelphia, Pennsylvania 19104*

There is a large volume of evidence supporting the idea that tumor cells express cell surface antigens that are not expressed on the corresponding nonmalignant cells (7,15). On the other hand, there is indication that many of these tumor-associated antigens are actually normal antigens expressed in an abnormal way (Table 1). Until recently analysis of tumor-associated antigens has depended on the production of antisera that react specifically with tumor cells and not with normal cells. Most antisera are complex collections of antibodies of various classes, specificities, and affinities, and it took an extensive amount of work and a large amount of sera to define whether the sera were against a single antigen or several antigens and whether the serum's reactivity with one cell type represented reactivity with the same antigen or set of antigens as did the reactivity with a second cell type. Serologists longed for a way to remove from such a complex antiserum one of the component antibodies reacting with a specific antigenic determinant so that they could work with that reagent apart from all the other background components. This was particularly true of investigators who work with human cells and necessarily inject these cells into other species for the production of antisera. Such an immunization usually resulted in a large amount of antibody against general species differences. These heterospecific antibodies reacting with all human cells had to be removed by absorption before the antibodies reacting specifically with the human cell type of interest could be obtained. In spite of these difficulties, much work was done because of the great potential seen for antibodies which react with tumor cells and not other human cells (Table 2).

It was found that many of the apparently tumor-specific antigens defined by antisera turned out to be after sufficient analysis either differentiation antigens expressed on a small proportion of normal cells represented as an expanded clone by the tumor or fetal antigens that are "re-expressed" in the malignant cell. Often interpretation of the antigen's distribution on different cell types was complicated by the probability that the antisera contained more than a single type of antibody and possibly several antibodies against different antigens.

In 1975 Köhler and Milstein (12) reported a procedure for obtaining a clonal

TABLE 1. *Possible origins of "tumor-specific" antigens*

Origin	References
Viral antigens expressed after active infection	14
Mutation to new cellular gene product	7,15
Normal cellular gene product altered by *interaction* with other cell surface components or uncovered as a result of rearrangement	5
Abnormal expression of *differentiation antigens*	1
or *fetal antigens*	3,11

antibody component of the immune response (Fig. 1). They immunized a mouse with sheep red blood cells (SRBCs) and fused the spleen cells from the immunized mouse with a cultured mouse plasmacytoma line. In the culture conditions employed, only hybrids between the tumor line and the spleen cells survived and grew into colonies. Many of these plasmacytoma hybrids (hybridomas) were making antibody against SRBCs and continued to grow and make antibody which could be collected from the culture supernatant in concentrations on the order of 100 μg/ml. The hybrids could be injected into mice and the tumor-bearing mouse then exhibited concentrations of the antibody produced by the hybrid on the order of 1 mg/ml. Each antibody represented a clonal anti-SRBC antibody response of the cell which was fused with the plasmacytoma. Thus Köhler and Milstein provided with their procedure the coveted mechanism for obtaining, in a purified form, an antibody against a single antigenic determinant apart from the background of immunoglobulins and other antibodies normally found in an antiserum. Many investigators have taken advantage of this observation and have produced hybridomas making antibodies against a wide variety of antigens (13). Among these, antibodies against several human cell types have been reported including human B cells, melanomas, neuroblastomas, and antibodies against specific human cell surface molecules such as a blood group antigen, a human species antigen on chromosome 11, and HLA antigens (9).

TABLE 2. *Potential uses of "tumor-specific" antibodies*

Tumor identification
  Diagnosis
  Detection of metastasis

Specific delivery of covalently bound cytotoxic drugs to tumor cells

Cytolysis of tumor cells

Labeling of cells with fluorescent dye so that they can be separated from normal cells by a fluorescent-activated cell sorter

HYBRIDOMA PRODUCTION

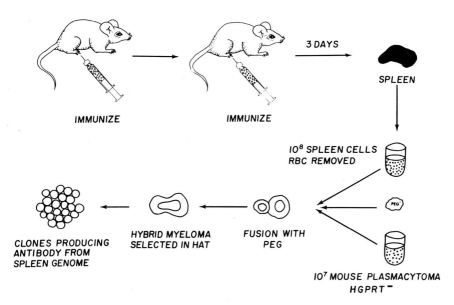

FIG. 1. *Hybridoma production.* Spleen cells from an immunized mouse are fused with a mouse plasmacytoma line. Polyethylene glycol or Sendai virus is used as fusing agent. The fused cells are plated into several wells and grown in hypoxanthine, aminopterin thymidine (HAT) medium. The cell line lacking the enzyme hypoxanthine-guanine-phosphoribosyl transferase (HGPRT) will not grow in this selective medium. The spleen cells have a limited life span in culture and do not form visible colonies. Hybrid cells grow to form visible colonies within 2–3 weeks. Supernatants are tested for antibody, and those hybrids making antibody with the desired specificity are grown and recloned. The monoclonal antibody can then be obtained from the supernatant of these hybrid cells. The cells can also be injected into a mouse and ascites fluid or serum containing the antibody in mg/ml amounts obtained from the mouse (9). (Figure by Kendra Eager).

Because of the increased discrimination and limited specificity of monoclonal antibodies compared to antisera, we have produced monoclonal antibodies against several types of human cell surface antigens including antigens on human neuroblastomas. We will describe here the isolation and characterization of several of these antibodies and discuss how they are useful in the detection of and possibly therapy for human neuroblastoma.

MATERIALS AND METHODS

Cells

As reported previously (10), most of the cultured cell lines were obtained from the Human Genetics Cell Center of the University of Pennsylvania, the Wistar Institute, or Children's Hospital of Philadelphia. REH was obtained from Dr. M. Greaves, University College, London. Acute lymphocytic leukemia (ALL) cells were obtained from Children's Hospital. Chronic lymphocytic leukemia (CLL) cells were obtained from Drs. D. Rowland and P. Nowell, Department of Pathology, University of Pennsylvania. The myeloma line P3X63Ag8 was derived by Dr. C. Milstein (12), SP2/0 by Drs. M. Shulman and G. Köhler (16).

Production of Hybridomas

Hybrid plasmacytomas were produced as reported previously (10). Mice were given two injections of cells treated with a mouse antiserum against human species antigens or two injections of concentrated supernatant from cultured cells. Spleen cells were removed for fusion 3 days after the second injection. The splenic lymphocytes were fused with 10^7 myeloma cells using polyethylene glycol 1000 (Baker) as a fusing agent. Cells were grown in Dulbecco's Modified Eagle's Medium (DMEM) with high glucose plus 10 to 20% calf serum.

Assay of Antibodies—Detection of Antigens

Cytotoxicity and binding assays of antibody in the hybridoma supernatants were done as previously reported (10). For the binding assay the cells to be assayed were incubated with the supernatant and washed twice in medium (DMEM or RPMI 1640) plus 0.5% bovine serum albumin (BSA). Any antibodies which attached to the cells were detected with ^{125}I-rabbit antimouse immunoglobulin (Ig) or by rabbit anti-mouse Ig conjugated to peroxidase (Cappell). In the case where enzyme-linked antibody was used, orthophenyldiamine (Sigma) was used as a substrate at 1 mg/ml in 0.1 M citrate buffer, pH 4.5. Detection of antigen using peroxidase-labeled antibodies and diaminobenzidine (DAB) was carried out by a modification of the procedure reported by Bross et al. (2).

RESULTS AND DISCUSSION

Antineuroblastoma Antibodies

We have reported previously the production of monoclonal antibodies against the human neuroblastoma IMR6. One of these antibodies, PI153/3, reacts with human neuroblastomas, retinoblastomas, a glioblastoma, fetal brain, and none of the several other cell types tested including adult brain (11). Table 3 shows the reactivity of PI153/3 with various fetal tissues.

With this specificity in mind, we began to screen for neuroblastoma in the marrow of neuroblastoma patients with the intention of being able to detect tumor cells. This is particularly important when marrow is being assessed for the presence of tumor cells prior to its harvest and preservation for future therapy. Even in those cases where neuroblastomas are detected, it is potentially

TABLE 3. *Reaction of PI153/3 antibody with fetal tissues*

Fetal tissue	Specific cpm 125I anti-fab bound
Brain	21,394
Adrenal	1,244
Liver	797
Pancreas	179
Thymus	165
Spleen	942
Testis	—
Kidney	787
BJAB-cells	—
IMR-6 neuroblastoma	6,005

Tissues were homogenized gently and equivalent packed cell volumes incubated with PI153/3 supernatant. Bound antibody was detected with 125I anti-mouse Fab. 500–1,000 cpm background was subtracted from each. No counts indicate nothing bound above this background.

possible to use the antibody to remove the tumor cells from the bone marrow either by taking advantage of the cytolytic property in the presence of complement or by using it to fluorescently label the cells and remove them from the marrow using a fluorescent-activated cell sorter (FACS) (8).

We determined that by treating the marrow cells with the PI153/3 antibody and then peroxidase-linked antimouse Ig followed by DAB and osmium tetraoxide, we could detect cells expressing this antigen by a dense black precipitate at the membrane. Control marrow samples taken from two marrow transplant donors showed no labeled cells, nor did neuroblastoma marrows without addition of the specific PI153/3 antibody. The cells identified were larger and often appeared in clumps and thus confirmed that the cells characterized as neuroblastomas in the marrow of patients thought to be positive for metastasis actually are neuroblastomas expressing the oncofetal antigen detected by the monoclonal antibody PI153/3 (Fig. 2). In addition, we could also occasionally detect large single cells also expressing the antigen which using standard methods of visualization would have gone undetected.

The Antigenic Determinant Detected by PI153/3 Is Expressed on Immature Lymphocytes and Some Leukemias

As we screened more bone marrow samples, we began to observe that occasionally some samples showed a significant number of small cells labeled. Also, a non-Hodgkin's lymphoma marrow was found to have a significant number of large cells that were labeled and thus expressed the antigen. Another monoclonal

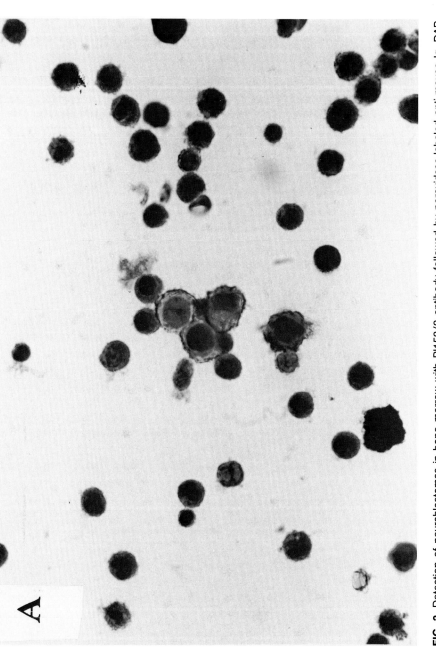

FIG. 2. Detection of neuroblastomas in bone marrow with Pl153/3 antibody followed by peroxidase-labeled anti-mouse Ig, DAB, and OsO₄. Cells expressing the antigen show a dark precipitate around the cell (A). Controls without Pl153/3 or with another antibody of the same class (IgM) show no precipitates (B).

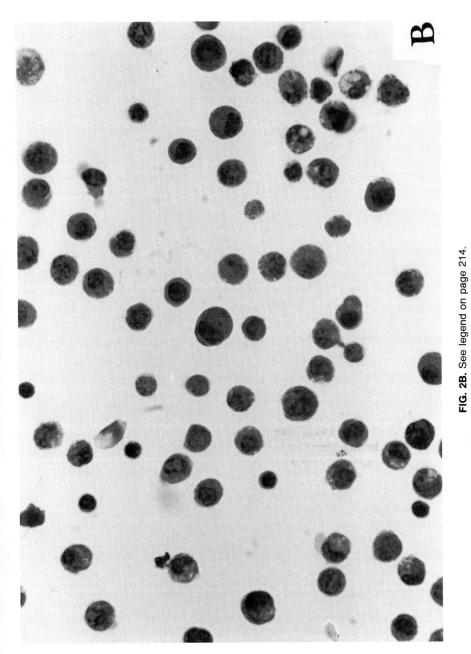

FIG. 2B. See legend on page 214.

antibody of the same class (IgM) made against a mouse antigen on mouse neuroblastoma 1300 was used in place of PI153/3, and in no case were any labeled cells detected.

We then screened peripheral blood from several leukemia patients and found that several ALL and CLL patients had cells which reacted with PI153/3 (Table 4). This led us to postulate that the antigen detected by PI153/3, in addition to being suppressed in fetal brain and tumors derived from neural crest cells, is also expressed on some form of immature lymphocyte. We checked for the expression of this antigen on REH, a cell line derived from a null cell leukemia patient. This cell line, like many of the peripheral blood cells from null ALL patients, reacted with PI153/3. This leaves us with the question of whether the same antigen is present on both types of cells or whether two different antigens, a neuroblastoma-oncofetal antigen and a lymphocyte differentiation antigen, share a common antigenic determinant recognized by the mouse. The second possibility could result, for example, from the same specific antigenic sugar sequence being attached to two different glycoproteins or from the same antigenic three-dimensional array of amino acids being present in two different proteins. Which of these possibilities exists here can be defined only by continuation of the work of Drs. Momoi and Glick, who have begun to characterize the antigen present on neuroblastoma and fetal brain (see p. 177, *this volume*).

The ability to distinguish early lymphocytes or lymphoblasts from neuroblasts is particularly important since it has been reported that in some children with

TABLE 4. *Cytolylic reactivity of monoclonal antibodies against leukemia peripheral blood*

	Cells	PI153/3	P3B13C2
REH	Null ALL line	+	+
ALL-1	Null ALL	+	+
ALL-2	T-ALL	−	−
ALL-3	Null-ALL	+	+
ALL-4	Null-ALL	+	+
ALL-5	Null-ALL	−	−
ALL-6	Null-ALL	−	−
ALL-7	B-ALL	+	+
CLL-259		−	−
CLL-248	B	+	+
CLL-262	T	−	−
CLL-253	B	−	−
CLL-249	B	+	+
AML-1	Monocytic AML	−	+

Cytolytic activity of monoclonal antibodies PI153/3 and P3B13C2 against leukemia cells. Cells were incubated with the antibodies and then rabbit serum added as a C' source. Viability was determined by phase microscopy and then trypan blue dye exclusion. P3B13C2 reacts with 20–30% of normal peripheral blood lymphocytes (B cells). PI153/3 reacts with no detectable normal peripheral blood lymphocytes. P3B13C2 + > 50%; PI153/3 + > 20%.

neuroblastoma the bone marrow may be infiltrated with primitive lymphocytes which could be mistaken for primitive neuroblasts (6).

Antileukemia Antibodies

In parallel with the antineuroblastoma antibodies, we have produced monoclonal antibodies against leukemia cells and against human B cells. Our initial studies have resulted in obtaining antibodies against two different antigens which have bearing on our study of neuroblastoma antigens (Table 5): (a) two of these antibodies react with the same cell types as our original PI153/3, confirming that there is an antigenic determinant in common; (b) the second type of antibody reacts with the leukemia cells that react with PI153/3 and also reacts with human B cells. P3B13C2, which has this pattern of reactivity, has been shown to react specifically with human immune response associated antigens which are expressed on B cells, B cell precursors, and null cells (10).

The use of this second type (anti-Ia) of antibody against a human lymphocyte differentiation antigen allows us to distinguish between lymphocytes which express the PI153/3 antigen and tumor cells such as neuroblastomas which express the antigen. Thus when cells expressing the neuroblastoma antigen are detected by peroxidase-linked antibody assay in bone marrow, we will determine whether they are lymphocytes by using a fluorescein-linked antibody against the lymphocyte antigen to determine whether or not the cell is a lymphocyte.

In principle, this will also work for removal of cells by the FACS. If one of the antibodies is labeled with rhodamine and the second with fluorescein, sorting of cells on the basis of two colors will allow discrimination of neuroblastoma cells from lymphocytes because the lymphocytes will be labeled with both fluorescent dyes. Whether the PI153/3 would be effective in removing neuroblastoma by its cytolytic effect or effective in delivering covalently linked drugs to the tumor cells (4) would depend on the possible detrimental effects of deleting from the lymphocyte population those cells reacting with PI153/3 at any given time. Such questions could best be asked in a mouse model using the C1300 neuroblastoma, and it is with this in mind that we have begun to produce monoclonal antibodies against this tumor and to define their reactivity with other mouse cell lines and primary cell types.

The results with these monoclonal antibodies do raise some general questions about tumor antigens that are both interesting and of practical importance. The first is the question of whether tumor-specific antigens actually do exist. It is of course difficult and often impossible to assay for the presence of the antigen on all possible types of normal cells—both fetal and adult. The real question becomes: Is the antigen present on normal cells that are present in significant quantities when the antibody will be used to react specifically with the tumor cells for either detection or therapy?

We consider the production of monoclonal antibodies against specific human tumors and differentiated cell types as the approach which for the moment

TABLE 5. *Reactivity of monoclonal antibodies with different human cell types*

Antibody	Immunizing cell	Reactivity = cytotoxicity and binding activity						
		IMR6 neuroblastomas	REH null ALL	B-cell lines	T-cell lines	Fibroblasts	HT/080 fibrosarcoma	SK Hep hepatoma
PI153/3	IMR6	+	+	−	−	−	−	−
PAD10/2	B-CLL	+	+	−	−	−	−	−
PAD28	B-CLL	+	+	−	−	−	−	−
SPAR14/1	REH	−	+	+	−	−	−	−
SPAR20.8	REH	−	+	+	−	−	−	−
SPARII.2	REH	−	+	+	−	−	−	−
P3B13C2	B-cell supernatant (10)	−	+	+	−	−	−	−

Reactivity of 7 monoclonal antibodies selected for reactivity against the indicated immunizing cell were screened by cytotoxicity and binding assays against a panel of human cell types. Several B-cell lines, T-cell lines, and fibroblasts were used with identical results. Two reaction patterns are seen. One set of antibodies reacts like PI153/3 with neuroblastomas and null ALL but not B-cells, and the other with null ALLs and B-cells but not neuroblastomas.

seems the most likely to result in obtaining truly tumor-specific reagents. If that is found, upon further analysis, to be impossible, then the monoclonal antibodies can be used in combinations which allow, as shown here, discrimination between certain tumor cells and subpopulations of normal cells.

ACKNOWLEDGMENTS

We thank Jean Haas, Barbara Meyer, Rosemary Horton, and Harriet Davis for excellent technical assistance. This work was supported by grants from NSF—PCM 76–82997, and NIH—CA 24263, CA 09140, CA 10815, and GM 23892.

REFERENCES

1. Boyse, E. A., and Old, L. J. (1969): Some aspects of normal and abnormal cell surface genetics. *Annu. Rev. Genet.*, 3:269–290.
2. Bross, K. J., Pangalis, G. A., Staatz, C. G., and Blome, K. G. (1978): Demonstration of cell surface antigens and their antibodies by the peroxidase anti-peroxidase method. *Transplantation*, 25:331–334.
3. Castro, J. E., Hunt, R., Lance, E. M., and Medawar, P. G. (1974): Implications of the fetal antigen theory for fetal transplantation. *Cancer Res.*, 34:2055–2060.
4. Davies, D. A. L., and O'Neill, G. J. (1975): Method of cancer immunochemotherapy (DRAG and DRAC) using antisera against tumor specific membrane antigens. In: *Proceedings of the International Cancer Congress*, XI, Florence, edited by P. Baccalssi, U. Veronesi, and N. Cascinelli, pp. 218–221. American Elsevier, New York.
5. Doherty, P., and Zinkernagel, R. (1975): A biological role for the major histocompatibility antigens. *Lancet*, 1:1406–1409.
6. Evans, A. E., and Hummeler, K. (1973): The significance of primitive cells in marrow aspirates of children with neuroblastoma. *Cancer*, 4:906–912.
7. Friedman, J. M., and Fialkow, P. J. (1976): Cell marker studies of human tumorigenesis. *Transplant. Rev.*, 28:2–13.
8. Julius, M., Masuda, T., and Herzenberg, L. A. (1972): Demonstration that antigen binding cells are precursors of antibody producing cells after purification with a fluorescent-activated cell sorter. *Proc. Natl. Acad. Sci. U.S.A.*, 69:1934–1938.
9. Kennett, R. H. (1979): Monoclonal antibodies. Hybrid myelomas—A revolution in serology and immunogenetics. *Am. J. Human Genet.*, 31:539–547.
10. Kennett, R. H., Denis, K. A., Tung, A. S., and Klinman, N. R. (1978): Hybrid plasmacytoma production: Fusions with adult spleen cells, monoclonal spleen fragments, neonatal spleen cells, and human spleen cells. *Curr. Top. Microbiol. Immunol.*, 81:77–91.
11. Kennett, R. H., and Gilbert, F. (1979): Hybrid myelomas producing antibodies against a human neuroblastoma antigen present on fetal brain. *Science*, 203:1120–1121.
12. Köhler, G., and Milstein, C. (1975): Continuous cultures of fused cells making antibody of predefined specificity. *Nature*, 256:495–497.
13. Melchers, F., Potter, M., and Warner, N. L. (1978): Lymphocyte hybridomas: Workshop on Hybridomas, April 3–5, 1978. *Curr. Top. Microbiol. Immunol.*, 81.
14. Risser, R., Stockert, E., and Old, L. J. (1978): Abelson antigens: A viral tumor antigen that is also a differentiation antigen of Balb/c mice. *Proc. Natl. Acad. Sci. U.S.A.*, 75:3918–3922.
15. Robins, R. A., and Baldwin, R. W. (1977): Immune markers on cancer cells. *Cancer Immunol. Immunother.*, 2:205–207.
16. Shulman, M., Wilde, C. D., and Köhler, G. (1978): A better cell line for making hybridomas secreting specific antibodies. *Nature*, 276:269–270.

Advances in Neuroblastoma Research,
edited by Audrey E. Evans.
Raven Press, New York © 1980.

Potential of Monoclonal Antibodies as Tools for the Study of Human Neuroblastoma

Lois Alterman Lampson

Howard Hughes Medical Institute Laboratories and the Department of Medicine, Stanford University Medical Center, Stanford, California 94305

Monoclonal antibodies are potentially ideal reagents for the study of human cell surface antigens. The essence of the antibody production is that the murine immune response to a human cell is cloned out *in vitro,* so that each culture contains the progeny of a single antibody-forming cell. This means that the monoclonal antibody products are, by definition, monospecific, and no absorption or other purification is necessary to obtain pure reagents. This technique is particularly valuable for raising antibodies to human cell surface antigens, because in this case the traditional serological approaches—controlled immunizations between inbred strains and purification by absorption against cells from inbred strains—are not available. Further, the technique of monoclonal antibody production is particularly well suited to the study of human tumors and their derivative cell lines, because these materials can provide sources of homogeneous material in quantities sufficient for screening large numbers of antibodies. The human neuroblastomas and neuroblastoma cell lines would seem to be ideal tissues to study in this way, and, indeed, the production of monoclonal antibodies to the human neuroblastoma line IMR6 has already been described (1). In assessing the final potentials of this approach, three general questions arise.

The first question concerns the mouse antibody repertoire. Will the mouse indeed produce antibodies to determinants as narrowly defined as a human alloantigen—or will the overwhelming majority of the antibodies be directed against "species" determinants? The second question concerns the screening process. Among the great number of antibodies that can be generated against a single cell, the task of finding antibody of a particular desired specificity can be a formidable one. Are there screening techniques that can simplify this process? The third question concerns the ability of this technique to reveal new specificities and new heterogeneity among previously defined molecules. Each monoclonal antibody will be specific not only for a single molecule, but for a particular determinant on that molecule. Conceivably, then, new heterogeneity will be revealed among molecules that have been previously defined by whole antisera. How can this possibility best be exploited? In order to approach these questions, the human histocompatibility antigens, some of which are on all nucleated human cells, and are already well defined, were chosen as a model.

MATERIALS AND METHODS

The techniques used have been published in detail elsewhere.[1] To raise monoclonal antibodies to the human B cell line 8866, Balb/c mice were primed and boosted with 8866 cells, and the antibody-forming cells in the recipient spleen were cloned out using either a fragment culture technique (6) or by PEG-mediated fusion to the mouse plasmacytoma variant NSI/1-AG4-1 (2). Antibody binding to target cells was measured in an indirect binding assay in which ^{125}I-goat antimouse κ antibody was used as the detecting reagent (5). For immunoprecipitation studies, cell membranes were labeled externally, using lactoperoxidase and hydrogen peroxide. Membranes were then solubilized with NP-40. *Staphylococcus aureus* (Staph A) was used to precipitate antigen-antibody complexes. Material was eluted from the Staph A by boiling in 2-ME/SDS, and electrophoresed on SDS-polyacrylamide gels by the technique of Laemmli (3).

RESULTS AND DISCUSSION

In order to address the questions of the mouse repertoire and of efficient screening, the murine response to the human histocompatibility alloantigen HLA-A2 (A2) was studied. The response to an A2+ lymphoblastoid cell line, 8866, was cloned out using a fragment culture system. The antibodies produced by 167 cultures were studied for their ability to bind to each of two cell lines: the A2+ immunizing cell, 8866, and an A2− loss variant of that line, clone 1–2. This variant had been isolated from the A2+ wild type line by immunoselection with an anti-A2 alloantiserum, and appears to differ from the wild type line only (or primarily) at the A2 locus (7).

Of the 167 cultures screened, 141 produced antibody to 8866, and the great majority of these antibodies showed identical binding to the two cell lines. However, three of the cultures produced antibody that discriminated between the two cell lines. The binding of these three discriminators is illustrated in Fig. 1. In each case, there is much greater binding to the A2+ wild type than to the A2− loss variant. The specificity of these three antibodies was confirmed in two ways. First, the antibodies also showed much greater binding to a second A2+ cell line, T5-1, than to an A2− loss variant of that line, clone 6.6.5. Second, the specificity of the antibodies was confirmed in the complement-dependent microcytotoxicity assay, using panels of normal human peripheral blood

---

[1] Lampson, L. A., Warnke, R., and Levy, R. (1980): Two subpopulations of Ia-like molecules on a human B-cell line. *Submitted for publication.*

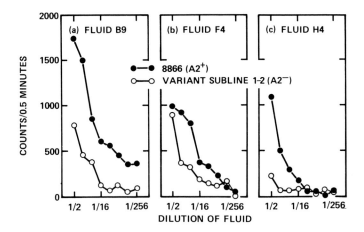

FIG. 1. Binding of discriminator culture fluids to A2+ and A2− cell lines. Antibody binding activity of supernatant medium from cultures B9, F4, and H4 was measured by radioimmunoassay: 2 × 10⁵ target cells were incubated with 25 μl of serial dilutions of culture fluid, followed by ¹²⁵I-goat anti-mouse κ antibody (4,5). Graphs show (counts bound per 2 × 10⁵ target cells with test fluid)-(mean of counts bound with 8 control fluids). Mean control binding for 8866 cells was 188; for 1-2 cells, 214. Reprinted by courtesy of Nature.

lymphocytes as the target cells. This is the conventional test for anti-HLA activity. The cytotoxic analysis confirmed that each of the cultures produced antibody that lysed A2+ cells, but not cells bearing any of the other non-cross-reactive HLA-A specificities (4).

These experiments demonstrate two important points. The first is that the mouse can indeed recognize a well-defined human cell surface alloantigen. The second is that the combination of loss-variant and wild type cell lines is an efficient and powerful screening tool. Many interesting human cell surface antigens, including a number of human neuroblastoma antigens, have already been defined by zenoantisera (Seeger and Kemshead, *this volume*). This study, then, suggests an approach to screening for monoclonal antibodies to those molecules.

The question of using monoclonal antibodies to identify new antigenic determinants and new levels of heterogeneity was approached in a second type of experiment. In this case, somatic cell hybridization was used to obtain a series of monoclonal antibodies to a different set of human histocompatibility antigens, the Ia-like molecules. Two of the anti-Ia antibodies had an identical cell and tissue distribution when tested against a large number of human cells (see footnote 1). Thus, if these two antibodies had been present in a whole antiserum, it would not have been possible to separate the antibodies from each other by the traditional technique of absorbing the serum against a cell which bears the determinant recognized by one antibody but not the determinant recognized by the other—no such cell has yet been found. However, two types of studies show that the two antibodies are directed against different antigenic determinants, and possibly different molecules.

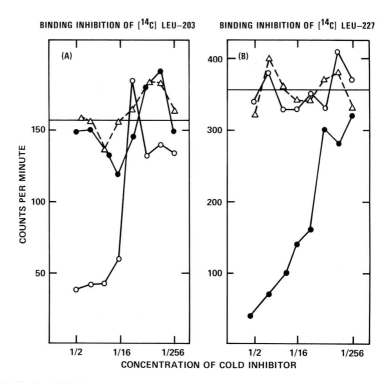

BINDING INHIBITION OF [^{14}C] LEU–203   BINDING INHIBITION OF [^{14}C] LEU–227

FIG. 2. Binding inhibition assays. First, 25 μl of serial dilutions of (unlabeled) antibody was incubated with 2.5 × 10^5 8866 target cells for 1.5 hr at room temperature. Then 10 μl of biosynthetically labeled antibody ([^{14}C]leu-203 or ^{14}C[leu]-227; see footnote 1) was added, and the cells were incubated for a further 2 hr. The target cells were then washed and transferred to vials of scintillant for counting. Figure shows inhibition of ^{14}C[leu]-203 **(A)** and of ^{14}C[leu]-227 **(B)** by anti-Ia antibody 203 (○), or anti-Ia antibody 227 (●). To indicate level of nonspecific inhibition, binding seen when an anti-HLA antibody was used as inhibitor is also shown (△). Base line: mean of 8 values obtained when no anti-human inhibitor was present.

Binding inhibition studies show that the two anti-Ia antibodies, numbered 203 and 277, do not cross-inhibit each other. This is illustrated in Fig. 2, and implies that the antibodies are recognizing different antigenic determinants. Furthermore, when the two antibodies were used to immunoprecipitate their antigens from the surface of the B cell line Raji, two different banding patterns were seen, implying that the two antibodies may be recognizing different forms of Ia-like molecules (Fig. 3). The banding pattern seen with 227 has not been seen before in studies in which conventionally raised antisera have been used to study the human Ia-like molecules.

SUMMARY

The experiments described above illustrate three points about the potential of using monoclonal antibodies to study human cell surface antigens. The first

A   B

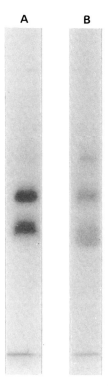

FIG. 3. SDS-PAGE analysis of material immunoprecipitated by anti-Ia antibodies. Cells from the human B cell line Raji were externally labeled with ^{125}I and the membranes solubilized with NP-40. Two anti-Ia antibodies, 203 and 227, were used to precipitate their antigens from aliquots of the same labeled extract. Precipitates were solubilized in SDS/2-ME and electrophoresed on a 10% acrylamide gel under reducing conditions. Figure shows banding patterns of material precipitated by antibody 203 **(A)** and by antibody 227 **(B)**.

is that the mouse is indeed able to recognize a well-defined human cell surface alloantigen. The second is that pairs of wild type cell lines and single loss variants provide a powerful screen for monoclonal antibodies to antigens that have already been defined by whole antisera. The third point is that monoclonal antibodies can define new determinants and reveal new heterogeneity among known molecules. The availability of neuroblastoma-derived cell lines and the difficulties of studying human cell surface antigens by conventional serological techniques make human neuroblastoma particularly suitable for study by monoclonal antibodies.

ACKNOWLEDGMENTS

I thank Dr. Ronald Levy for productive discussion and material support, and Mr. A. Bravo for preparing the manuscript. This work was supported in part by funds from the USPHS. The author holds an NIAID Immunobiology Postdoctoral Fellowship.

REFERENCES

1. Kennett, R. H., and Gilbert, F. (1979): Hybrid myelomas producing antibodies against a human neuroblastoma antigen present on fetal brain. *Science,* 203:1120–1121.

2. Kohler, G., and Milstein, C. (1976): Derivation of specific antibody-producing tissue culture and tumor lines by cell fusion. *Eur. J. Immunol.,* 6:511–519.
3. Laemmli, U. K. (1970): Cleavage of structural proteins during the assembly of the head of bacteriophage T4. *Nature,* 227:680–685.
4. Lampson, L. A., Levy, R., Grumet, F. C., Ness, D., and Pious, D. (1978): Production *in vitro* of murine antibody to a histocompatibility alloantigen. *Nature,* 271:461–462.
5. Lampson, L. A., Royston, I., and Levy, R. (1977): Homogeneous antibodies directed against human cell surface antigens: I. The mouse spleen fragment culture response to T and B cell lines derived from the same individual. *J. Supramol. Struct.,* 6:441–448.
6. Levy, R., and Dilley, J. (1977): The *in vitro* antibody response to cell surface antigens. II. Monoclonal antibodies to human leukemia cells. *J. Immunol.,* 219:394–400.
7. Pious, D., Hawley, P., and Forrest, G. (1973): Isolation and characterization of HL-A variants in cultured human lymphoid cells. *Proc. Natl. Acad. Sci. U.S.A.,* 70:1397–1400.

Advances in Neuroblastoma Research,
edited by Audrey E. Evans.
Raven Press, New York © 1980.

Differential Expression of Surface Antigens on Human Neuroblastoma Cells

*,**John T. Kemshead, *Melvin F. Greaves, †Jon Pritchard, and
**,‡John Graham-Pole

*Department of Membrane Immunology, Imperial Cancer Research Fund; **Department
of Medical Oncology, St. Bartholomew's Hospital; and †Department of Haematology,
The Hospital for Sick Children, London, England*

Metastatic infiltration of neuroblasts into the bone marrow presents a considerable problem clinically as identification of such cells relies on relatively insensitive cytological analysis of biopsy samples. Administration of highly cytoxic drugs to patients has to be balanced against the side effects of treatment, and therefore a more sensitive method of detecting cellular infiltration is required. An immunological approach to this problem has been attempted.

Antisera were raised in rabbits against human neuroblastoma lines, and the serum obtained showed similar specificities to those described by Casper (2) and Kennett (4). Evidence is presented that the neuroblastoma lines investigated are antigenically different and that this observation correlates with our initial studies on neuroblasts found in bone marrow. The significance of these observations in relation to immunological diagnosis of neuroblastoma is discussed.

MATERIALS AND METHODS

Cell Lines

All cell lines (Table 1) were grown in 6% CO_2 at 37°C using Dulbecco's Modified Eagle's Medium (EDM) [Flow Lab. Cat. No. 12-332-54 (1-001) M] supplemented with 10% fetal calf serum (FCS), 100 Iu/ml penicillin, 100 μg/ml streptomycin, and 2 mM glutamine. For immunofluorescence studies cells were washed ×2 in serum-free medium and the viability (80%+) determined prior to assay.

---

‡ Department of Paediatric Oncology, Rainbow Babies and Children's Hospital, Case Western Reserve University, Cleveland, Ohio.

TABLE 1. *Surface phenotype of neuroblastoma lines Platt and Holmes*

	Neuroblastoma line	
Antisera	Platt	Holmes
Anti-Ig	−	−
Anti-Ia	−	−
Anti-T cell	−	−
Anti-Thy	−	−
Anti-white cell[a]	+	ND
Anti-β_2 microglobulin[a]	+	+
Anti-HLA[a]	+	+
Anti-ALL	−	−
Anti-myeloid cell	−	−
Fcγ receptors	−	−

Assays were undertaken by indirect immunofluorescence using fluorescein-conjugated F(ab′)$_2$ goat anti-rabbit F(ab′)$_2$ as a second antibody. Fc receptors were assayed by rosette formation with ox red blood cells coated with immunoglobulin.

[a] Monoclonal antisera from hybridomas.

Antisera

Rabbits were injected with either 10^7 Holmes or 10^7 Platt cells intravenously (i.v.) followed by a boosting injection (10^7 cells) 14 days later. Animals were bled on days 21 and 28 and the serum heat inactivated at 56°C for 30 min. F(ab′)$_2$ preparations were made by pepsin digestion following the method of Welsh and Turner (6). All other antisera used in typing neuroblastoma cells were reagents used in our laboratory for the immunological analysis of human leukemia.

Indirect Immunofluorescence

First, 10^6 cells were incubated with rabbit antisera of defined specificity for 30 min at 4°C in serum-free E.D.M. After centrifugation and washing, ×2 cells were resuspended in 50λ of E.D.M., 10% FCS containing 0.02% sodium azide, and 5λ of fluorescein-conjugated F(ab′)$_2$ goat anti-rabbit F(ab′)$_2$. Following incubation for 30 min cells were washed ×3 before examination using a Zeiss fluorescent microscope with incident illumination and by flow cytofluorimetry using a fluorescence-activated cell sorter (FACS-I, Becton Dickinson, California).

RESULTS

Initial experiments established that neuroblastoma cell lines Platt and Holmes expressed HLA and β_2 microglobulin antigens. With the exception of one hybridoma detecting a white cell antigen, they shared no other antigenic markers with hemopoietic cells (Table 1). These results indicate that neuroblastoma cells in marrow might be distinguishable immunologically from hemopoietic cells.

Prior to an examination of the efficacy of binding to neuronal tissue, the specificity of antisera raised against the human neuroblastoma lines Platt and Holmes was determined by assay against a panel of cultured lymphoid lines and fresh human tissue. Even prior to absorption, following dilution to 1:200, antisera raised against these lines were found almost specific for neuronal tissue (Table 2). At any concentration of antisera assayed, only traces of activity against the B cell line Raji and myeloid line HL-60 were found by indirect immunofluorescence, and this pattern was reflected on assay of fresh tonsil and bone marrow (Table 2). No reactivity was detected against human T cell lines, the histiocytic line (U937), acute lymphocytic leukemia (ALL) cells, thymus, or peripheral blood (Fig. 1). To ensure specificity for neuronal tissue antisera, 200 μl aliquots were therefore diluted 1:50, absorbed ×3 with equal numbers of Raji and HL-60 cells (5 × 10^7/absorption), and used in all subsequent assays at a final dilution of 1:250.

TABLE 2. *Specificity of antineuroblastoma antisera*

	Rabbit antisera raised against:			
Cell type	Platt 1:10	Platt 1:200	Holmes 1:10	Holmes 1:200
Raji (B cell)[a]	+ → ++ Some −	+/− → + Some −	20%+	V. faint → −
HPB-T-ALL (T cell)[a]	−	−	−	−
KM3 (cALL cell[b])[a]	−	−	−	−
U937 (histiocytic cell)[a]	−	−	−	−
HL-60 (myeloid cell)[a]	+	+/−	V. faint	VV. faint → −
ALL cells	−	−	−	−
Peripheral blood	−	−	−	−
Tonsil	30% faint; rest v. faint	V. faint	ND	ND
Bone marrow	10% +/− rest faint → −	−	ND	ND
Fetal brain[c]		Strong		Strong
Adult brain[c]		Weak		Weak

For each cell type, 10^6 cells were assayed against antineuroblastoma antisera at 2 concentrations by indirect immunofluorescence. Controls of normal rabbit serum and second layer of antibody alone were performed on each cell type.

[a] Cell lines established from hemopoietic malignancies.

[b] cALL, common acute lymphoblastic leukemia, unreactive with T and B cell markers, reactive with antiserum to ALL (considered a lymphocyte precursor).

[c] Reactivity of antineuroblastoma antisera to fetal and adult brain determined against neuroblastoma cells following absorption with the respective tissue.

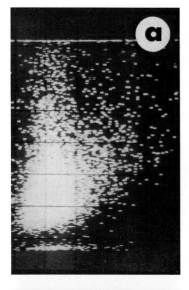
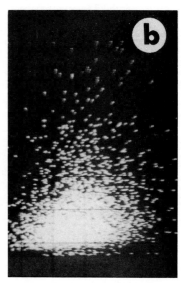
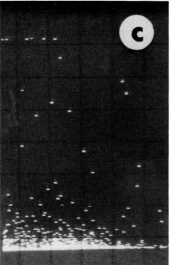

FIG. 1. Example of fluorescence-activated cell sorter: analysis of cell lines with anti-neuroblastoma antisera. Binding determined by indirect immunofluorescence using fluorescein-conjugated F(ab')₂ goat anti-rabbit F(ab')₂. Axes: Horizontal, relative cell size; vertical, relative cell fluorescence. **a:** Platt cells binding with Platt antiserum, dilution 1:100. **b:** Holmes cells binding with Platt antiserum, dilution 1:100. **c:** KM3 (cALL, see legend Table 2) cells binding anti-Platt antiserum, dilution 1:100.

Preparations of antineuroblastoma antisera raised against individual cell lines were tested for their ability to react with other neuroblastoma lines. Although antisera raised against Platt cells and tested at a dilution of 1:250 showed strong reactivity to this line by immunofluorescence (+++), less reactivity was detected against the neuroblastoma lines Holmes (+) and CHP 100 (+/−) (Table 3, Fig. 1). This differential binding could reflect either the presence of different antigens on the surface of neuroblastoma lines or quantitative differences in the expression of antigenic determinants. Evidence favoring the former explanation comes from

TABLE 3. *Reactivity of rabbit antineuroblastoma antisera against different neuroblastoma cell lines*

Cell line	Rabbit anti-Platt 1:200	Rabbit anti-Holmes 1:200
Platt	+++	+
Herne	++	ND
Holmes	+	+++
Ozieh	+++	ND
CHP 100	+/−	+/−
Mouse neuroblastoma Neuro-2a	+++	+/−

Against each rabbit antineuroblastoma antiserum, 10^6 cells of each line were assayed by indirect immunofluorescence.

analysis of the binding of antisera raised against the lines Platt and Holmes. The two antisera show reciprocal binding specificities against the lines used for induction and the mouse neuroblastoma line Neuro-2a (Table 3, Fig. 1). This result would not be expected if the different binding spectra were due to quantitative differences in the expression of a single antigenic determinant. Absorption studies and a biochemical analysis of surface proteins/glycoproteins should further resolve the question.

The antisera raised against either Platt or Holmes cell lines were also found to bind strongly with fetal brain and to a lesser extent adult brain (Table 2). As difficulty was encountered in obtaining these tissues in a viable form, these studies were performed by absorption, so it has not been possible to determine accurately quantitative differences in the binding of antisera.

The differences in the binding of antineuroblastoma antisera to different cell

TABLE 4. *Analysis of bone marrow samples with suspected neuroblastoma infiltration*

Patients	Cytological analysis	F(ab')₂ rabbit anti-Platt 1:100	F(ab')₂ rabbit anti-Holmes 1:100
12 patients	−ve	−ve	−ve
F	Neuroblastoma cells present	20% cells ++	−ve
CM	"	10% cells v. faint	ND
NH	"	5% cells +/−	ND

Where possible, bone marrow samples were assayed on the day of biopsy, against F(ab')₂ rabbit antineuroblastoma and controls of F(ab')₂ NRS and second layer antibody only as check against nonspecific fluorescence. Red cells were removed from the samples by ficoll triosil.

lines suggest that no one such antiserum will necessarily stain all neuroblast-infiltrated bone marrow. From the limited number of patients screened, this appears to be the case as anti-Platt antiserum reacted only weakly with two of three bone marrow samples heavily infiltrated with neuroblasts (Table 4). However, the marrow containing blasts binding anti-Platt antibodies avidly did not bind antiserum raised against the neuroblastoma line Holmes. Obviously, a more detailed analysis of children with neuroblastoma is necessary to confirm these results, and this work is continuing as patients present with the disease.

DISCUSSION

Typing of a number of cell lines established from patients with neuroblastoma has shown that these cells fulfill criteria for being classified as neuronal. Chromosomal analysis, histology, catecholamine content, differentiation studies, and—with the exception of HLA—the absence of common lymphoid markers (Table 1) or fibroblastoid characteristics all suggest neuronal origin of the lines. Antisera raised in rabbits against some of the neuroblastoma lines have been shown to be relatively specific for neuronal tissue prior to absorption (Table 2) and have similar specificities to the reagents raised by Casper (2) and Kennett (4).

Despite similarities in the binding of the two antineuroblastoma antisera to non-neuronal tissue (Table 2), differences were detected upon assay against a panel of neuroblastoma cell lines (Table 3, Fig. 1), suggesting that the phenotypic expression of antigens on the surface of the lines *in vitro* is considerably different. Should this situation be paralleled *in vivo,* this would indicate that neuroblastoma may be heterogeneous and involve either cells of different origin or cells in different stages of maturation. Preliminary observations on neuroblasts in bone marrow biopsies suggest that these are antigenically different as they show different binding spectra to antisera raised against the neuroblastoma cell lines Platt and Holmes (Table 4).

Evidence for the differential expression of antigens during differentiation comes from studies of murine neuroblastoma (1,5), and our studies on the induced differentiation of Platt cells using sodium butyrate indicate that at least quantitative differences in antigenic expression occur between differentiated and nondifferentiated cells *(unpublished observations).* Neuroblastoma is also a malignancy with a high rate of spontaneous maturation of cells to a nondividing state (3). This hypothesis that neuroblastoma represents a complex malignancy involving cells of either different lineage or different differentiation states thus considerably complicates the possibilities of an immunological diagnosis of metastatic spread. Studies to resolve the putative spectrum of antigenic markers on neuroblastoma cells *in vivo* and *in vitro* are continuing.

ACKNOWLEDGMENTS

We wish to thank Mr. D. Bicknell and Ms. P. Warne for their excellent technical assistance, and Ms. J. Riggs for secretarial work.

REFERENCES

1. Akeson, R., and Herschman, H. (1974): *Nature,* 249:620.
2. Casper, J. T., Borella, L., and Sen, L. (1977): *Cancer Res.,* 37:1750.
3. Jaffe, N. (1976): *Cancer Treatment Rev.,* 3:61.
4. Kennett, R. H., and Gilbert, F. (1978): *Science,* 203:1120.
5. Schubert, D., Humphries, S., Baroni, C., and Cohn, M. (1969): *Proc. Natl. Acad. Sci. U.S.A.,* 64:316.
6. Welsh, K., and Turner, M. W. (1976): *Tissue Antigens,* 8:197.

Advances in Neuroblastoma Research,
edited by Audrey E. Evans.
Raven Press, New York © 1980.

Studies of Immunity to a Transplantable Murine Neuroblastoma

Richard Epstein and William Elkins

*Department of Pathology, University of Pennsylvania School of Medicine,
and the Children's Cancer Research Center of the Children's Hospital of Philadelphia,
Philadelphia, Pennsylvania 19104*

The clinical course of neuroblastoma varies widely, ranging from complete spontaneous remission to relentless progression in the face of therapy. The possibility that an immune response of the host to a tumor-associated antigen is one determinant of the clinical course has been under consideration for some time (7). If an animal model could be developed for the study of immunity to neuroblastoma, considerable insight might be gained concerning the importance of tumor immunity in the natural history of this disease. We here report on some studies of the immunogenetic determinants of resistance to a transplantable murine neuroblastoma, C1300.

C1300 is a transplantable neuroblastoma that arose spontaneously in an inbred strain A mouse in 1940 (5). It has been extensively utilized for studies of cellular differentiation, and has impeccable credentials as a neuroblastoma (13). We have utilized a subline of tumor adapted both for *in vitro* and *in vivo* growth. This subline retains its virulence *in vivo* and metastasizes widely in strain A/J hosts (1).

Graded doses of tumor cells were injected under the dorsal skin. The resulting local growth was observed and scored 3 × weekly for each mouse, and the survival time of tumor-bearing mice recorded. In most experiments it was necessary to give at least 10^4 cells to cause $\geq 90\%$ tumor take in adult A/J hosts, but there was considerable variability from one batch of cells to another in this respect.

We found that individual A/J and F_1 mice inoculated with C1300 distribute themselves into two groups. In some cases the tumor grows progressively and kills the host within about 80 days. Alternatively, the tumor either does not grow to palpable size or else grows and then regresses. These animals survive for observation periods up to a year in an apparently tumor-free state. Mice in the latter group can be considered resistant provided that the same dose of tumor cells was lethal for the majority of strain A mice in the experiment. We can thus express strain-associated resistance in terms of overall survival as computed by life table analysis (12).

RESISTANCE TO C1300 IS REGULATED BY NON H-2 GENES IN THE HOST

In order to determine whether resistance to C1300 might be under genetic control, we transplanted the tumor into various F_1 hybrids derived by outcrossing from A/J. Such F_1s should not respond to the alloantigens, e.g., $H\text{-}2^a$, which the tumor shares with normal cells of strain A, but the genome contributed by the other parental strain might confer a superior capacity to respond to tumor-associated antigens.

The results of an experiment in which graded doses of C1300 were injected into 2- to 3-month-old panels of male $(C_{57}Bl/6J \times A/J)F_1$, hereafter abbreviated $(B6 \times A)F_1$, and female A/J are shown in Table 1. $(B6 \times A)F_1$ are seen to be significantly more resistant to the lethal growth of C1300 than strain A in the dose range $10^4 - 5 \times 10^6$ tumor cells. Subsequent experiments indicated that the critical determinant of resistance in this experiment was the strain, not the sex, of the host.

Similar experiments utilizing tumor cell doses of 10^4, 10^5, and 10^6 were carried out with other types of F_1 hosts. Six to ten hosts of each type were injected with each dose. Where we encountered statistically significant ($p \le 0.05$) prolongation of survival of F_1 compared to A strain hosts injected with an equal number of the same batch of tumor cells, the F_1 was classified as a resistant strain. Thus in addition to $(B6 \times A)F_1$, $(C_{57}/Bl\ 10.A \times A)F$ mice are resistant, but $(A.By \times A)F_1$, $(BALB/_c \times A)F_1$, and $(CBA \times A)F_1$ are susceptible. The data from these tests will be published at a later date, but the results are summarized in Table 2, which gives the $H\text{-}2$ alleles for each strain. It is apparent that resistance to C1300 is not primarily determined by $H\text{-}2$. Rather strong resistance seems to be associated with the $C_{57}Bl$ background. More data would be required to eliminate a possible contributory effect of $H\text{-}2^a$, and to establish critically the genetic basis for resistance to this tumor.

TABLE 1. *Survival of (B6 × A)F₁ and A hosts after injection of graded doses of C1300*

| Dose | (B6 × A)F₁ hosts | | A hosts | | Probability that difference is not due to chance |
	s/n[a]	mst[b]	s/n	MST	
5×10^6	1/8	28.6	0/8	18.6	*[c]
10^6	1/8	38.5	0/8	26.5	**
10^5	5/8	—	1/8	39.1	**
10^4	6/8	—	1/8	49.1	**
10^3	8/8	—	8/8	—	—

[a] Fraction of mice surviving tumor free at ≥ 80 days.
[b] Median survival time.
[c] $p \le 0.05$; ** $p \le 0.01$, based on log rank test.

TABLE 2. *Resistance to C1300 is not correlated with H-2 allele of host*

Host strain	H-2	Resistance
A	a/a	Low
(B10.A × A)F$_1$	a/a	High
(B6 × A)F$_1$	b/a	High
(A.By × A)F$_1$	b/a	Low
(CBA × A)F$_1$	k/a	Low
(BALB/c × A)F$_1$	d/a	Low

ADAPATIVE IMMUNITY TO C1300

Other studies of resistance to parental strain tumors by F$_1$ hybrid mice have indicated that resistance is often nonadaptive, i.e., not enhanced by prior exposure to antigens of the tumor (reviewed in 3,10). This natural immunity may be mediated by a subclass of spontaneously cytotoxic lymphocytes which are usually called "natural killer" cells (NKCs) (3,8,10).

By contrast, we find that there is an adaptive immune response to C1300. Many mice which survive the primary injection of 10^5 to 10^6 C1300 cells do not manifest a palpable local tumor, nor do they succumb to metastatic disease following a second challenge with C1300 that grows in and kills mice not previously exposed. This statement applies to the very few surviving mice of the susceptible strains, including A/J, as well as to the far more numerous survivors among the resistant hybrids.

In other experiments it was possible to show that resistance could be adoptively conferred on sublethally irradiated (B6 × A)F$_1$ hosts by T cells from long-term (B6 × A)F$_1$ survivors of a primary inoculum of 10^5 to 10^6 C1300 (Table 3).

TABLE 3. *Adaptive transfer of immunity to irradiated (B6 × A)F$_1$ hosts*

	Cells transferred	No. surviving tumor-free/No. injected
Experiment 1	75 × 10^6 immune spleen	6/6
	75 × 10^6 immune spleen T cell depleted	0/6
Experiment 2	90 × 10^6 immune spleen	3/4
	90 × 10^6 immune spleen T cell depleted	0/8
	26 × 10^6 immune spleen T cell enriched	6/8
	No cells	0/8

Recipient mice received 450 r whole-body irradiation prior to inoculation with 5 × 10^4 C1300 and i.v. inoculation of immune spleen cells. T cell depletion was accomplished by incubation with ascites fluid containing anti-Thy 1.2 followed by guinea pig complement. Control immune cells were incubated in the latter only. T cell enrichment was accomplished by nylon wool filtration to yield final suspension containing 92% Thy 1.2 positive cells. Donors of immune spleen cells had survived 1–3 doses of 10^5–10^6 C1300 cells over a period of about 5–12 months and were grossly tumor free at sacrifice.

We interpret the above as strong evidence that adaptive immunity develops in mice that do not succumb to a primary inoculum of 10^5 to 10^6 tumor cells and that the resulting heightened resistance is T cell dependent. This leaves open the question whether resistance to the primary challenge depends on this same T cell response, or whether the latter develops only in those mice which have survived by virtue of effective natural immunity capable of restraining progressive tumor growth until such time as adaptive immunity can develop.

POSSIBLE ROLE OF NATURAL RESISTANCE AND NATURAL KILLER CELLS

The work of several independent groups has suggested the possible correlation between resistance of certain F_1 mice to a variety of transplantable parental strain neoplasms and the presence of NKC (3,10). The latter are detected by their capacity for *spontaneous* cytotoxic activity against tumor target cells *in vitro*. The level of NKC activity against a particular tumor is under genetic control, and both *H2* and non-*H2* factors have been implicated as determinants of the efficiency of this barrier to tumor growth (3,10). We thus sought to determine whether there were NKCs for C1300 and whether the level of NKC activity correlated with *in vivo* resistance.

Spleen cells from 12- to 13-week-old (B6 × A)F_1 and (B10A × A)F_1 mice were found to contain NKC for C1300 as well as YAC lymphoma cell targets. The latter were included as a control cell known to be sensitive to NKCs. In our studies spontaneous cytotoxicity was greater for YAC than C1300, but whenever the spleen cell suspension was spontaneously cytotoxic for YAC some killing of C1300 also occurred. Since spleen cells from A mice did not kill those targets, one might suspect that *in vivo* resistance was mediated through these cells. The correlation breaks down, however, when results with 29- to 38-week-old mice are considered. We did not detect NKCs for YAC or C1300 in (B6 × A)F_1 or (B10A × A)F_1 mice at this age, but such mice are at least as resistant to lethal growth of C1300 as 10- to 12-week-old mice. These data will be presented elsewhere.

RESISTANCE IN T DEPLETED MICE

NKCs are generated from precursors in bone marrow, and their activity (or number) is at least normal in T cell deprived or athymic mice (3,10). We made use of this fact to investigate further the nature of resistance to C1300 in the nonimmunized mouse.

In order to generate mice which would be putatively T cell deficient but well endowed with NKCs, panels of (B6 × A)F_1 were thymectomized or sham operated when 3 weeks old. One month later, these mice were subjected to 800 r whole-body irradiation and reconstituted with syngeneic bone marrow that had been depleted of T cells by treatment with anti-Thy 1.2 serum and complement. The mice were challenged with C1300 35 days later, and survival of the thymectomized and sham-operated controls was determined as above. All 16 T deprived hosts died with progressively growing tumors (median survival 34 days). Four of 16 sham operated and 3 of 16 normal controls (age, sex matched) survived tumor-free for over 80 days (median survival 48 days). The difference in survival between the T deprived mice and each control group is significant at the 0.025 level. Thus resistance in mice not previously immunized with C1300 appears to be T cell dependent.

STUDIES OF *IN VITRO* T CELL MEDIATED CYTOTOXICITY

When lymphocytes are stimulated for 4 to 6 days by tumor cells *in vitro*, a population of cytotoxic T cells may be generated from antigen-sensitive precursors. In order to determine whether genetic resistance might be expressed as a difference between resistant and susceptible strains with respect to the capacity of their lymphocytes to generate cytotoxicity, we studied the capacity of spleen cells from individual mice to give rise to cytotoxic T cells after *in vitro* stimulation with irradiated tumor cells. Since the development of significant cytotoxicity to non-*H-2* antigens may be dependent on prior *in vivo* immunization, we injected some of these mice with tumor up to 35 days before the *in vitro* assay. For positive controls we utilized cells from individual mice proven to be resistant to C1300 by long-term disease-free survival following two successive challenges with at least 10^5 C1300 cells (tumor immune controls). For negative controls we used spleen cells cultured in the absence of C1300. Specificity of killing was checked by use of PHA-stimulated A lymphoblast targets. Spleen cells from 20 of 28 mice of resistant F_1 type gave rise to detectable cytotoxicity against C1300 at 100:1 killer:target ratio, whereas only 4 of 12 A/J spleens had precursors which could generate such activity ($p \leq 0.005$). Although the T cell identity of the killers was not proven in these particular experiments, it is inferred from other experiments in which killing of C1300 was completely abolished by pretreatment of the *in vitro* stimulated cells with anti-Thy 1.2 antisera and guinea pig complement.

DISCUSSION

Classic genetic tolerance of F_1 mice for parental tissue grafts is seen in situations such as orthotopic transplantation of skin in which the target histocompatibility antigens are codominantly expressed. However, the work of Cudkowicz and his colleagues (2) with murine bone marrow transplantation has revealed that certain histocompatibility antigens on hematopoietic cells are recessive, and as a result engraftment of parental bone marrow may be resisted by certain irradiated F_1 mice. This type of hybrid resistance can also be demonstrated to affect parental strain leukemias and lymphomas (3,10,11). We doubt that it is important in resistance to C1300 neuroblastoma, because hybrid resistance to normal and malignant cells of hematopoietic origin is typically nonadaptive, T independent, radiation resistant, and dependent on an *H-2* region difference between donor and host (2,3). Hybrid resistance to C1300 neuroblastoma displays none of these features.

On the contrary, we obtained evidence which implicates conventional, i.e., adaptive, T cell dependent immunity as the basis for resistance to C1300. As a result we suspect that IR genes in the $C_{57}B1$ background may determine effective resistance in the F_1 hosts generated by outcrossing strain A to $C_{57}Bl/6$ or $C_{57}B1/10.A$. These genes may regulate T cell recognition of tumor-associated antigens (see below), but more work is needed to establish this hypothesis more firmly, especially since all known IR genes that regulate T cell function map with *H-2*.

The alternative possibility that the trait *susceptibility* is determined by the presence of serum blocking factors is suggested by the studies of Hellström et al. (7) with neuroblastoma and other neoplasms. Under this hypothesis each strain would be about equally endowed with T cell mediated capacity for resistance, but would differ with respect to presence or absence of blocking. We cannot rule out this possibility, but there is one relevant piece of evidence against it. Strain-associated resistance appears to be reflected by increased capacity of spleen cells from resistant type F_1 relative to A/J to become cytotoxic for C1300 *in vitro,* and these assays were all run in the presence of normal mouse serum. Thus resistance appears to be determined by a property inherent in the T cells themselves.

Unfortunately, the source of the antigen(s) which elicit this immunity is unknown. Among the alternatives are a true neuroblastoma-specific transplantation antigen, a neural differentiation antigen (9,14), or an inappropriately expressed transplantation antigen normally expressed by some strain(s) other than A/J (6). The last seems quite unlikely in view of the susceptibility of $(C \times A)F_1$, $(CBA \times A)F_1$, and $(A.By \times A)F_1$ in addition to A/J. Also to be considered is the possibility that the antigenic targets are some artifactual product of the long laboratory life span of this tumor. If so, our studies are not instructive as to the role of immunity to neuroblastomas in general. We badly need new tumors with which to continue these studies.

If it could be established that recently derived spontaneous murine neuroblastomas express tumor-associated antigens, which elicit resistance similar to that seen in the C1300 system, the hypothesis that the natural history of neuroblastoma is determined in part by the capacity of the host to respond to tumor antigens will be strengthened.

ACKNOWLEDGMENTS

We wish to thank Drs. Klaus Hummeler and Harvey Schlesinger for generous gifts of the tumor and Dr. Jonathan Sprent for gifts of anti-Thy 1.2 antiserum. This work was supported by USPHS Grants CA 158222, 14489, and GM 07170, and, in part, by Grant CA 14489, awarded by the National Cancer Institute, DHEW.

REFERENCES

1. Buck, B., McAlack, R., and Schlessinger, H. (1976): Metastatic characterization of murine neuroblastoma. A model for the human disease. *Fed. Proc. Abstracts,* p. 1086.
2. Cudkowicz, G., and Bennett, M. (1971): Peculiar immunobiology of bone marrow allografts. I. Graft rejection by irradiated responder mice. *J. Exp. Med.,* 134:83.
3. Cudkowicz, G., and Hochman, P. S. (1979): Do natural killer cells engage in regulated reactions against self to ensure homeostasis? *Immunol. Rev.,* 44:13.
4. Cudkowicz, G., and Warner, J. F. (1979): Natural resistance of irradiated 129-strain mice to bone marrow allografts: Genetic control by the H-2K region. *Immunogenetics,* 8:13.
5. Durham, L. C., and Stewart, H. L. (1955): A survey of transplantable and transmissible animal tumors. *J. Natl. Cancer Inst.,* 13:1299.
6. Gibson, T. J., Imamura, M., McGregor, A. C., and Martin, W. J. (1978): Lung tumor-associated depressed alloantigen coded for by the K region of the H-2 major H complex. *J. Exp. Med.,* 147:1363.
7. Hellström, I., Hellström, K. E., Bill, A. H., Pierce, G. E., and Yang, J. P. S. (1976): Studies on cellular immunity to neuroblastoma cells. *Int. J. Cancer,* 6:172.
8. Herberman, R. B., and Holden, H. E. (1978): Natural cell mediated immunity. *Adv. Cancer Res.,* 27:305.
9. Kennett, R. H., and Gilbert, F. (1979): Hybrid myeloma producing antibodies against a human neuroblastoma antigen present on fetal brain. *Science,* 203:1120.
10. Kiesling, R., and Wigzell, H. (1979): An analysis of the murine NK cell as to structure, function, and biological relevance. *Immunol. Rev.,* 44:165.
11. Klein, G., Klein, G. O., Karre, K., and Kiessling, R. (1978): Hybrid resistance against parental tumors: One or several genetic patterns? *Immunogenetics,* 7:391.
12. Peto, R., Pike, M. C., Armitage, P., Breslow, N. E., Cox, D. R., Howard, S. V., Mantel, N., McPherson, K., Peto, J., and Smith, P. G. (1977): Design and analysis of randomized clinical trials requiring prolonged observations of each patient. II. Analysis and examples. *Br. J. Cancer,* 35:1.
13. Prasad, K. (1975): Differentiation of neuroblastoma cells in culture? *Biol. Rev.,* 50:129.
14. Seegar, R. C., Zeltzer, O. N., and Razner, S. A. (1979): Onconeural antigen: A new neural differentiation antigen expressed by neuroblastoma, oat cell carcinoma, Wilms' tumor and sarcoma cells. *J. Immunol.,* 122:1548.

Advances in Neuroblastoma Research,
edited by Audrey E. Evans.
Raven Press, New York © 1980.

Prospects for Immunotherapy of Neuroblastoma

Irwin D. Bernstein

*Pediatric Oncology, Fred Hutchinson Cancer Research Center, Seattle, Washington
98104; and Department of Pediatrics, University of Washington School of Medicine,
Seattle, Washington 98105*

The possibility of treating cancer by immunologic means has been of considerable interest since the turn of the century. Immunologic treatment of neuroblastoma has been of particular interest since clinical evidence points to a role of host immune responses against neuroblastoma, as, for example, the high incidence of spontaneous regression (1). During the past decade there have been numerous clinical immunotherapy trials for a variety of tumors including neuroblastoma. Results of these trials, which have been reviewed elsewhere (1,2), have not been encouraging. Nevertheless, there are recent findings, both clinical and experimental, suggesting the future to be more promising. These include the clinical use of intralesional BCG; the possibility of "programming" the immune response to achieve heretofore unobtainable antitumor responses; and the development of methods to produce large quantities of biologically potent immune cells or serum for passive immunotherapy. In this chapter, we will briefly review these recent exciting approaches to immunotherapy. Recent data from our laboratory suggesting a potential role for passive therapy using monoclonal antibodies will be described in more detail.

INTRATUMORAL ADMINISTRATION OF INFLAMMATORY AGENTS

The intralesional injection of BCG has been shown to cause regression of injected tumor nodules in animals (3) and humans (4,5). In perhaps the most notable study of this approach, McKneally et al. (6) injected BCG intrapleurally following resection of carcinoma of the lung. They observed that patients with completely resected tumors who receive BCG show prolonged survival; whether an increased cure rate is also achieved remains unanswered. Currently, a large cooperative effort is aimed at defining the efficacy of this approach in lung cancer. There are also efforts to inject BCG directly into lung tumors prior to resection.

The intratumoral injection of BCG or other agents also lends itself to other tumors, e.g., those of the bladder, where tumor nodules can be visualized and easily injected. Although the value of this approach for neuroblastoma is not readily apparent, there are situations where it may prove useful. Patients in whom clinical remission has been induced reveal, upon a "second look" operation, residual neuroblastoma at the primary intra-abdominal site. It may be that injection of BCG into remaining tumor would inhibit subsequent metastases and also induce immunity effective against undetectable micrometastases. However, a trial of this sort must await more information about the biology of neuroblastoma in treated patients.

IMMUNOLOGIC PROGRAMMING

There have been recent laboratory studies which suggest that the failure to immunize individuals against tumor antigens effectively may not be due to the lack of expression of such antigens, but may result from the action of suppressor T lymphocytes. Under certain experimental conditions, antigens appear unable to elicit a detectable immune response. Recent evidence indicates that these antigens do, however, evoke the generation of suppressor T lymphocytes which result in the inhibition of the otherwise expected immune response. Evidence that suppressor T cells may inhibit antitumor responses *in vivo* come from recent experiments by Green et al. (7). In these studies, the activity of suppressor cells was abrogated by pretreatment of mice *in vivo* with an antiserum specific for antigens expressed by suppressor cells (I-J determinants). Treatment with anti-I-J serum led to significant inhibition of tumor growth in treated as compared to control animals. Presumably, the elimination of suppressor cells allowed the host to mount an effective antitumor response.

Thus it may be possible to "program" the immune system to respond in the desired fashion by deleting suppressor activity or, alternatively, increasing helper activity. Use of "selected" lymphocyte populations from neuroblastoma patients may enable the demonstration of reactivity against the tumor. If this proves to be the case, then immunization of patients with tumor antigens following deletion of suppressor activity could then be considered. Of course, such studies in humans must await the expected availability of antisera which will selectively eliminate functional subclasses of human lymphocytes.

PASSIVE IMMUNOTHERAPY

There is much renewed interest in passive immunotherapy using immune cells or serum. This interest stems from the development of new techniques for the *in vitro* production of potent preparations of immune cells or serum. Included among these approaches are techniques involving immunizing lymphocytes to tumor antigens *in vitro* and establishing long-term cultures of killer lymphocytes, as well as the development of techniques for production of monoclonal antibody. With respect to the former, it is now known that T lymphocytes cytotoxic for tumor cells can be generated *in vitro*. Immune cells stimulated *in vitro* have been observed by us to confer effective systemic antitumor immunity on nonimmune rats (8); their use in mice in combination with chemotherapy by Fefer and colleagues (9) has led to successful treatment of a transplantable virus-induced lymphoma. Of current interest is the possibility of establishing these *in vitro* generated cytotoxic cells in long-term culture in the presence of growth factors elaborated by stimulated T cells. These cells can be cloned and grown in relatively large numbers. Such clones have been established by Baker, Gillis, and Smith (10), who are currently evaluating their *in vivo* antitumor activity. There is also evidence suggesting that cells cytotoxic for human leukemias can also be generated *in vitro* (11,12); it will be important to learn whether such cells can be established as *in vitro* lines and possibly tested in a therapeutic setting.

MONOCLONAL ANTIBODY TREATMENT OF CANCER

Although the treatment of malignant disease with antibody has been of considerable interest, significant therapeutic effects have been achieved only rarely. Limitations in the effectiveness of sera may have been due to lack of sufficiently high titered antibodies of the appropriate class and specificity. With recent advances in somatic cell hybridization techniques, it is now possible to produce large quantities of antibody of defined class and specificity. These monoclonal antibodies can then be tested for therapeutic effects. The production of monoclonal antibody is based on techniques described by Köhler and Milstein (13), who fused mouse myeloma cells with mouse spleen cells from immunized donors. Resultant hybrids secreting an antibody defined by the immune B cells reactive against a cell surface antigen were selected and cloned; these clones could be maintained indefinitely in culture or as ascites tumor *in vivo*. In the studies reviewed below, we utilized monoclonal antibodies directed against a T cell differentiation antigen, Thy-1.1, to treat successfully a transplantable mouse lymphoma. These experiments, which were done in collaboration with Drs. R. Nowinski and M. Tam, are also presented in greater detail elsewhere (14).

The methods used to establish the anti-Thy-1.1 monoclonal antibody have been described (15). In brief, spleen and lymph node cells were obtained from 129 mice immunized with a transplantable AKR/J SL3 leukemia. NS/1 myeloma cells and lymphocytes were fused with polyethylene glycol and the hybrid cells selected by growth in HAT medium, which inhibits growth of the unfused myeloma cells. The antibody products of the hybrid cells were tested by an antibody-binding assay utilizing ^{125}I-labeled protein A. For these assays cell membrane fragments that were exfoliated by AKR/J SL3 cells into the culture medium were used as a source of Thy-1.1 antigen. Hybrid cells whose culture fluids were reactive in the antibody binding assay were cloned twice by limiting dilution.

Cells from these cloned cell lines were inoculated intraperitoneally (i.p.) in syngeneic $(129 \times BALB)F_1$ mice; the resultant ascites fluid which contained high-titered antibodies was used in the experiments that follow. In these studies, the monoclonal anti-Thy-1.1 antibodies of the IgG_{2a} class were used. They were designated 19-A10, 19-E12, and 19-F12(M). The ascites fluid 19-A10 showed a complement-dependent cytotoxic titer of 5×10^{-5} (50% endpoint) and a cell-dependent titer of 1.25×10^{-5} (20% endpoint); the 19-E12 antibody, a titer of 8×10^{-6} and 2×10^{-6} in the two cytotoxic assays, respectively; and F12(M) titers of 1.2×10^{-7} and 4×10^{-6}. Target cells were ^{51}Cr-labeled AKR/J SL2 transplantable spontaneous lymphomas.

Initially, three experiments were performed testing the 19-A10 and 19-E12 antibodies for their *in vivo* activity against transplants of the AKR/J SL2 spontaneous leukemia. Results of a single experiment (Table 1) showed that administration of ascites fluid in combination with rabbit serum as a source of complement prolonged survival and resulted in the cure of a significant proportion of the mice. Additional control mice received complement alone; they behaved exactly as did the untreated controls. Mice which received antibody and no complement also showed an improvement in their median survival (experiment I), although none of these mice were permanently cured. These results suggest that complement treatment can be used to amplify the effect of antibody against the subcutaneous solid lymphoma.

In the above experiments, solid lymphomas grew at the site of tumor inoculation in most of the treated mice. In fact, treated mice lived longer and grew tumors larger than those seen in control mice before the leukemia was observed. This observation suggested antibody to be more effective in preventing metastases as compared to a local, established mass. Based on this observation, we are presently using combinations of surgery and antibody therapy to achieve an increased cure rate. In one experiment, (C57BL/6 × AKR)F$_1$ were challenged with 3×10^6 leukemia cells. They were then treated with 19-A10 antibody and complement as in the above experiments on days 0,3,5, and 7. Certain of the mice had the tumor at the inoculation site removed on day 10. Results showed that 4 of 6 mice challenged with 3×10^6 leukemia cells were cured by antibody and complement treatment combined with surgery. None of the mice which did not receive antibody and complement, including control mice from whom the tumors were excised, survived.

The above experiments suggested that antibody treatment can affect the growth of syngeneic leukemia cells; and that this effect is increased by the addition of exogenous complement. The antibody most likely causes direct lysis of the tumor cells, but there was the possibility that the anti-T-cell antibody acted by modifying the host antileukemia immune response. Experiments were therefore accomplished using AKR/Cum mice. These mice are genetically similar to AKR mice, except that they express the Thy-1.2 and not Thy-1.1 T cell surface antigen. Thus, if anti-Thy-1.1 antibody were effective against the AKR leukemia cells in these mice, we would conclude that the direct action of antibody on tumor is sufficient for a therapeutic effect. The anti-Thy-1.1 antibody, F12(M), was administered to AKR/Cum mice that had been challenged with a lethal dose of the AKR/J SL2 (Thy 1.1) leukemia. Inhibition of tumor was seen in

TABLE 1. In vivo activity of antibodies against transplants of the AKR/J SL2 spontaneous leukemia

Recipients	Inoculum dose[a]	Antibody[a]	Dose schedule[b]	Median survival		No. survivors/ total no. mice	
				Treated	Control	Treated	Control
I (129 × AKR/J)	10^6	19-A10	0, 2, 4, 7	33	23	3/8	0/7
II (C57BL6 × AKR/J)	3×10^6	19-A10	0, 3, 7, 10, 14	33	19	0/8	0/8
"	3×10^6	19-E12	0, 3, 7, 10, 14	33	19	0/8	1/8
III AKR/J	10^5	19-A10	0, 3, 7, 10, 14	—	21	6/6	0/8

[a] Antibody was administered at a dose of 100 μl i.v. on day 0 and 50 μl i.p. on the remaining days. Rabbit serum as an exogenous source of complement was injected along with antibody by the same route in a volume of 100 μl.
[b] Tumor cells were injected subcutaneously on day 0 prior to administration of antibody.

each of the treated mice. Thus a direct effect of antibody on tumor can affect tumor growth. Whether there is, in addition, an antitumor effect of antibody mediated by host T cells is currently being studied.

These experiments are of particular interest since the therapy was directed at a normal differentiation antigen analogous to those expressed by certain human leukemias and lymphomas. We believe careful analysis of spontaneous and transplantable AKR/J lymphoma will provide guidelines for future clinical studies (e.g., selection of antibody class, requirement for exogenous complement, existence of sanctuary sites) and hopefully avoid the pitfalls inherent in past empirical approaches to clinical immunotherapy.

CONCLUSION

Although immunologic approaches to the treatment of cancer have not to date proved highly successful, there are new approaches which may fulfill some of the early promises. At least one approach, in which BCG is administered intradermally, appears effective in certain defined instances. Newer experimental evidence suggests that (a) host responses might be altered to allow stimulation of effective antitumor responses; or (b) individuals could be passively immunized with potent antitumor immune cells or antibody produced *in vitro*. The next decade should offer the development of sound approaches to immunotherapy based on rigorous laboratory investigations. Thus there remains great expectation that successful immunologic approaches to cancer therapy will emerge in the near future.

ACKNOWLEDGMENT

This investigation was supported by Grant CA26386, awarded by the National Cancer Institute, DHEW.

REFERENCES

1. Bernstein, I. D., and Wright, P. W. (1976): Immunology and immunotherapy of childhood neoplasia. *Pediatr. Clin. North Am.,* 23:93–109.
2. Terry, W. D., and Windhorst, D. (eds.) (1978): *Immunotherapy of Cancer; Present Status of Trials in Man.* Raven Press, New York.
3. Zbar, B., Bernstein, I. D., Bartlett, G. L., Hanna, M. G., Jr., and Rapp, H. J. (1972): Immunotherapy of cancer: Regression of intradermal tumors and prevention of growth of lymph node metastases after intradermal injection of living *Mycobacterium bovis. J. Natl. Cancer Inst.,* 49:119–130.
4. Morton, D. L., Eilber, F. R., Malmgren, R. A., et al. (1974): Immunological factors which influence response to immunotherapy in malignant melanoma. *Surgery,* 68:158–164.
5. Bast, R. C., Zbar, B., Borsos, T., and Rapp, H. J. (1974): BCG and cancer. *N. Engl. J. Med.,* 290:1458–1469.
6. McKneally, M. F., Maver, C. M., and Kausel, H. W. (1976): Regional immunotherapy of lung cancer with intrapleural BCG. *Lancet,* i:377.
7. Greene, M. I., Martin, E. D., Pierres, M., et al. (1977): Reduction of syngeneic tumor growth by an anti I-J alloantiserum. *Proc. Natl. Acad. Sci. U.S.A.,* 74:5118–5151.

8. Bernstein, I. D. (1977): Passive transfer of systemic tumor immunity with cells generated in vitro by a secondary immune response to a syngeneic rat Gross virus-induced lymphoma. *J. Immunol.,* 118:122–128.
9. Cheever, M. A., Greenberg, P. D., and Fefer, A. (1977): Tumor neutralization immunotherapy and chemoimmunotherapy of a Friend leukemia with cells secondarily sensitized in vitro. *J. Immunol.,* 119:714–718.
10. Baker, P. E., Gillis, S., and Smith, K. A. (1979): Monoclonal cytolytic T-cell lines. *J. Exp. Med.,* 149:273–278.
11. Sondel, P. M., O'Brien, C., Porter, L., Schlossman, S. F., and Chess, L. (1976): Cell-mediated destruction of human leukemic cells by MHC identical lymphocytes: Requirement for a proliferative trigger in vitro. *J. Immunol.,* 117:2197–2203.
12. Zarling, J. M., Raich, P., McKrough, M., and Bach, F. H. (1976): Generation of cytotoxic lymphocytes in vitro against autologous human leukemia cells. *Nature,* 262:691–693.
13. Köhler, G., and Milstein, C. (1975): Continuous cultures of fused cell secreting antibody of predefined specificity. *Nature,* 256:495–497.
14. Bernstein, I. D., Tam, M. R., and Nowinski, R. C. (1980): Mouse leukemia: Therapy with monoclonal antibodies against a thymus differentiation antigen. *Science,* 207:68–71.
15. Nowinski, R. C., Lostrom, M. E., Tam, M. R., Stone, M. R., and Burnette, W. N. (1979): The isolation of hybrid cell lines producing monoclonal antibodies against the p15(E) protein of ecotropic murine leukemia viruses. *Virology,* 93:111–126.

Advances in Neuroblastoma Research,
edited by Audrey E. Evans.
Raven Press, New York © 1980.

Systemic and *In Situ* Natural Killer Activity in Patients with Neuroblastoma

*,**James M. Gerson and *Ronald B. Herberman

*Laboratory of Immunodiagnosis, National Cancer Institute, Bethesda, Maryland 20205;
and **Division of Oncology, Children's Hospital of Philadelphia,
Philadelphia, Pennsylvania 19104

Natural killer (NK) cells are attracting considerable interest for their possible role in host defenses against cancer, and have been proposed as contributors to immunosurveillance against neoplastic transformation (14). In mice, levels of NK activity have been shown to vary according to the strain and age of the mice tested (16,23), to be inherited as an autosomal dominant (26), and this effector function appears to have an *in vivo* role in tumor rejection (15). In man, only limited information on the genetics of expression of NK activity is available (32), the levels of activity remain fairly stable over prolonged periods of time and thus appear to be independent of age (21,29), and direct evidence for the role of NK cells *in vivo* is lacking. Both murine and human NK cells are nonadherent and nonphagocytic, have receptors for the Fc portion of IgG, and contain markers characteristic of the T-cell lineage (14). A recent important finding has been that the activity of mouse, rat, and human NK cells is augmented by interferon or interferon inducers (4,5,13,19).

NK activity has been shown to be depressed in mice bearing primary virus-induced tumors or transplantable tumors (1,9). There have been few studies on NK activity in cancer patients, and these have focused on systemic or peripheral blood leukocyte (PBL) activity. NK activity in the patients studied appeared to be inversely correlated with tumor burden (28,30). However, systemic activity may not reflect immunological events at the tumor site, and there is little available information on NK activity *in situ*. The few studies of *in situ* NK activity have been negative (31,33).

We have tested 11 neuroblastoma patients prior to therapy for NK activity of their PBLs, and have also tested six primary tumors for NK activity *in situ*. The following report describes our studies of NK activity in the PBLs of 11 patients with neuroblastoma and six primary tumors prior to the initiation of treatment.

MATERIALS AND METHODS

Peripheral Blood Leukocytes

PBLs were obtained by centrifugation of heparinized whole blood on Ficoll-Hypaque (3). The PBLs were suspended in RPMI 1640 medium (Biofluids, Inc., Rockville, Md.) plus 10% heat-inactivated fetal bovine serum (Grand Island Biological Co., Grand Island, N.Y.) supplemented with 1 mM glutamine, 100 units/ml penicillin, 100 μg/ml streptomycin, and 10 mM HEPES buffer (complete medium).

Tumor Cell Suspensions

Biopsy specimens were received on wet ice in complete medium. Necrotic tissue was debrided, the specimen was dissociated with scalpels into fragments 2 to 3 mm in diameter, which were then sequentially digested with 125 mg% collagenase (Sigma, Type I, St. Louis, Mo.) and DNAse. The cell-rich supernatants were pooled, washed, and passed through double-layered gauze to remove clumps. The single cell suspension (SCS) obtained was then separated by several procedures in an attempt to obtain an enriched or pure lymphocyte population.

Discontinuous Sucrose Gradients

We applied the method developed by Fauci (6) to obtain lymphocytes from human bone marrow. Sucrose was layered by pipette in 2 ml aliquots at 5% increments from 15 to 35% sucrose on a 17 × 100 Falcon plastic tube. Two milliliters SCS was overlayed by pipette at a concentration of 25 to 30 × 10⁶ cells/ml, and the gradient was centrifuged for 7 min at 100 g at 24°C. The fractions were removed by pipette from above, washed, and tested for NK activity.

Linear Density Gradient (LDG) of Ficoll

A linear isokinetic gradient of Ficoll, ranging from 2.7 to 5.5%, has been shown by Pretlow et al. (27) and Blazar and Heppner (2) to be effective in separating lymphocytes from tumor cells and stromal cells. We have previously characterized PBLs separated by this method for NK activity (7). In brief, the LDG was made utilizing a two-chambered gradient maker (Lido Glass, Sterling, N.J.) and a peristaltic pump with a flow rate of 1 ml/min. The gradient was layered over a 5.5 ml cushion of 43% Ficoll (Pharmacia, Piscataway, N.J.) in a siliconized 100 ml polycarbonate tube and ranged from 2.7% at the sample gradient interface to 5.5% at the gradient cushion interface. Linearity was monitored by refractive index determination. Then 30 to 50 × 10⁶ viable cells in 7.0 ml were layered onto the gradient and spun at 97 g at 4°C for 17 min.

Twenty-four fractions were then collected by displacement with 40% sucrose via a tapping cap (Halpro, Rockville, Md.). The cells were washed in complete medium and fractions tested for NK activity.

Plastic Adherence and Nylon Column Passage

The SCSs were incubated in plastic Petri dishes for 45 min at 37°C–5% CO_2 at a concentration of 2×10^6 cells/ml. The loosely adherent and nonadherent cells were removed, washed, and then either directly tested for NK activity or first passed through a nylon wool column according to the method of Julius et al. (22) to remove loosely adherent cells and to enrich for T-lymphocytes

Cell Counts and Differentials

All counts were done by hemocytometer and viability was assessed by trypan blue staining. Cytospin (Shandon-Southern, Sewickley, Pa.) preparations were made, stained by Wright-Giemsa (Dif-Quik, A. H. Thomas, Philadelphia, Pa.), and 200 cells counted to obtain differential counts. Macrophages were also enumerated by nonspecific esterase (NEAE) staining according to the method of Koski et al. (24)

Cytotoxicity

NK activity was assayed in a 4 hr chromium-51 release assay (CRA) using the human myeloid line, K-562, as target cells. The assay was run in microplates (Linbro, Hamden, Conn.), in triplicate, and at attacker to target ratios of 100:1, 50:1, and 25:1. Percent cytotoxicity was calculated by the formula $\frac{[(A - B) - (C - B)]}{T - B} \times 100$, where A = mean counts per minute (cpm) released in test combinations, B = mean cpm of machine background, C = mean cpm of autologous control, and T = mean cpm of total ^{51}Cr incorporated into 5×10^3 target cells.

Competitive Inhibition Assay

This assay has been previously described in detail (17). Briefly, tumor cell suspensions were tested for their ability to inhibit or suppress the cytotoxicity of normal PBLs against ^{51}Cr-labeled K-562 target cells in a 4 hr assay. The assay was run in triplicate, in 12 × 75 mm glass tubes in a 1.0 ml volume. The effector to target ratio was kept constant at 50:1, and the number of inhibitors added was varied from fourfold excess to 6% of the normal PBL. The percent inhibition was determined by the formula $\left[1 - \frac{E}{C}\right] \times 100$, where E = experimental and C = control % cytotoxicity without inhibitors present.

RESULTS

NK Activity of Peripheral Blood Lymphocytes

The NK activity of PBL of neuroblastoma patients was appreciably lower than that of normal donors (Table 1). In this small series of patients, there was no apparent correlation of NK activity with stage or tumor burden. A recent study of patients with lung or breast cancer demonstrated the presence of suppressor cells in the PBL (20). We therefore tested 3 patients and found that depletion of adherent cells resulted in enhanced cytotoxicity.

Tumor Cell Suspensions

The viability of the SCS ranged from 39 to 98% by trypan blue determination. The yield of viable cells per gram of tissue also had a wide range from 0.5 to 4.8×10^8 cells.

Differential cell count. Differential analysis of 200 cells in cytospin smears as well as calculation of the % NEAE positive cells in the SCS was made (Table 2). The lymphocytes present ranged from 7.1 to 17.6%, and the macrophages present from none to 9.0%.

TABLE 1. *Natural killer activity against K-562 by peripheral blood leukocytes of untreated neuroblastoma patients*

			% Cytotoxicity		
Patient	Stage		60 [a]	30	10
JR	I	NA [b]	50.7	45.2	41.2
HJ	I		22.5	45.2	41.2
DP	II		3.6	2.1	2.6
BJ	II		12.1	8.7	5.2
MH	IV		8.0	5.6	−11.6
DD	IV		14.6	8.1	4.0
		NA	22.0	19.1	11.0
KS	IV–S		32.8	13.4	4.3
TI	IV–S		3.2	2.9	3.2
		NA	8.2	3.6	2.5
EC	GNBL [c]		6.9	5.6	1.5
RR	GNBL		4.1	0.2	0.3
YL	GN [c]		14.6	11.3	3.3
Mean					
Patients (11)			15.7	12.2	3.3
Normals (12)			31.1	23.2	12.9

[a] Effector:target cell ratio.
[b] Cells nonadherent to plastic and/or nylon column.
[c] GNBL, ganglioneuroblastoma; GN, ganglioneuroma.

TABLE 2. *Cells in suspensions (SCS) of human neuroblastomas*

	Differential count		
Cells	% Lymphocytes	% Macrophages	% Tumor cells
SCS-1	7.1	8.9[a]	84
SCS-2	10.2	3.2	84.7
SCS-3	8.8	9.0[a]	82.2
SCS-4	17.6	0.0	82.4
SCS-5	12.5	1.0	86.5

[a] Determined by esterase staining.

Cytotoxicity. As shown in Fig. 1, none of the effector cell fractions tested had detectable NK activity. It should be noted that the fraction selected as representative of enriched lymphocytes was based on data obtained using PBL separated by the same methods.

Cold target inhibition. Since there was always > 30% tumor cells in the effector populations, one possible explanation for the negative cytotoxicity results was that the tumor cells were able to inhibit lysis of the labeled target cells. Therefore, some of the tumor suspensions were tested for cold target inhibition (Fig. 2). Significant inhibition by the SCS of the NK activity of normal PBLs was evident, particularly at high concentrations of SCS. At low concentrations of SCS, augmented cytotoxicity was frequently observed.

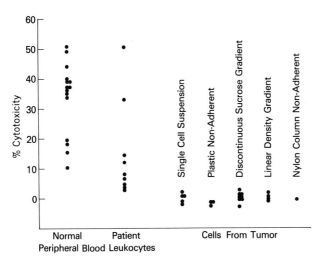

FIG. 1. Systemic versus in situ natural killer cytotoxicity against K-562 target in patients with neuroblastoma.

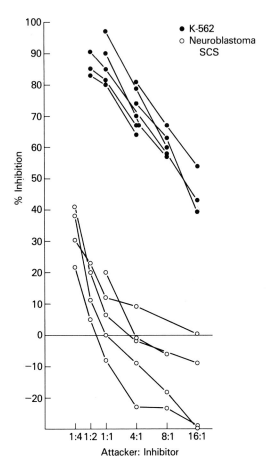

FIG. 2. Competitive inhibition of natural killer activity against K-562 by single cell suspensions (SCS) from human neuroblastomas.

DISCUSSION

Many of the unusual features of the clinical course of patients with neuroblastomas have been attributed to immune responses of the host against his tumor. This subject was reviewed in a prior publication (8). Surprisingly, there has been a paucity of data concerning *in vitro* correlates of immune function and clinical course. In earlier studies the Hellstroms (11,12) reported that nearly all patients tested had lymphocytes reactive against autologous and/or allogeneic neuroblastoma target cells. These studies were done using either a colony inhibition or microcytotoxicity assay. These assays measure some unknown combination of lysis, stasis, and cell detachment, and the nature of the effector cells cannot be defined. In particular, the possible role of NK cells, which have been a confounding factor in many clinical cytotoxicity studies, was not considered (18).

Our data show that PBL or systemic NK activity is present but depressed in neuroblastoma patients relative to normal donor controls. The mechanism of this suppression is not clear, but our results suggest that an adherent suppressor cell may in part be responsible. It has been reported that tumor cells can share antigens with K-562 and thus inhibit NK activity (25). Furthermore, data presented by Seeger et al. (this volume) demonstrated that their monoclonal anti-NMT antibody against neuroblastoma was partially absorbed by K-562, lending further support to the possibility that neuroblastomas share antigens with K-562 and thereby might be able to competitively inhibit cytotoxicity. The lack of *in situ* NK activity most likely can be explained by cold target inhibition by tumor cells due to the large number of tumor cells present, although one cannot exclude the possibilities that: (a) NK cells fail to enter and/or persist in these tumors, (b) suppressor cells or factors were present, and (c) nonrepresentative tissue sampling or extraction occurred. Of interest in this regard, we have found that adherent, phagocytic cells from murine sarcoma virus-induced progressor tumors in CBA mice will inhibit NK activity (10). There is a need to further determine the nature of cells inhibiting cytotoxicity—tumor cells or host cells—by better separation procedures. It should be realized that we have examined only one facet of host defenses in neuroblastoma, and further studies clarifying the role of T-cell immunity, macrophages, and antibody are also needed.

REFERENCES

1. Becker, S., and Klein, E. (1976): Decreased "natural killer"—NK—Effect in tumor bearing mice and its relation to the immunity against oncorna virus determined cell surface antigens. *Eur. J. Immunol.,* 6:892–898.
2. Blazar, B. A., and Heppner, B. H. (1978): In situ lymphoid cells of mouse mammary tumors. I. Development and evaluation of a method for the separation of lymphoid cells from mouse mammary tumors. *J. Immunol.,* 120:1876–1880.
3. Boyum, A. (1968): Separation of leukocytes from blood and bone marrow. *Scand. J. Clin. Invest.,* 21:1.
4. Djeu, J. Y., Heinbaugh, J. A., Holden, H. T., and Herberman, R. B. (1979): Augmentation of mouse natural killer cell activity by interferon and interferon inducers. *J. Immunol.,* 122:175–181.
5. Einhorn, S., Blomgren, H., and Strander, H. (1978): Interferon and spontaneous cytotoxicity in man. I. Enhancement of the spontaneous cytotoxicity of peripheral lymphocytes by human leukocyte interferon. *Int. J. Cancer,* 22:405–412.
6. Fauci, A. S. (1975): Human bone marrow lymphocytes. I. Distribution of lymphocyte subpopulations in the bone marrow of normal individuals. *J. Clin. Invest.,* 56:98–110.
7. Gerson, J. M., Chiapella, C., and Ortaldo, J. (1979): Enrichment of natural killer (NK) and killer (K) cytotoxicity by cells separated on a linear isokinetic Ficoll gradient. *Fed. Proc.,* 38:1278.
8. Gerson, J. M., and Evans, A. E. (1976): Neuroblastoma and host defense mechanisms. In: *Oncologic Medicine,* edited by A. I. Sutnick and P. F. Engstrom, pp. 61–70. University Park Press, Baltimore.

9. Gerson, J. M., Holden, H. T., Bonnard, G. D., and Herberman, R. B. (1979): Natural killer activity in murine and human solid tumors. *Proc. Am. Assoc. Cancer Res.,* 20:238.
10. Gerson, J. M., Varesio, L., and Herberman, R. B. (1979): In preparation.
11. Hellstrom, I., Hellstrom, K. E., Bell, A. H., Pierce, G. E., and Yang, J. P. S. (1970): Studies on cellular immunity to human neuroblastoma cells. *Int. J. Cancer,* 6:172.
12. Hellstrom, I., Hellstrom, K. E., Pierce, G. E., and Bell, A. H. (1968): Demonstration of cell bound and humoral immunity against neuroblastoma cells. *Proc. Natl. Acad. Sci. U.S.A.,* 60:1231–1238.
13. Herberman, R. B., Djeu, J. Y., Ortaldo, J., Holden, H. T., West, W. H., and Bonnard, G. D. (1978): Role of interferon in augmentation of natural and antibody-dependent cell mediated cytotoxicity. *Cancer Treatment Rep.,* 62:1893–1896.
14. Herberman, R. B., and Holden, H. T. (1978): Natural cell-mediated immunity. *Adv. Cancer Res.,* 27:305–377.
15. Herberman, R. B., and Holden, H. T. (1979): Natural killer cells as antitumor effector cells. *J. Natl. Cancer Inst.,* 62:441–445.
16. Herberman, R. B., Nunn, M. E., and Lavrin, D. H. (1975): Natural cytotoxic reactivity of mouse lymphoid cells against syngeneic and allogeneic tumors. I. Distribution of reactivity and specificity. *Int. J. Cancer,* 16:216–229.
17. Herberman, R. B., Nunn, M. E., and Holden, H. T. (1976): Cytotoxicity inhibition analysis of specificity of cell-mediated ^{51}Cr release cytotoxicity. In: *In Vitro Methods in Cell Mediated and Tumor Immunity,* edited by R. B. Bloom and J. R. David, pp. 489–495. Academic Press, New York.
18. Herberman, R. B., and Oldham, R. K. (1975): Problems associated with study of cell mediated immunity to human tumors by microcytotoxicity assays. *J. Natl. Cancer Inst.,* 55:749–753.
19. Herberman, R. B., Ortaldo, J. R., and Bonnard, G. D. (1979): Augmentation by interferon of human natural and antibody-dependent cell mediated cytotoxicity. *Nature,* 277:221–223.
20. Jerrells, T. R., Dean, J. H., Richardson, J. L., McCoy, J. L., and Herberman, R. B. (1978): Role of suppressor cells in depression of in vitro lymphoproliferative responses of lung cancer and breast cancer patients. *J. Natl. Cancer Inst.,* 61:1001–1009.
21. Jondal, M., and Pross, H. (1975): Surface markers on human B and T lymphocytes. VI. Cytotoxicity against cell lines as a functional marker for lymphocyte subpopulations. *Int. J. Cancer,* 15:596–605.
22. Julius, M. H., Simpson, E., and Herzenberg, L. A. (1973): A rapid method for the evaluation of functional thymus-derived murine lymphocytes. *Eur. J. Immunol.,* 3:645–649.
23. Kiessling, R., Klein, E., and Wigzell, H. (1975): "Natural" killer cells in the mouse. I. Cytotoxic cells with specificity for mouse Moloney leukemia cells. Specificity and distribution according to genotype. *Eur. J. Immunol.,* 5:112–117.
24. Koski, I. R., Poplack, D. G., and Blaese, R. M. (1976): A nonspecific esterase stain for the identification of monocytes and macrophages. In: *In Vitro Methods in Cell-Mediated and Tumor Immunity,* edited by B. Bloom and J. R. David, p. 359. Academic Press, New York.
25. Ortaldo, J., Oldham, R. K., and Herberman, R. B. (1977): Specificity of natural cytotoxic reactivity of normal human lymphocytes against a myeloid leukemia cell line. *J. Natl. Cancer Inst.,* 59:77–82.
26. Petranyi, G. G., Kiessling, R., and Klein, G. (1975): Genetic control of "natural" killer lymphocytes in the mouse. *Immunogenetics,* 2:53–61.
27. Pretlow, T. G., II, Jones, M., and Pretlow, T. (1976): Separation of tumor cells by density gradient centrifugation: Recent work with human tumors and a discussion of the kind of quantitation needed in cell separation experiments. *Biophys. Chem.,* 5:99–106.
28. Pross, H. F., and Baines, M. G. (1976): Spontaneous human lymphocyte mediated cytotoxicity against tumor target cells. I. The effect of malignant disease. *Int. J. Cancer,* 18:593–604.
29. Takasugi, M., Mickey, M. R., and Terasaki, P. I. (1973): Reactivity lymphocytes for normal persons in cultured tumor cells. *Cancer Res.,* 33:2898–2902.
30. Takasugi, M., Ramseyer, A., and Takasugi, J. (1977): Decline of natural nonselective cell mediated cytotoxicity in patients with tumor progression. *Cancer Res.,* 37:413–418.
31. Totterman, T. H., Hayry, P., Saksela, E., Temonen, T., and Eklund, B. (1978): Cytological and functional analysis of inflammatory infiltrates in human malignant tumors. II. Functional investigations of the infiltrating inflammatory cells. *Eur. J. Immunol.,* 8:872–875.

32. Trinchieri, G., Santoli, D., Zmijewski, C. M., and Koprowski, H. (1977): Functional correlation between antibody-dependent and spontaneous cytotoxic activity of human lymphocytes and possibility of HLA-related control. *Transplant. Proc.,* 9:881–884.
33. Vose, B. M., Vanky, F., Argov, S., and Klein, E. (1977): Natural cytotoxicity in man: Activity of lymph mode and tumor infiltrating lymphocytes. *Eur. J. Immunol.,* 7:353–357.

Advances in Neuroblastoma Research,
edited by Audrey E. Evans.
Raven Press, New York © 1980.

Discussion: Immunology

Dr. Franz (Boston) asked Dr. Bernstein about the effect of his antisera and complement on normal T-cell numbers in AKR mice. Dr. Bernstein replied that he is studying its effect on T-cell numbers, function, and on autoimmune responses. Dr. Franz also questioned the mechanism whereby the animals died. Dr. Bernstein replied that the animals developed very large local tumors which tend to metastasize through lymphoid tissue and they presumably die from systemic disease. He was not sure whether death is ultimately due to bleeding or infection, but the presence of metastatic tumor indicates the difference between the animals that die and live.

Dr. Green (Memphis) asked if Dr. Bernstein had any data on the dispersion of monoclonal antibody to other compartments in the body. Dr. Bernstein replied that such studies need to be done to elucidate whether there are sanctuary sites and what is the pharmacology of the antibody. He has set up an animal model for the tumor growing in the appropriate host so that these questions may be studied.

Dr. Kemshead (London) cautioned investigators about using mouse and rat monoclonal antibodies clinically and noted that we are a long way from injecting mouse and rat antibodies into humans for treatment. Human monoclonal antibodies are needed which will probably take a long time. Dr. Bernstein pointed out that if a monoclonal mouse antibody of certain potency exists, its use could be considered in the same way that patients with aplastic anemia are treated with horse anti-thymocyte globulin.

Dr. Lampson (Stanford) suggested that the real problem with using human antibodies is the different repertoire of specificity. Mouse antibodies recognize differentiation antigens, but human anti-human antibodies will only recognize polymorphic specificities.

Dr. Prasad (Denver) asked Dr. Kemshead whether there is a possibility that drug treatment may change the antigen profile of neuroblastoma cell. Dr. Kemshead indicated that anything affecting the genetic makeup of the cells may affect their expression of antigens.

Dr. Reynolds (Dallas) asked Dr. Kemshead whether he had ruled out the possibility that the antisera are not reacting with fetal calf serum antigens. Dr. Kemshead responded that they have studied that question and the sera are not reacting with fetal calf serum antibodies.

Dr. Rajewsky (Essen) asked Dr. Bernstein if he had used fluorescent monoclonal antibodies and the cell sorter in the AKR system to sort the cells that are not binding the antibody and determined if these cells continue to produce tumors. Although Dr. Bernstein agreed that the question was important, he did not believe that the cell-sorter analysis would allow one to reach conclusions if the population was a minor one (one in 10^5 or 10^6 cells). The only real approach is to ask the biological question: what success do we have with treating spontaneous AKR leukemia?

Dr. Anderson (Denver) asked Dr. Epstein if he had ruled out macrophages as a possible mediator of cell-mediated immunity in his system. *Dr. Epstein* responded that the resistance mechanism to C1300 neuroblastoma is radiation sensitive (sublethal doses) and the macrophage would probably not be affected. Dr. Anderson asked if he had ever tried antimacrophage agents like silica or carrageenan and Dr. Epstein replied he had not.

Dr. Anderson stated that he had some preliminary evidence that murine neuroblastoma cells inhibit macrophage functions which could be an important means of subverting the immune response. He asked if there is any other evidence that neuroblastomas inhibit immune cells or macrophages. Dr. Epstein replied that they have not looked at the question of suppressors in vivo with, for example, anti-suppressor sera (anti I-J) as have Green et al. In their in vitro system, he noted, restimulation of spleen cells from mice with very large progressively growing tumors results in generation of killer cells against the tumor, suggesting suppressor are not active.

Dr. D'Angio (Philadelphia) asked whether there are any lymphocytic infiltration in the C1300 tumors, but this aspect had not been studied by any members of the panel.

Dr. Elkins (Philadelphia) asked Dr. Gerson if he had succeeded in isolating NK cells from any tumors. He replied that groups in Sweden and Finland have attempted to detect NK activity in situ in human tumors and were unable to do so. In murine MSV induced progressor tumors, NK activity cannot be detected. In studying spontaneous mammary tumors in C3H mice, Dr. Gerson found NK activity in small tumors, but not in larger ones.

Dr. Green (Memphis) asked how we are to proceed to sort through the diverse antigens on the surface of the neuroblastoma cell and come up with an antibody to neuroblastoma. He questioned whether the cell membrane should be cleaved into proteins or antigens to start with a single protein to make an antibody or whether it was best to start with the whole cell. Dr. Lampson replied that if you start with a whole cell, at least the resultant antibody will recognize a cell surface determinant that will be in its native form. When considering the use of antibody for diagnosis or therapy, this is very desirable.

Dr. Kennett (Philadelphia) remarked that the only way of picking out specific molecules at the moment is with monoclonal antibodies and many are lost when membranes are chopped into small segments. The secret in making monoclonal antibodies that are useful is to design screening procedures that detect with a minimum of effort the kind of antibody that is wanted. The antibody can then be used to purify the antigen of interest.

Dr. Seeger (Los Angeles) remarked that we are not compelled to obtain an antibody against tumor-specific antigen. Antibodies to numerous antigens can be useful. For example, antibodies to cell surface fetal antigens, differentiation antigens, histocompatibility antigens, and blood group antigens may all be valuable. It is unlikely that tumor specific antigens will be unequivocally defined; thus, we should be pragmatic in developing antibodies to antigens that are useful. Dr. Green suggested that directing the antibody response of the mouse should help to get the kinds of monoclonal antibodies that are wanted. For example, masking undesirable antigens with heterologous antibodies before immunization may be beneficial. Dr. Kemshead believed that such an approach is appropriate. An alternative is to "tolerize against one cell line and immunize against another" to decrease the number of antigenic determinants the mouse will see.

Dr. Hann (Philadelphia) commented that Dr. Kennett's antigen on neuroblastoma cells is a glycoprotein and noted that ferritin is an α 2 glycoprotein. She asked if his antigen was similar to ferritin. Dr. Kennett replied that, as Dr. Momoi had shown, the antigenic determinant recognized by P1 153/3 monoclonal antibody is the sugar. This sugar could be on various proteins of different kinds of cells. Obtaining a monoclonal antibody is the first step in defining antigens; the antigen then must be purified to characterize it biochemically.

Cytokinetics and Chemotherapy Models

Advances in Neuroblastoma Research,
edited by Audrey E. Evans.
Raven Press, New York © 1980.

Predictive Value of Cell Kinetic Studies in Neuroblastoma

F. A. Hayes and A. A. Green

St. Jude Children's Research Hospital, Memphis, Tennessee 38101

In order to utilize cell kinetics in the design of therapy, one must first develop a data base for the tumor under study. In 1974 we initiated a program of cell kinetic studies in children with disseminated neuroblastoma admitted to St. Jude Children's Research Hospital. The high frequency of bone marrow metastases in this tumor provides an easily accessible site for the procurement of tumor cells for study in the unperturbed state and sequentially during perturbation by chemotherapy. The results of these studies have provided objective parameters by which we can identify patients who will not respond to planned chemotherapy and in whom response, if it occurs, will be of short duration.

METHODS AND MATERIALS

From August 1974 through December 1978, there have been 69 children with disseminated neuroblastoma admitted to St. Jude Children's Research Hospital. These children form the patient population from whom cell kinetic data of tumor obtained at diagnosis, second look surgery, and relapse have been derived. All patients were initially treated with cyclophosphamide 150 mg/m²/ day for 7 days followed on day 8 by adriamycin 35 mg/m². This sequential therapy was repeated every 14 to 21 days for a 4-month induction period. Mitotic (MI) and labeling (LI) indices of primary and metastatic tumor were done by methods previously described (1). Sequential bone marrow aspirates for tumor cell MI and LI were obtained before treatment and, during the first course of therapy, after 7 days of cyclophosphamide, and 4, 24, and 48 hours after the first dose of adriamycin. Samples of tumor for cell kinetics were also obtained from marrow and solid tumors at varying times during the patient's disease.

RESULTS

Cell kinetic evaluation of tumor cells in children with neuroblastoma metastatic to bone marrow has proven value in predicting response to therapy with sequential cyclophosphamide and adriamycin (1). Since the initial publication of these studies, further patients have been evaluated and the correlation between changes in the LI and MI occurring with the first course of therapy and the remission status of the patient at 4 months continues to be positive.

The pretreatment LI of bone marrow tumor cells obtained in 32 patients ranges from 1 to 33% (median 14.4%) and does not correlate with the patient's response to treatment. However, of the 14 children over the age of 1 year at diagnosis who attained complete remission (CR) at 4 months, the median time to relapse and median survival were significantly longer in those with initial LI of < 15% than those with a higher percent of labeled cells (10.5 versus 6.4, 18+ versus 11 months). Of the 7 children with LI of < 15%, 3 are alive without disease 12+, 17+, and 57+ months, whereas none of the 7 with an initial LI of > 15% survive free of disease. The LI of cell suspensions of primary tumors (as distinct from marrow) obtained at diagnosis in patients with disseminated disease ranged from 0.4 to 26.3% (median 10%) and also had no correlation with response to therapy.

Patients who attained complete clinical remission were evaluated at a "second look" surgical procedure 4 months after diagnosis. Four patients in whom the LI of residual tumor was < 10% at this time have all remained in remission for at least 5 months after surgery, whereas six patients with an LI of > 10% all relapsed within 3 months of surgery.

Although there was no correlation between the height of the LI and attainment of remission at diagnosis, there was a definite correlation between these two factors at relapse. Of the 21 patients evaluated at relapse, 5/5 with a low LI of primary or marrow tumor attained second remissions of at least 5 months' duration. In contrast, of the 16 patients with high tumor cell LI at relapse, none attained second remissions.

Preliminary studies comparing LI, the ability of tumor to establish sustained growth in culture, and the response of the tumor to therapy are providing interesting results. Currently, 27 solid tumors and 37 bone marrow samples have been obtained simultaneously at diagnosis, second look surgery, or relapse for cell kinetic evaluation and growth in culture. Of these 64 tumor samples, 18 have established sustained growth in culture. All 18 were obtained from patients whose tumor had a high LI and demonstrated resistance to therapy. Thus 18/33 samples from nonresponding patients established sustained growth in culture while none of the 31 attempts from responding patients were successful.

DISCUSSION

With these cell kinetic studies, we are able to identify during the first week of therapy the child with bone marrow metastases who will not respond to initial treatment. In the child who does attain remission, the duration of that remission correlates with the height of the initial LI.

A high LI of residual solid tumor obtained at second look surgery appears to predict a short remission, and a high LI of solid or bone marrow tumor at relapse has been uniformly associated with failure to attain second remission. It is possible that these correlations will be present regardless of previous therapy and could be utilized to identify the children in whom different maintenance therapy or aggressive alternate reinduction therapy is needed to maintain or attain clinical remission.

These studies appear to provide objective prognostic data to aid in therapeutic decisions which may benefit the individual child. They also provide insight into the biological variability of this tumor, not only from child to child, but also in the same child at varying times during the course of the disease. When utilizing human tumor cell lines for the study of biological markers, *in vitro* response to drugs, immunological studies, etc., one must realize that the tumor used to establish these lines is biologically different from the majority of tumors, and is highly resistant to therapy *in vivo*.

ACKNOWLEDGMENTS

This work was supported by Grants CA 15956, CA 23099, the Ruby Levi Fund, and ALSAC.

REFERENCE

1. Hayes, F. A., Green, A. A., and Mauer, A. M. (1977): Correlation of cell kinetic and clinical response to chemotherapy in disseminated neuroblastoma. *Cancer Res.,* 37:3766–3770.

Advances in Neuroblastoma Research,
edited by Audrey E. Evans.
Raven Press, New York © 1980.

FMF Analysis of the Cell Cycle: Membrane and Nucleic Acid Stainings

C. Nicolini

Division of Biophysics, Department of Physiology/Biophysics, Temple University Health Science Center, Philadelphia, Pennsylvania 19140

In recent years, microfluorometry has become extremely popular among cell biologists, causing a chain reaction of scattered papers in a variety of related fields (9,24). Regardless of these efforts, a review (18) of all pertinent literature of both static and flow microfluorometry reveals little awareness of: (a) the optimal staining conditions; (b) the physicochemical mechanisms and macromolecular organization, *in situ,* determining given spectral emission and fluorescence quantum yield; (c) the different binding processes between the various dyes commonly utilized and cell components, such as RNA, chromatin-DNA, protein, and outer membrane; and (d) the unique spectrofluorometric properties of each dye when interacting with double- or single-stranded nucleic acid and proteins, as functions of ionic strength.

This review is aimed to address the above points to prove that, under proper staining conditions, it is possible to study differentially chromatin (17), membrane (8), and RNA (17) *in situ* with dyes such as ethidium bromide (14,15), acridine orange (17,18), and fluorescamine (5,6). Specifically, extending our original quantitative work with ethidium bromide (14) and acridine orange (16–18), in this overview we have the goal of establishing a bridge between nucleic acid and cell membrane staining, which, combined with traditional cell size evaluation, constitutes a uniquely powerful means for objectively characterizing cell cycle phase in perturbed and unperturbed populations.

MULTIPARAMETER FLOW CYTOMETRY

Cell fluorescence (green, red, and total) and low-angle forward light scatter are measured on a flow microfluorometer using an ion laser of various powers (between 35 mW and 4 watt) at various wavelengths, ranging from the far ultraviolet to the visible (18). Usually a sample of fluorescently tagged cells may be injected into the center of a flowing stream. The stream after emerging from the nozzle tip is about 50 μm in diameter. As previously shown (18), as cells pass through the laser beam, different cells give different but characteristic signals, both in fluorescence and in scattering.

In order to perform multiparameter analysis with our flow systems (either an Orthocytofluorograf or a B-D cell sorter) on-line with our PDP11/40 computer, various electronic modifications were made to allow multiple fluorescent and/or scatter measurement on each cell (22). After collection, the data are sorted and stored in a two-dimensional 50 × 50 array on a Deck Disc for further analysis. To process the acquired data, various software routines have been written which allow for easy manipulation of the data (22). This routine includes the capability of plotting the two-dimensional cytogram of any specified window on the data as well as the simultaneous plotting of the 2 one-dimensional histograms obtained by projecting the cytogram on each axis. The statistics on each window are available along with the capability of storing projections for the different windows, to allow the analysis to be performed by our computer in *real time*. Unfixed cell suspensions properly stained are utilized in these studies.

FLUORESCENCE STAINING

Chromatin-DNA and RNA

Ethidium bromide is a specific intercalating dye for nuclei acids, both RNA and DNA, which has been extensively studied both in *solution* (7,19,21) and *in situ* (14,15,18).

In order to discriminate between the binding processes (primary or secondary) of DNA or RNA, we evaluate the mean fluorescence per cell as a function of added dye (14,18). This could allow us to determine the amount of bound and free dye at any concentration of ethidium bromide (EB). By analogy with the Scatchard plot analysis (14,18), we can then determine the association constant and the number of primary binding sites in the intact cell, by staining the cell with EB $= 10^{-5}$ M final concentration and $R = \dfrac{(\mu\text{M added EB})}{(\mu\text{M DNA-P})}$ ranging between 0.1. and 10. Under our experimental conditions (unifixed cells), the chromosomes maintain their conformation intact, such that mainly at low $R(< 1.0)$, a variation in conformation can be reflected in variation of fluorescence per cell (14,18). However, even free EB, outside weakly bound EB and EB bound to RNA, does yield orange red fluorescence even if with lower quantum yield, requiring perfect instrument calibrations, lengthy and complex analysis of broad multiband (15) peak to detect subtle differences in chromatin conformation (14,15).

Because frequently cell death has been correlated with EB uptake, we like to comment on such correlation, even if cell death (eventually occurring in unfixed cells during the procedure) is not at issue here, since it does not alter DNA organization and subsequent fluorescence emission within the short time between cell staining and analysis (18). A careful time sequence on *in vitro* cells, directly stained on their coverslip with EB at saturation, shows (18) that within 2 to 6 min (depending on cell concentration) all viable cells exhibit clear orange fluorescent nuclei while preserving their morphology. Furthermore, when stained at R = 4 and absolute EB concentration of 4×10^{-5} M (staining condition utilized in this report), not only do viable cells pick up the dye, but they maintain their capability to grow after quick dye removal (18).

The other dye frequently utilized is acridine orange (AO), both for flow microfluorometric (FMF) studies and for static fluorescense (SF) studies of the intact cells. However, until recently (17) we were lacking a rigorous approach to the AO staining, where, even if we are dealing with cells and not with nucleotides in solution, we have a comparably good control and understanding of the entire dye-cell interaction and subsequent fluorescence emission. For both FMF and SF studies there are in the literature either empirical protocols (2,20) or quantitative but misleading approaches. For this reason, we have explored (17) a large range of R $\frac{\text{(total dye)}}{\text{(total DNA)}}$ ratios and final AO concentrations, and found that the results *in situ* even if more approximate are essentially in agreement with those of the studies in solution, for either fixed or unfixed cells (18). Specifically, at final AO concentration of 2.5×10^{-5} M and at different molar ratios R, the nucleus and the cytoplasm are both green at R = 0.16, respectively green and reddish orange at R = 4, and respectively yellow-orange and red at R = 10. Similar dependence on molar ratios R (ranging between 0.1 and 23) are found in a wide range of final AO concentrations (10^{-4} to 10^{-7} M) as previously shown (17,18).

At AO concentration of 2.5×10^{-5} M and R = 4 (experimental conditions utilized here), while the nuclear green fluorescence is selectively affected (80 to 90% reduction in intensity) by DNAse, the cytoplasmic reddish-orange fluorescence is drastically reduced by RNAse digestion (17). These studies, confirmed in other cell lines (as CHO and M3), gave identical results with or without cell pretreatment by Triton X-100 and chelating agents at various pHs (2,18). It is therefore apparent that the differential spectral emission, i.e., nuclear DNA versus cytoplasmic RNA, strongly depends on the dye/DNA ratio compatible with the critical EB dependence of the same ratio; particular attention to the mass action law (17) must be paid to obtain reproducible FMF data. Table 1 summarizes the relevant parameters and computed association constants for the primary and secondary sites of nuclear DNA and cytoplasmic RNA *in situ* for both ethidium bromide and acridine orange, explaining in terms of mass action law and ready AO polymer formation (18) how differential staining of chromatin DNA and RNA are possible with AO and not with EB.

Membrane

Fluorescamine is a fluorescent dye which combines covalently with primary amines. This covalent reaction occurs optimally at pH 9 with a half-time in the order of milliseconds to a second. Excess fluorescamine is hydrolyzed to a nonfluorescent form in a time range of the order of seconds (5,6).

TABLE 1. *Association constant for AO-nucleic acids interactions*

	Dye-DNA		Dye-RNA	
	Primary	Secondary	Primary	Secondary
Solution (AO) (at high ionic strength)	1.3×10^5	0.8×10^4	1.3×10^5	—
In situ (AO) Acridine orange	2.6×10^5	0.7×10^4	2.6×10^5	4.3×10^4
In situ (EB) Ethidium bromide	4×10^5	6.5×10^4	4×10^5	6.5×10^4

Binding constants (1 mol^{-1}) for AO-DNA and AO-RNA interaction in solution (at high ionic strength, i.e., 0.2 M) and *in situ* for AO and ethidium bromide. For AO primary sites refer to the green emission, whereas secondary sites refer to dimer and higher aggregate formation outside nucleic acids. For ethidium bromide (EB) both primary and secondary sites are orange-red.

On this assumption it is expected that all labeled molecules will be in the outer membranes in intact cells. This was checked on a preliminary basis (6) through monitoring two cytoplasmic proteins found to be nonfluorescent. Recently, however, it was shown that the inner and nuclear membranes are stained (8).

The staining procedure used by Hawkes et al. consisted of a 30 sec exposure of living proliferating cells grown in a monolayer to a fluorescamine concentration of 500 μg/ml in 0.5% acetone and 0.2 M borate buffer at pH 9. Concentration of cells was unknown. Examination by fluorescent microscopy revealed a uniformly stained cell population with the exception of mitotic cells that fluoresced more intensely.

Uncorrected emission and excitation spectra show a single excitation peak at 415 nm and a single emission peak at 480 nm (8).

In the experiment here reported, rough calculation of the saturation concentration needed for staining yielded a concentration of 0.33 μg/ml. As this was several orders of magnitude lower than what had been used in previous work with the dye, and we wanted to be sure to saturate all available sites, we used routinely instead a value of 600 μg/ml; free excess fluorescamine is indeed hydrolyzed in a nonfluorescent form in a few seconds. The exact staining procedure is as follows:

1. Cells are grown in 75 cm^2 Falcon bottles.
2. These cells are rinsed once with Hanks, twice with 0.2 M borate buffer adjusted to pH 9.
3. Fluorescamine 3 mg is dissolved in 0.1 ml of acetone.
4. Then 5 ml of warm borate buffer is added to this acetone solution, and immediately the entire mixture is added to the Falcon bottle.
5. After 30 sec this solution is removed, the cells washed with Hanks, and then scraped from its plastic surface.

Under our experimental condition, we utilize a B-D cell sorter at the excitation wavelength of 454.5 nm and 375 mW. At this wavelength the excitation spectrum has a value slightly larger than half its peak value. The filter for the fluorescamine emission is 480 ± 3 nm.

Double Staining

Double staining of nucleic acids and cell membrane using our B-D cell sorter with laser excitation at 454 nm is accomplished in two steps: cells are stained with fluorescamine as shown above, then cells are scraped and suspended in buffered Hanks (Ca = Mg free) and finally EB is added to reach R = 9 and 10^{-5} M concentration (at saturation).

The blue fluorescence emission of the membrane-bound fluorescamine peaks at 480 nm, whereas the orange fluorescence emission of the chromatin-DNA ethidium bromide peaks at 590 nm. With proper filter, i.e., red (650 ± 50 nm) for EB and blue (480 + 3 nm) for fluorescamine, membrane and nucleic acids can be differentially and simultaneously stained without any overlap.

RESULTS

Human Lymphocytes

The peripheral blood (Ficoll-Hypaque) cells from a healthy donor were incubated with phytohemagglutamin (PHA) in order to stimulate proliferation of the previously resting lymphocytes. Lymphocytes suspension were prepared from the cell culture 0, 24, 48, and 72 hr after PHA stimulation (12). The scattergrams (scatter versus green fluorescence) and green fluorescence histograms obtained by FMF after AO staining are shown in Figs. 1 and 2. It has been shown frequently in lymphocytes (2,12) that DNA synthesis, under these conditions, does not increase until 48 hr after PHA stimulation. Therefore, in the first 48 hr when the scatter profiles remain practically invariant, any change indicated by the increased green fluorescence (peak skew toward larger fluorescence already at 24 hr) is related to the G0 (resting)–G1 (cycling) transition. These data on unfixed cells, stained directly by AO, confirm previous findings (2) on the same system obtained with an unnecessarily complex staining procedure that involved cell pretreatment with Triton X-chelating agent (2). A population with lower green fluorescence, for the same scatter, is also apparent. This fraction (which could refer to Q cells irreversibly out of cycle) increases with time after stimulation. The entire log phase population (G0, G1, S, and G2 + M) can be easily found in the histogram of PHA-stimulated lymphocytes after 72 hr (Fig. 2). Figure 2 shows that the G0 peak (similar scatter as G1 but lower green fluorescence) progressively decreases and the G1 peak (higher fluorescence for same scatter as G0) increases after PHA stimulation.

These effects of PHA stimulation on lymphocytes have been recently (12)

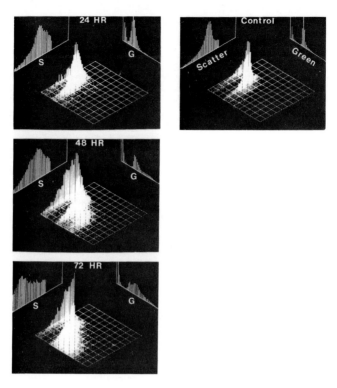

FIG. 1. Scattergram of AO-stained PHA-stimulated lymphocytes for 0, 24, 48, and 72 hr by laser flow microfluorometry on line with a PDP11/40 computer.

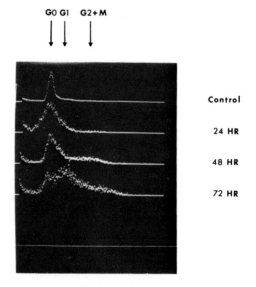

FIG. 2. As Fig. 1, but green fluorescence histogram of fixed human lymphocytes at 0, 24, 48, and 72 hr after PHA stimulation. Lymphocytes were fixed in alcohol.

TABLE 2. *PHA-stimulated lymphocytes*

	FMF		Image analysis	
	Noncycling cells (%)	Cycling cells (%)	Noncycling cells (%)	Cycling cells (%)
Unstimulated	88	12	89	11
24 hr	45	55	53	47
48 hr	25	75	40	60
72 hr	9	91	15	85

Estimated data (within 15% SE) from two-parameter distribution of scatter vs green fluorescence (FMF) of unfixed cells and integrated optical density vs average optical density of Feulgen-stained nuclei (11,12).

demonstrated also by automated image analysis of Feulgen-stained cell smears, indicating that the nuclear chromatin of stimulated G1 cells becomes more dispersed (smaller average optical density) than in unstimulated G0 cells (12), similar to other cell system such as WI-38 (11) and melanoma B16 tumor in mice (16).

Both studies of cell suspensions (FMF) and smears (image analysis) present indeed (12) a striking similarity in these results, when the fractions of noncycling cells decrease and those of cycling cells increase with time after PHA stimulation (Table 2).

Human Fibroblasts

The most striking example, which confirms both the existence of a differential emission for RNA versus DNA at the proper AO molar ratio and our previous EB data on the G0–G1 transition of WI-38 fibroblast (15), is shown in Fig. 3. WI-38 human diploid fibroblasts have been grown up to 23 days into "deep" confluency with weekly changes of the medium. Two days after plating, WI-38 cells show a log-phase distribution for the green fluorescence with a population of cells having the same scatter (respect to G1) but quite lower chromatin primary sites (green) and lower amount of RNA (red): this subpopulation, likely relating to noncycling cells (which, after plating, even if adherent to the plastic, did not start growing), is drastically reduced at 5 days (5%) and then progressively increases at 12 days (~30%) and 23 days (up to 95%). This reduced lack of proliferation is apparent also from the red versus green cytograms, where the red fluorescence (RNA), under the same staining and instrument conditions, progressively decreases with time after plating, going below the minimum threshold at 23 days. It is reassuring that at 2 days G2 cells with twice as much DNA (green) show also twice as much RNA (red) in respect to G1. At the same time, the green fluorescence distribution shows the constant presence of a G1 peak (around channel 20) progressively decreasing in amplitude at the expense of a lower fluorescence Q peak (constantly around channel 5). These

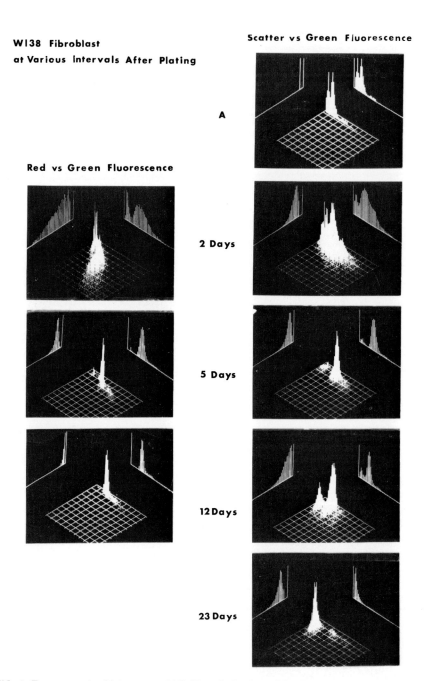

FIG. 3. Two-parameter histograms of WI-38 at 2, 5, 12, and 23 days after plating (phase II, grown in parallel). Cells were stained with AO = 3 × 10⁻⁵ M (final) and R = 4. All cytograms were obtained with green PMT = 4.6 and red PMT = 4.8. Scatter = medium in cytofluorograph on line with PDP11/40. Cytogram A was obtained when channel 3 on the scatter axis was isolated from the 2 days after plating cytogram. The medium was changed weekly ~95–98% of the WI-38 cells are viable, as shown by trypan blue exclusion (see ref. 18).

WI 38 FIBROBLASTS 10 DAYS AFTER PLATING

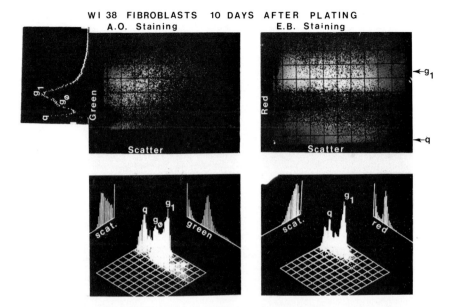

FIG. 4. Lower panels: As Fig. 3, but for phase III WI-38 fibroblasts 10 days after plating, and logarithmic compressed scale for the scatter signal. Unfixed cells are stained with either AO *(left)* or ethidium bromide *(right)*. Upper panels: As the lower panels, only acquired in linear scale, using the Becton-Dickinson cell sorter. For EB, red fluorescence is acquired; and for AO, green fluorescence. Sorted subpopulations with very low dye uptake display viability identical to those with higher fluorescence.

findings are compatible with previous observations, using EB, that the transition between proliferating G1 and nonproliferating Q + G0 cells is not a continuum, but rather a quantum jump (15). An intermediate chromatin AO uptake appears at 12 hr when WI-38 cells already have reached confluency. This could refer to a chromatin difference between readily reversible (G0) and deeper G0 (or irreversible Q) noncycling cells (1).

The cells were examined after removal of the medium (which removes also dead cells that are not adherent to the glass). Indeed, the trypan blue exclusion test indicated that almost 100% of the remainder were viable. Consequently, the reduction in Q compartment could be either recruitment or simple loss of Q cells due to the collection process (between 2 and 5 days).

The existence of three levels of chromatin condensation (G1, G0, Q) for 2C DNA WI-38 fibroblasts at confluency has been recently demonstrated by automated image analysis of intact nuclei (1). Their existence is also evident in Fig. 4 where WI-38 cells at confluency, 10 days after plating, for an identical cell size (scatter), exhibit three levels of AO uptake at R = 4 and 10^{-5} M AO final concentration, in both the linear scale (using the Becton-Dickinson) and the logarithmic compressed scale (using the cytofluorograph).

Without two-parameter acquisition and log-scale in the scatter, the cells with (Q) dye uptake could be easily confused with cell debris or PMT noise, by

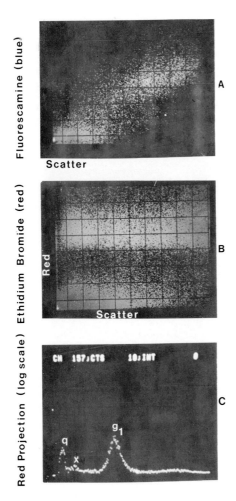

FIG. 5. Phase III WI-38 cells (42nd passage) 10 days after plating. Unfixed cells were simultaneously stained with ethidium bromide (red fluorescence) and fluorescamine (blue fluorescence), and two separate scattergrams were acquired: scatter vs blue fluorescence **(A)**, scatter vs red fluorescence **(B)**. **(C):** The red fluorescence distribution of all cells with large scatter signal (from compressed scale).

analyzing only the fluorescence frequency distribution (see Figs. 1 and 3) (17,18). Actually, double staining WI-38 fibroblasts with EB and fluorescamine indicates that these (G0, G1, Q) cells have not only similar size, but also the same number of bound fluorescamines, i.e., similar membrane properties (see Fig. 5). Indeed, the frequency distribution for cells with the same blue emission or with the same scatter yields three levels of chromatin-DNA uptake, followed by a few cells in S, G2 + M (Fig. 5).

Melanoma B16: Bulk Tumor and Its Variants
with Different Metastatic Potentials

Previously we have shown, by a combined utilization of flow and static cytometry, that melanoma B16 tumor growing in mice contains about 30% of noncycling cells (Q + G0) characterized by both a lower acridine orange uptake and higher chromating condensation (16), compared to G1 cycling cells, with the same amount of 2C DNA (18). Since then we have established a primary line *in vitro* from the same B16 primary tumor growing in mice and maintained it in tissue culture, Falcon flasks with Eagle's minimum essential medium supplemented with 10% calf serum (8). Two-parameter acquisition of scatter versus green fluorescence (Fig. 6) of unfixed cells stained with AO at R = 4 and 10^{-5} M revealed that the fraction of cells with very low dye uptake Q (noncycling cells) dramatically decreases with the number of passages, being 17% at the 15th passage and 2% at the 59th passage. It is interesting that low (F1) and high (F10) metastatic potential (3,4) B16 cells derived from the same primary tumor (courtesy of Dr. I. J. Fidler at the NCI-Frederick Cancer Center, Bethesda, Md.) reveal high (F10) and low (F1) growth fractions; i.e., F10 has about 3% of cells with low dye uptake (Q compartment), while F1 has about 20%. In all the B16 tumors, G0 cells (intermediate green fluorescence between G1 and Q) appear absent, but they are present in both human fibroblasts (Fig. 4) and human lymphocytes (Figs. 1 and 2).

Two-parameter acquisition of scatter (compressed logarithmic scale) and fluorescence reveal that identical FMF distribution may be obtained for the same primary melanoma tumor (which apparently does not have cells with intermediate G0 fluorescence uptake) either with EB staining of unfixed or

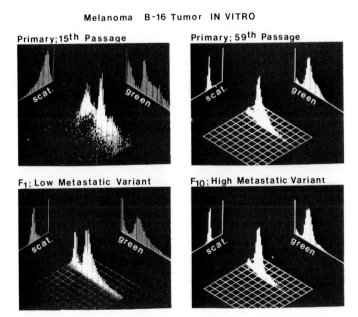

Melanoma B-16 Tumor IN VITRO

Primary; 15th Passage   Primary; 59th Passage

F1: Low Metastatic Variant   F10: High Metastatic Variant

FIG. 6. Computer-drawn two-parameter histograms of scatter vs green fluorescence for the primary melanoma tumor cells (15th and 59th passages *in vitro*), its F1 and F10 clone variants. Cells are AO stained as described in the text.

fixed cells at R = 4 and 10^{-5} M or with AO staining of unfixed cells at R = 4 and 2.5×10^{-5} M (not shown).

A careful analysis of the two-parameter scattergram (using the Becton-Dickinson with a high laser power, 375 mW) reveals that all unfixed cells (either melanoma or WI-38) are quite heterogeneous in scatter signal, even for the same green fluorescence level (either G1 or Q). The scatter heterogeneity is due to a large heterogeneity in cell size (as apparent by sorting) and also to (a) elongated cells, as fibroblasts, flowing at different orientation with respect to incoming laser light; (b) broken cell membrane but intact nuclei; and (c) cellular debris and photosensor noise (close to origin).

We have acquired two-parameter distribution of scatter versus blue fluorescence (Fig. 7) for cells double stained with EB (nucleic acid) and fluorescamine (an independent probe of cell membrane related also to cell size). It appears that although cells with lowest scatter also have lowest fluorescamine uptake (mostly broken cells), cells display similar fluorescamine uptake for a large range of scatter values: the very high scatter population contains, in addition to Q and G1 cells, also S, G2, and M phase cells, with more bound fluorescamine per cell. It is reassuring, however, to note that both low and large scatter F1

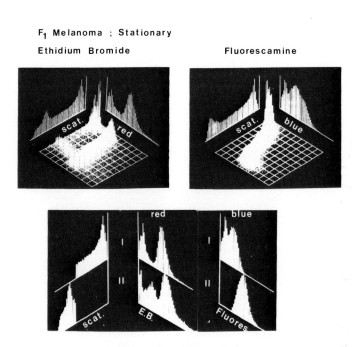

F₁ Melanoma ; Stationary

Ethidium Bromide   Fluorescamine

FIG. 7. Computer-drawn two-parameter distribution of scatter vs red fluorescence *(upper left)* and scatter vs blue fluorescence *(upper right)* for F1 melanoma cells double stained with ethidium bromide and fluorescamine, as described in the text. The lower panel represents the red and blue fluorescence distribution for the same F1 cells with low (I) and high (II) scatter.

cells (Fig. 7, *lower panels*) have discrete values of blue fluorescence with two (low scatter) or more distinct levels of ethidium bromide uptake.

The red fluorescence frequency distribution of F1 cells with large scatter displays two distinct levels of EB uptake followed by a typical log-phase distribution (G1, S, G2 + M), whereas the blue fluorescence for the same large scatter cells is distributed around a large mean value as a gaussian curve skewed toward higher fluorescence (mitotic cells) (see also ref. 5).

Cells with very low dye uptake (Q cells) do therefore represent cells with cell membranes organization indistinguishable from that of the cell with G1 dye uptake. Incidentally, preliminary sorting indicates that the large F1 cells with EB fluorescence intermediate between Q and G1 appear to be mitotic cells, rather than G0: indeed, they have a large and homogeneous scatter signal and higher fluorescamine uptake.

CONCLUSIONS

The data presented on various cell systems *in vivo* and *in vitro* confirm that cells with the same DNA but in a different functional state (cycling G1 versus noncycling G0 or Q) can be discriminated in terms of differential dye uptake, as previously shown (17,18), by the proper utilization of the mass action law governing dye-nucleic acid binding both in solution and in the intact cell. By means of simultaneous acquisition of scatter and chromatin-DNA fluorescence, or cell membrane versus nucleic acid fluorescence, our data permit us to monitor both G0 cells (reversibly out of cycle) and Q cells (differentiated or irreversibly out of cycle), which are present in normal and transformed cell lines. In addition, this method permits us to identify the mechanism governing the differential fluorescence emission, i.e., the alteration in higher order chromatin structure (10) as shown by independent and parallel automated image analysis of intact nuclei (1,11–13,16).

The nuclear morphometric data obtained by means of automated image analysis of the smears of PHA-stimulated lymphocytes (12) or serum-stimulated fibroblasts (1,11) show two distinct peaks of average optical density distribution at diploid DNA content, in striking analogy with parallel findings obtained for melanoma B16 tumor growing in mice (16): in all systems the chromatin of the cycling G1 cells is more dispersed and convoluted than the chromatin of the noncycling (G0 and Q) cells. It can then become possible to determine objectively the growth fraction (number of all proliferating cells/total number of cells) in human peripheral blood, human fibroblasts, and animal tumor. Cell sorting has shown (16,18) that lower average optical density of the nuclear chromatin corresponds to higher numbers of chromatin-DNA/primary binding sites for acridine orange in intact cells (G1 cells), while higher average optical density corresponds to lower binding sites (G0 and Q cells) for the same (2C) DNA content. At the same time the membrane properties of these cell populations are rather invariant, yielding similar fluorescamine uptake.

Analysis of the multidimensional distributions of green fluorescence versus light scatter (size) or blue fluorescence (fluorescamine) versus red fluorescence (ethidium bromide) indicates that fractions of the cell population (G0, Q, G1, S, G2, M) can be readily identified. This may be especially important to the cancer therapist for diagnosis, prognosis, and assessment of therapeutic response (9).

This multiparameter FMF analysis permits the acquisition of cell kinetic information in real time, for unperturbed or drug-perturbed populations (23), discriminating also between cell synchrony and cell recruitment (from noncycling compartment), as induced in a given population by a given chemotherapy regimen (23). A high degree of cell heterogeneity has been recently detected (3,4) in a melanoma B16 tumor due to variants presumably arising through mutation and selection or epigenetic mechanisms. Clones derived *in vitro* from a parent culture of murine malignant melanoma cells varied greatly in their ability to produce metastatic colonies in the lungs, suggesting also that highly metastatic tumor cell variants exist in the parental population. Recently we have attempted (Fig. 8) to identify the variant by labeling cell surfaces of the F1 (low metastatic potential) versus F10 (high metastatic potential) melanoma tumor cells with fluorescamine to selectively label membrane proteins, which have been involved in the expression of cell malignant transformation. If as preliminary

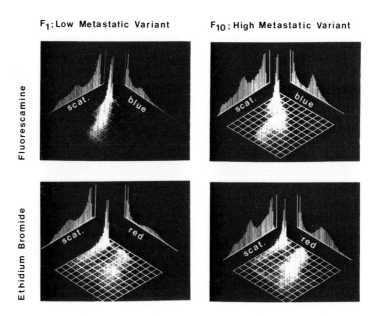

FIG. 8. As Fig. 7, but for F1 *(left panels)* and F10 *(right panels)* melanoma tumor cells. Although the scatter vs red fluorescence is similar for both cell lines (with the exception of higher fraction of low EB uptake for F1), it appears evident that the blue fluorescence (fluorescamine binding) for F10 is significantly larger than for F1, mainly for intermediate scatter cells.

studies suggest we can discriminate the variants apparently existing in the melanoma tumor in terms of differential fluorescamine uptake, we can then simultaneously monitor, by multiparameter flow microfluorometry of double-stained cells (Fig. 8), the kinetic response (EB uptake) of each subpopulation, with particular attention to the one containing the most highly metastatic variant (fluorescamine uptake) cells. Efforts to design alternative therapeutic procedures will then be directed toward the few albeit fatal metastatic subpopulations within the primary tumor itself before lung metastases occur. We hope that by this review we will convince the scientific community that the development of rigorous physicochemical staining combined with multiparameter acquisition and adequate mathematical techniques (24) are important and rewarding endeavors, which permit one to take full advantage of all capabilities of flow microfluorometry.

ACKNOWLEDGMENTS

This work constitutes a summary of parallel research efforts recently conducted at Temple University with cooperation of members of my group: A. Abraham, A. Belmont, S. M. Fang, S. Lessin, and S. Zietz. Human lymphocytes were provided by Dr. E. Vonderheid, Dermatology Department, School of Medicine. This work was supported by Grant CA20034 from the National Cancer Institute.

REFERENCES

1. Beltrame, F., Kendall, F. M., and Nicolini, C. (1979): New growth parameters of mammalian cells in suspension and a substrate. In: *Pittsburg Conference on Modeling and Simulation,* edited by G. Voyt and M. Mickle, 10:77–86. Instrument Society of America, Pittsburgh.
2. Darzynkiewicz, Z., Treganos, F., Sharpless, T. K., and Melamed, M. R. (1977): Cell cycle-related changes in nuclear chromatin of stimulated lymphocytes as measured by flow cytometry. *Cancer Res.,* 37:4635–4640.
3. Fidler, I. J. (1973): Selection of successive tumor lines for metastasis. *Nature* [*New Biol.*], 242:248–250.
4. Fidler, I. J. (1977): Metastasis results from preexisting variant cells within a malignant tumor. *Science,* 197:893–895.
5. Hawkes, S. P., and Bartholemew, J. C. (1977): Quantitative determination of transformed cells in a mixed population by simultaneous fluorescence analysis of cell surface and DNA in individual cells. *Proc. Natl. Acad. Sci. U.S.A.,* 74:1626–1630.
6. Hawkes, S. P., Meechan, T., and Bissel, T. (1976): The use of fluorescamine as a probe for labeling the outer surface of the plasma membrane. *Biochem. Biophys. Res. Commun.,* 68:1226–1233.
7. Le Pecq, J., and Paoletti, C. (1967): A fluorescent complex between ethidium bromide and nucleic acids: physical-chemical characterization. *J. Mol. Biol.,* 27:87–106.
8. Lessin, S., Abraham, S., and Nicolini, C. (1980): High versus low metastatic potential melanoma cells: biophysical cytological studies. Submitted.
9. Nicolini, C. (1976): The principles and methods of cell synchrony and cancer chemotherapy. *Biophys. Biochem. Acta Rev. Cancer,* 458:243–282.
10. Nicolini, C. (1979): Chromatin structure from angstrom to micron, and its relationship to mammalian cell proliferation. In: *Chromatin Structure and Function,* edited by C. Nicolini, pp. 613–666. Plenum Press, New York.

11. Nicolini, C., Desaive, C., Kendall, F. M., and Giaretti, W. (1977): The G0–G1 transition of WI-38 cells. II. Geometric and densitometric texture analysis. *Exp. Cell Res.,* 106:118–127.
12. Nicolini, C., Fang, S. M., Abraham, S., and Vanderheid, E. (1980): *J. Invest. Derm. (in press).* See also Fang, S. M., Masters thesis, 1979, Temple University, Philadelphia.
13. Nicolini, C., Grattorola, M., and Beltrame, F. (1979): Direct relationship between acridine orange uptake and nuclear morphometry in cycling versus confluent human fibroblasts. *Biophys. J.,* 25:4a.
14. Nicolini, C., Kendall, F. M., Desaive, C., et al. (1976): Physical-chemical characterization of cell cycle phases by laser microfluorometry in living cells. *Cancer Treatment Rep.,* 60:1819–1827.
15. Nicolini, C., Kendall, F. M., Desaive, C., Clarkson, B., and Fried, J. (1977): The G0–G1 transition of WI-38 cells. I. Laser flow microfluorometric studies. *Exp. Cell Res.,* 106:111–117.
16. Nicolini, C., Linden, W. A., Zietz, S., and Wu, C. T. (1977): Objective identification of non-proliferating cells in a melanoma B16 tumor in vivo. *Nature,* 270:163–176.
17. Nicolini, C., Parodi, S., Belmont, A., Abraham, S., and Lessin, S. (1979): Mass action and acridine orange staining. *J. Histochem. Cytochem.,* 27:102–113.
18. Nicolini, C., Parodi, S., Lessin, S., Belmont, A., Abraham, S., Zietz, S., and Grattorola, M. (1979): Chromatin study in situ. II. Static and flow microfluorometry. In: *Chromatin Structure and Function,* edited by C. Nicolini, pp. 293–323. Plenum Press, New York.
19. Parodi, S., Kendall, F. M., and Nicolini, C. (1975): A clarification of the complex spectrum observed with ultraviolet circular dichroism of ethidium bromide bound to DNA. *Nucleic Acids Res.,* 2:477–486.
20. Rigler, R. (1966): Microfluorometric characterization of intracellular nucleic acids and nucleoproteins by acridine orange. *Acta Physiol. Scand.* [Suppl. 267], 67:1–121.
21. Waring, M. J. (1965): Complex formation between ethidium bromide and nucleic acids. *J. Mol. Biol.,* 13:269–282.
22. Wu, S., Kendall, F. M., Linden, W., Toton, S., Zietz, S., and Nicolini, C. (1977): On line configuration PDP11/40—Laser flow microfluorometry and mathematical models for multiparameter cell proliferation studies. *Pulse Cytophotometry,* III:47–71.
23. Zietz, S., Grattorola, M., Desaive, C., and Nicolini, C. (1980): FPi analysis. II. Use of the method to monitor the in vivo kinetics. *Cell Tissue Kinet. (in press).*
24. Zietz, S., and Nicolini, C. (1978): Flow microfluorometry and cell kinetics: A review. In: *Biomathematics and Cell Kinetics,* edited by A. J. Valleron, pp. 357–395. North Holland Publishing Co., Amsterdam.

Advances in Neuroblastoma Research,
edited by Audrey E. Evans.
Raven Press, New York © 1980.

Flow Microfluorometric Analysis of Human Neuroblastoma DNA Distributions

*Yehuda L. Danon,[1] **,†Martin B. Epstein, †Michael M. Siegel, †Stuart E. Sicgcl, †Calvin P. Mycrs, ‡William F. Bcncdict, and *Robert C. Seeger

*Department of Pediatrics, UCLA School of Medicine, Los Angeles, California, 90024; **Physics Department, California State University, Los Angeles 90024; †Department of Radiological Sciences, UCLA School of Medicine 90024; ‡Department of Pediatrics, Division of Hematology/Oncology, Children's Hospital of Los Angeles, and USC School of Medicine, Los Angeles, California 90054*

Cytokinetic analysis may provide information which can be used to optimize chemotherapy for children with metastatic neuroblastoma. Such analysis would be facilitated if a rapid method for measuring the cell cycle distribution of tumor cells was available. Automated flow microfluorometry (FMF) with the use of appropriate cellular stains may provide such a method. This report details our investigations of cell cycle distributions of neuroblastomas utilizing FMF. First, the effects of cyclophosphamide on DNA distributions were studied using our recently developed *in vitro/in vivo* human neuroblastoma preclinical model for chemotherapy (11). Next, primary and metastatic tumors from patients were analyzed; one case was studied before and after cyclophosphamide. Finally, a method for simultaneous two-color analysis of DNA and of cell surface antigens with monoclonal antibodies was developed. This method may provide a means of identifying tumor cells in heterogeneous cell preparations for analysis of their DNA distributions and also should allow determination of the relationship between expression of cell surface antigens and the cell cycle.

MATERIALS AND METHODS

Cell lines. The human neuroblastoma cell lines LA-N-1 (10,13) and SK-N-MC (1) have been extensively characterized. LA-N-1 cells are relatively resistant whereas SK-N-MC cells are sensitive to the cytotoxic effects of cyclophosphamide *in vivo* and *in vitro* (4,11).

Preparation of neuroblastoma cells for FMF analysis of DNA distributions. Details of FMF analysis of neuroblastoma cells are presented elsewhere (2).

---

[1] Present address: Department of Pediatrics, Beilinson Hospital, Petah Tikva, Israel.

Briefly, cells grown *in vitro* were detached with trypsin-EDTA (Flow Laboratories, Rockville, Md.) and washed once with Eagle's minimal essential medium (MEM) containing 10% fetal calf serum (MEM-FCS). Tumors from nude mice and patients were minced into 1 mm³ fragments and treated with trypsin-EDTA in a trypsinizing flask to obtain single cells. If more than 10% nonviable cells were present, they were removed by filtering the suspension through 0.4 ml of loosely packed boiled cotton wool in a 5 ml syringe or by equilibrium centrifugation using Ficoll-Hypaque. Cells analyzed were greater than 90% viable as determined with trypan blue.

To stain DNA, 10^6 cells were pelleted and then resuspended in 2 ml of 0.1% citric acid containing 50 μg/ml of propidium iodide (7). Cells were incubated in propidium iodide for 15 min on ice and then were filtered through a 40 μm mesh filter to remove any debris and clumps of cells present. This preparation, which consisted of cells stripped of their cytoplasm, was analyzed with a multiparameter cell sorter/analyzer. In initial experiments, we compared the citric acid-propidium iodide method to other methods and demonstrated that it selectively stained DNA and that subpopulations of cells were not destroyed during the procedure.

Preparation of neuroblastoma cells for simultaneous fluorescence analysis of cell surface antigens and DNA. Cultured neuroblastoma cells were detached from culture flasks by shaking; they were further dispersed into single-cell suspensions by gentle pipetting and sonication (Heat Systems-Ultrasonics, Inc., 5 mV for 5 min, continuous cycle). Cells were not trypsinized. Cell surface antigens were labeled using indirect immunofluorescence with C10.115 monoclonal anti-neuroblastoma antibodies (9). Cells (2×10^6) were incubated with C10.115 antibody (0.2 ml of culture supernatant containing approximately 20 μg/ml antibody) for 30 min at 4°C, washed twice, incubated with fluoresceinated goat antimouse IgG (Meloy Labs, Springfield, Va.; diluted 1:10 and containing 0.1% azide) for 30 min at 4°C, and washed twice. The cells then were fixed at 4°C for 60 min in saline glucose medium containing 15 mM $MgCl_2$ and 25% ethanol (5). Fixed cells were treated with 1 mg/ml ribonuclease (Calbiochem, San Diego, Calif.) for 60 min at 37°C, washed, stained with propidium iodide (Calbiochem), 50 μg/ml in saline glucose medium for 30 min on ice, washed twice, and filtered through a 40 μm mesh filter to remove any debris and clumps of cells present (5). This preparation of single cells was analyzed with a multiparameter cell sorter/analyzer.

FMF analysis of DNA distributions. DNA analysis was performed using a multiparameter cell sorter/analyzer built according to the design of Steincamp et al. (12) modified as described by Pinkel et al. (8). The fluorescence intensity (DNA content) of greater than 10^4 cells was determined, and cell numbers in each of 256 fluorescence intensity channels were recorded using a PDP 11/10 minicomputer (Digital Equipment Corp., Maynard, Mass.). DNA distributions were analyzed with a PDP 11/10 minicomputer utilizing the functional form of Dean and Jett (3) as described before (2).

Dual color analysis. For dual color analysis with the multiparameter cell sorter/analyzer, the Glan-Thompson prism was used as a beam splitter. Wratten filters were inserted into the optical paths between the prism and photomultiplier tubes to attenuate green (Kodak #25) in one beam and red (Kodak #65A) in the other. Thus, fluorescence emitted by fluorescein (green) and propidium iodide (red) was detected simultaneously by two different photomultiplier tubes. DNA content of neuroblastoma cells (red fluorescence) was measured only if accompanied by fluorescence from the C10.115 monoclonal antineuroblastoma antibody (green fluorescence).

RESULTS

Effect of cyclophosphamide on SK-N-MC cells growing in vitro. Pulse treatment of SK-N-MC cells *in vitro* with Arochlor induced S-9 activated cyclophosphamide caused a fivefold decrease in the G2 + M population of SK-N-MC cells compared to control cells which were treated with either S-9 or cyclophosphamide alone (Table 1). This occurred at 24 and 48 hr after the cyclophosphamide pulse; by 72 hr the G2 + M population of these cells was not significantly different from that of untreated cells. In these experiments, cell counts demonstrated that cyclophosphamide (10 μg/ml) caused a 0, 32, 85, 54, and 60% decrease in viable cells at 9, 24, 48, 72, and 96 hr, respectively. With the colony forming assay, 85 and 100% cytotoxicity was demonstrated after 5 and 10 μg/ml, respectively (11). A dose of 100 μg/ml was so toxic that adequate numbers of cells were not obtainable for analysis of DNA distributions.

Effects of cyclophosphamide on SK-N-MC tumors growing in nude mice. One injection of cyclophosphamide (250 mg/kg) caused more than 50% regression

TABLE 1. *Effect of pulse treatment with liver S-9 activated cyclophospham-ide on DNA distribution of SK-N-MC cells* in vitro

Time in culture,[a] hr	G1 %	S %	G2 + M %
	Control[b]		
9	47.8 ± 4.0[c]	32.9 ± 6.8	17.8 ± 2.4
24	42.2 ± 16.9	42.9 ± 12.6	14.9 ± 2.9
48	38.4 ± 9.4	46.2 ± 10.8	18.7 ± 7.4
72	56.5 ± 3.7	26.9 ± 6.7	16.6 ± 2.9
	Cyclophosphamide[b]		
9	57.5 ± 6.9	26.8 ± 7.1	15.7 ± 1.0
24	43.9 ± 23.6	48.0 ± 8.8	3.2 ± 2.3
48	48.5 ± 16.3	38.4 ± 11.3	4.1 ± 3.3
72	46.3 ± 0.7	36.1 ± 0.0	14.0 ± 4.2

[a] Time in culture after pulse treatment.

[b] Control cells were pulsed with S-9 alone; cyclophosphamide-treated cells were pulsed with S-9 activated cyclophosphamide, 10 μg/ml; pulses were for 60 min.

[c] Mean ± 1 SD; each data point is the result of 3–5 experiments.

TABLE 2. *Effect of cyclophosphamide on DNA distributions of SK-N-MC cells growing as subcutaneous tumors in athymic nude mice[a]*

Days after cyclophosphamide	G1 %	S %	G2 + M %
0	65.3 ± 0.1 [b]	18.6 ± 0.2	16.2 ± 0.2
2	75.9 ± 4.5	21.0 ± 5.7	4.4 ± 0.6
4	88.0 ± 8.1	14.1 ± 12.2	3.8 ± 1.8
6	80.8 ± 5.3	12.6 ± 5.3	4.2 ± 4.8
8	74.2 ± 22.8	19.2 ± 17.7	8.5 ± 5.6
10	72.2 ± 3.9	15.7 ± 5.3	12.0 ± 1.6

[a] Mice were given one i.p. injection of cyclophosphamide (250 mg/kg) when tumor reached 10 mm diameter and were sacrificed at indicated times after cyclophosphamide.
[b] Mean ± 1 SD. Each data point is the result of analysis of 3–5 tumors.

of SK-N-MC tumor size in nude mice. Cell cycle parameters during this *in vivo* response were similar to those observed *in vitro* (Table 2). Two, four, and six days after cyclophosphamide, there was a five-fold decrease in the G2 + M cells and an increase in G1 cells. These populations returned to pretreatment levels by 10 days after therapy when tumors were beginning to regrow (11).

Effect of cyclophosphamide on LA-N-1 neuroblastoma cells growing in vitro. After pulse treatment with Arochlor induced liver S-9 activated cyclophosphamide (11), obvious changes in DNA distributions occurred (Table 3). Only 24 hr after 10 μg/ml of cyclophosphamide, the proportion of cells in G2 + M increased; by 48 hr this increase was maximal with 43% of cells being in G2 + M. Concomitantly, the proportion of G1 cells decreased with the most marked changes appearing at 48 hr after 10 μg/ml. The proportion of cells in S did not change significantly after treatment with cyclophosphamide. Cyclophosphamide at 10 μg/ml was moderately cytotoxic for LA-N-1 cells *in vitro;* counting viable cells at 9, 24, 48, 72, and 96 hr after pulse treatment demonstrated 0, 3, 54, 51, and 38% cytotoxicity, respectively. Assessment of cytotoxicity

TABLE 3. *Effect of pulse treatment with liver S-9 activated cyclophosphamide on DNA distribution of LA-N-1 cells[a]*

Time in culture, hr	G1 %	S %	G2 + M %
	Control		
9	68.2 ± 1.2	17.1 ± 3.4	12.3 ± 0.9
24	52.9 ± 5.5	31.9 ± 7.8	15.1 ± 3.3
48	58.3 ± 4.8	25.1 ± 9.5	15.2 ± 4.5
72	52.4 ± 6.0	31.5 ± 7.9	17.0 ± 0.8
	Cyclophosphamide		
9	61.5 ± 4.9	23.5 ± 5.0	15.1 ± 0.1
24	43.2 ± 8.9	26.0 ± 11.2	30.9 ± 5.3
48	34.9 ± 6.4	21.7 ± 8.1	43.4 ± 3.7
72	52.5 ± 12.2	19.8 ± 6.2	27.7 ± 8.3

[a] Footnotes as in Table 1.

TABLE 4. *Effect of cyclophosphamide on DNA distributions of LA-N-1 cells growing as subcutaneous tumors in nude mice[a]*

Days after cyclophosphamide	G1 %	S %	G2 + M %
0	73.1 ± 2.3	14.8 ± 1.1	12.2 ± 1.3
2	46.8 ± 2.7	34.1 ± 0.9	19.1 ± 3.7
4	29.9 ± 8.2	17.2 ± 1.4	53.1 ± 7.0
6	30.1 ± 9.1	18.1 ± 16.9	61.1 ± 23.1
8	55.7 ± 1.4	36.8 ± 0.7	9.5 ± 0.7
10	77.4 ± 2.3	9.2 ± 2.6	13.5 ± 0.3

[a] Footnotes as in Table 2.

with the colony forming assay demonstrated a 57% decrease in colony forming cells 2 weeks after pulse treatment with 10 μg/ml of cyclophosphamide (11).

Effect of cyclophosphamide on LA-N-1 tumors growing in nude mice. The response of LA-N-1 cells growing in nude mice to cyclophosphamide was similar although not identical to their response *in vitro* (Table 4). Two days after one dose of cyclophosphamide (250 mg/kg), cells in S and G2 + M were increased and those in G1 were decreased compared to untreated tumors. The proportion of cells in G2 + M increased to 55% and in G1 decreased to 33% four and six days after treatment; S phase cells again increased at 8 days. All cycle compartments returned to control levels by 10 days after therapy. Although these major changes in DNA distributions occurred after cyclophosphamide, the size of LA-N-1 tumors did not decrease significantly (4,11).

DNA content of neuroblastoma cells obtained from patients. The DNA content of cells within primary tumors and metastases was analyzed using the same methods as were used for tumors obtained from nude mice. Cytocentrifuge preparations of cells studied demonstrated greater than 90% tumor cells. Skin metastases from a 3-month-old with stage IV-S neuroblastoma were biopsied and studied before and during cyclophosphamide therapy (Fig. 1). Tumor cells

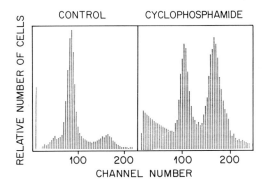

FIG. 1. Effect of cyclophosphamide on DNA distribution of skin metastases of a stage IV-S neuroblastoma. Tumor samples taken by skin biopsy were analyzed before (control) and during the second week of cyclophosphamide therapy (5 mg/kg/day; day 5 of the course).

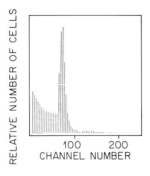

FIG. 2. DNA distribution of a primary human ganglioneuroma. This sample was obtained from the initial surgery before other therapy.

obtained during therapy (day 5 of the second 7-day course at 5 mg/kg/day) showed more than a fivefold increase in G2 + M cells compared to the pretherapy specimen. This clearly demonstrated that perturbations in tumor cell DNA distributions can occur in patients treated with cyclophosphamide.

Tumors from five additional patients were studied. The only ganglioneuroma analyzed consisted of all G1 (and possibly G0) cells (Fig. 2). The primary and omental metastatic tumors from a second infant with stage IV-S neuroblastoma were studied (Fig. 3). A pre-G1 peak of fluorescence intensity was present in both samples but was most prominent in the metastatic tumor; both samples had cells in S and G2 + M. The pre-G1 peak had the same fluorescence intensity (channel 50 to 60) as normal lymphocytes. Thus this peak may be due to normal cells mixed with tumor cells; alternatively, it may be tumor cells with less DNA or less readily stained DNA.

Neuroblastomas from three patients with stage IV disease all had G1, S, and G2 + M populations. The primary tumor and metastases were obtained at autopsy from one of these patients; viable cells from the periphery and center of the primary and from metastases to liver, lymph node, and lung were in all phases of the cell cycle.

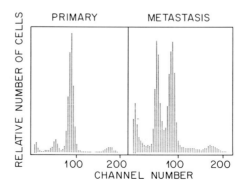

FIG. 3. DNA distribution of primary and metastatic lesion of stage IV-S neuroblastoma. Samples were obtained from the initial surgery before other therapy.

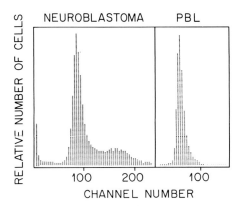

FIG. 4. DNA distribution of LA-N-1 neuroblastoma cells and normal peripheral blood lympho-cytes. Peripheral blood lymphocytes are all in G1/G0, whereas neuroblastoma cells are in G1, S, and G2 + M.

Simultaneous analysis of cell surface antigens (CSAs) and DNA. Identification of tumor cells mixed among normal cells is often needed in FMF analysis. For example, sequential studies of neuroblastoma cells which have metastasized to bone marrow could be performed with FMF if they could be identified or separated. Simultaneous analysis of CSA and DNA also would be useful for determining the relationship between expression of CSA and stage of the cell cycle. Therefore, we have begun developing a tumor cell identification system which uses antineuroblastoma monoclonal C10.115 antibodies and fluoresce-inated goat antimouse immunoglobulin. With this system, tumor cells can be identified by green fluorescence from their surface, and DNA can be simulta-neously analyzed by determining the orange fluorescence intensity due to propi-dium iodide staining.

We have preliminary results with a model system which demonstrate the feasibility of this approach. The DNA distribution of LA-N-1 neuroblastoma cells and normal peripheral blood lymphocytes is shown in Fig. 4. Peripheral blood lymphocytes only have a G1/G0 population whereas LA-N-1 cells are distributed throughout the cell cycle. These two cell types were mixed (1:1), incubated with monoclonal mouse antineuroblastoma antibody followed by fluo-resceinated goat antimouse immunoglobulin, fixed with ethanol, treated with ribonuclease, and finally stained with propidium iodide. Only the neuroblastoma cells had green fluorescence, whereas both cell types had orange fluorescence due to staining of DNA by propidium iodide. By means of electronic gating, the mixed cell populations were studied (Fig. 5). The DNA distribution for cells with green membrane fluorescence was essentially the DNA distribution of LA-N-1 neuroblastoma cells, whereas that of cells without membrane fluores-cence was that of lymphocytes. We conclude that this system can identify tumor cells mixed with normal cells and that the DNA distribution of both populations can then be determined.

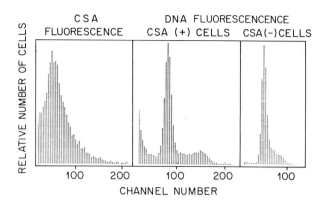

FIG. 5. Simultaneous fluorescence analysis of CSA and DNA. A mixed population of neuroblastoma and peripheral blood lymphocytes was analyzed. Left panel: indirect immunofluorescence (green) of CSA of LA-N-1 neuroblastoma cells using C10.115 monoclonal antibody and fluoresceinated antimouse immunoglobulin. Middle panel: DNA fluorescence (red) of cells with green surface fluorescence. Right panel: DNA fluorescence of cells lacking CSA recognized by C10.115 antibody (i.e., lacking green fluorescence).

DISCUSSION

This is one of the first studies of human neuroblastoma cells with automated FMF. Using both model systems and clinical materials, a number of points have been demonstrated. First, normal and perturbed DNA distributions can be readily quantitated. Second, the perturbations induced by cyclophosphamide are different for two neuroblastoma cell lines. Third, analysis of tumors from patients suggests that ganglioneuroma cells may have a different DNA distribution than neuroblastoma cells. Finally, by identifying neuroblastoma cells with antibodies against cell surface antigens, it is possible to analyze the DNA distribution of neurolastoma cells mixed with normal cells.

The effect of a single dose of cyclophosphamide on neuroblastoma cell lines LA-N-1 and SK-N-MC was markedly different. LA-N-1 as compared to SK-N-MC cells are relatively resistant to the cytotoxic effects of cyclophosphamide (11). Likewise, the effects of cyclophosphamide on the DNA distribution of these two cell lines are different. SK-N-MC cells surviving the effects of cyclophosphamide were mainly in G1 and S phase. This could be explained by an arrest in G1 or alternatively by a greater susceptibility of G2 + M cells to the lethal effect of cyclophosphamide.

DNA distributions of LA-N-1 cells were altered by one dose of cyclophosphamide. Whether growing *in vitro* or as subcutaneous tumors in nude mice, the proportion of LA-N-1 cells in G1 decreased two- to sixfold and in G2 + M increased fourfold following treatment with cyclophosphamide. The latter increase is interpreted to be primarily in G2 cells since no increase in M cells was appreciated from histological examination of treated tumors (11). The increased proportion of G2 cells could be due to a delay in progression or an arrest during G2 or to a selective cytotoxic effect against G1 cells. *In vivo,* the proportion of S phase cells was increased twofold 2 days after cyclophosphamide. The increased proportion of cells in S phase may reflect recruitment from G0 or G1 phases at 2 days and initial proliferative recovery at 8 days.

Detection of changes in DNA distributions of LA-N-1 cells in the absence of significant reduction in tumor size is significant for two reasons. First, this indicates that analysis of DNA distributions may be a sensitive means of monitoring therapeutic effects on tumors. Second, this suggests approaches to combination chemotherapy which otherwise might not be considered.

Data of Hayes et al. (6) suggest that perturbations in DNA distributions occur in some neuroblastomas in children after treatment with cyclophosphamide. Our study of skin metastases in one patient also demonstrated that cyclophosphamide can alter DNA distributions of neuroblastomas in children.

Our initial survey of tumors from patients included a ganglioneuroma, two stage IV-S neuroblastomas, and three stage IV neuroblastomas. The ganglioneuroma consisted of a homogeneous cell population with essentially all cells in G0 or G1. This DNA distribution is compatible with the highly differentiated, slow growing, and benign character of ganglioneuromas. Tumors from both patients with IV-S neuroblastoma had cells in all stages of the cell cycle. Of interest, the DNA distribution of cells from one of these tumors suggested the presence of both diploid (fluorescence intensity of normal lymphocytes) and hyperdiploid cells. These two populations may represent normal cells mixed with tumor cells or two different clones of tumor cells. The presence of a population with increased fluorescence intensity suggests chromosomal abnormalities and is compatible with the concept that stage IV-S neuroblastoma is a true neoplasm rather than delayed maturation of normal neuroblasts since normal neuroblasts should have a diploid amount of DNA.

Tumor cells from stage IV neuroblastomas were in all stages of the cell cycle. The primary tumor and multiple metastases which were obtained at autopsy from one patient had similar DNA distributions; viable cells from the edge and middle of the primary also had similar DNA distributions. These preliminary studies suggest heterogeneity between tumors from different patients (ganglioneuroma versus neuroblastoma) but considerable homogeneity for a tumor and its metastases in an individual patient.

The method described for simultaneous FMF analysis of CSA and DNA of the same cell has considerable potential value. First, with appropriate antibodies, neuroblastoma cells can be identified when they are mixed among normal cells; this allows determination of the DNA distribution of both populations. This should have general application to other cell systems where antibodies are available for marking one population or subpopulation. One difficulty with this approach was obtaining high titered specific antisera; this is circumvented by the availability of monoclonal antibodies. Now, the limiting factors are antigen density of the cell surface and the expression of antigen by more than one cell type. The method also allows analysis of CSA expression in relationship to the cell cycle. As demonstrated, the antigen identified by C10.115 antibody is expressed throughout the cell cycle. The ability to analyze CSA expression in this manner has considerable importance for biological studies as well as for immunodiagnosis and immunotherapy.

SUMMARY

DNA distributions of neuroblastoma cells were studied with automated flow microfluorometry. Using human neuroblastoma cell lines LA-N-1 and SK-N-MC *in vitro* and as subcutaneous tumors in nude mice, we showed that cyclophosphamide induces large perturbations in their DNA distributions. These perturbations were different for the two cell lines. Of importance, changes in the DNA distribution of LA-N-1 cells were detected even though a significant reduction in tumor size did not occur. Analysis of neuroblastoma cells from one infant who received only cyclophosphamide demonstrated that perturbations in DNA distributions also can occur in patients. Analysis of tumors from patients demonstrated that a ganglioneuroma had cells only in G1/G0 phase, whereas stage IV-S and stage IV neuroblastomas had cells in all stages of the cell cycle. A procedure was developed for simultaneous analysis of cell surface antigens and DNA. Initial results suggest that this should have considerable use both for analyzing DNA distributions of tumor cells which are mixed with normal cells such as in bone marrow and also for analyzing expression of CSA in relationship to the cell cycle.

ACKNOWLEDGMENTS

This research was supported in part by Grant CA22794, awarded by the National Cancer Institute, DHEW; contract EY-76-S-03-0034 awarded by the U.S. Department of Energy to the University of California; and the Stephanie Michelle Milkes Cancer Fund for Children. M.B.E. was partially supported by Associated Western Universities. M.M.S. was supported by an American Cancer Society Junior Faculty Fellowship. Research Career Development Awards from the National Cancer Institute, DHEW, are held by W.F.B. (CA70996) and R.C.S. (CA00069). Y.L.D. is the recipient of International Research Fellowship TW02565, awarded by the National Institute of Health, DHEW, and is a Fulbright Scholar.

REFERENCES

1. Biedler, J. L., Helson, L., and Spengler, B. A. (1973): Morphology and growth, tumorigenicity, and cytogenetics of human neuroblastoma cells in continuous culture. *Cancer Res.,* 33:2643–2652.
2. Danon, Y. L., Epstein, M. B., Siegel, M. M., Rucker, N., Myers, C. P., Norman, A., Benedict, W. F., and Seeger, R. C. (1980): Cyclophosphamide induced changes in DNA distribution of human neuroblastoma cells. Submitted for publication.

3. Dean, P. N., and Jett, J. H. (1974): Mathematical analysis of DNA distributions derived from flow microfluorometry. *J. Cell Biol.,* 60:523–527.

4. Harlow, P. J., Siegel, M. M., Siegel, S. E., and Benedict, W. F. (1980): Antitumor activity of chemotherapeutic agents alone or in combination using a human neuroblastoma model system. *Prog. Cancer Res. Ther.,* 319–325.

5. Hawkes, S. P., and Bartholomew, J. C. (1977): Quantitative determination of transformed cells in a mixed population by simultaneous fluorescence analysis of cell surface and DNA in individual cells. *Proc. Natl. Acad. Sci. U.S.A.,* 74:1626–1630.

6. Hayes, F. A., Green, A. A., and Maurer, A. M. (1977): Correlation of cell kinetic and clinical response to chemotherapy in disseminated neuroblastoma. *Cancer Res.,* 37:3766–3770.

7. Krishan, A. (1975): A rapid flow cytofluorometric analysis of mammalian cell cycle by propidium iodide staining. *J. Cell Biol.,* 66:188–193.

8. Pinkel, D., Epstein, M., Udkoff, R., and Norman, A. (1978): Fluorescence polarimeter for flow cytometry. *Rev. Sci. Instrum.,* 49:905–912.

9. Seeger, R. C., Danon, Y. L., Zelter, P. M., and Rayner, S. A. (1980): Expression of fetal antigens by human neuroblastoma cells. *Prog. Cancer Res. Ther., this volume.*

10. Seeger, R. C., Rayner, S. A., Banerjee, A., Chung, H., Laug, W. E., Neustein, H. B., and Benedict, W. F. (1977): Morphology, growth, chromosomal pattern, and fibrinolytic activity of two new human neuroblastoma cell lines. *Cancer Res.,* 37:1364–1371.

11. Siegel, M. M., Chung, H. S., Rucker, N., Siegel, S. E., Seeger, R. C., Isaacs, H., and Benedict, W. F. (1980): In vitro/in vivo preclinical chemotherapy studies of human neuroblastoma. *Cancer Treat. Reps. (in press).*

12. Steincamp, J. A., Romero, A., Horan, P. K., and Crissman, H. A. (1974): Multiparameter analysis and sorting of mammalian cells. *Exp. Cell Res.,* 84:15–23.

13. West, G. J., Uki, J., Herschman, H. R., and Seeger, R. C. (1977): Adrenergic, cholinergic, and inactive human neuroblastoma cell lines with the action-potential Na^+ ionophore. *Cancer Res.,* 37:1372–1376.

Advances in Neuroblastoma Research,
edited by Audrey E. Evans.
Raven Press, New York © 1980.

Experimental Chemotherapy of Human Tumors Heterotransplanted in Nude Mice

Beppino C. Giovanella and John S. Stehlin

Cancer Research Laboratory, St. Joseph Hospital, Houston, Texas 77002

The discovery in 1969 by Pantelouris (42) that the nude mouse described in 1966 by Flanagan (12) was congenitally thymusless has opened new perspectives in the field of heterotransplantation. Very soon, his finding was utilized by Rygaard and Povlsen (51) to transplant human tumors into the nude mouse. The nude accepted such transplants which developed into tumors closely resembling the tumor of origin (18,23). Rapidly accumulating evidence demonstrated that a high percentage of human tumors derived from primary human neoplasms, from metastasis of such neoplasms, and from human tumor-cultured cells (26) could grow indefinitely in the nude mouse and could be passaged serially from mouse to mouse (18,23,45).

For the first time, the oncologist had at his disposal a practical and reliable research tool that allowed him to remove human malignant neoplasms out of the body of the patient and to grow them as tumors in the mouse. The limitations, together with the possibilities of the system, are evident. Human tumors growing in the nude mouse do have a mouse stroma, and the metabolism of the organism in which they are living and growing is the metabolism of a mouse, not of a human. However, even with such limitations, there was a vast progress over the previous period in which human tumors could be grown only as tissue culture, i.e., as monolayers or suspensions of cells in an artificial medium outside any living metabolic environment or as temporary xenografts rapidly rejected by the hosts, as in the cheek pouch of the hamster. Another great advantage of the heterotransplantation of human tumors into the nude mouse is a relatively high rate of takes of the majority of the tumors considered. Excluding a few tumors such as breast carcinoma, prostate carcinoma, and Hodgkin's disease, a majority of the remaining neoplasms exhibit a rate of positive takes of 50% or more when transplanted in the subcutaneous tissue of the nude mouse (18,23).

Morphologically and biochemically, for every case in which it has been possible to analyze such tumors, the resemblance between the neoplasms growing in the nude mouse and the tumor growing in the patient of origin has been striking (15,18,36,59). Karyotypically, such tumors are human, as has been proven by various authors (17,25,26,56). Certain of these tumors have been, by now, pas-

299

saged 50 to 75 times over a span of over 7 to 8 years with no apparent change in their characteristics, even when they were rather differentiated at the beginning (45). Metastatic spread of human tumors in the nude mouse was proved for the first time by Giovanella et al. (25) and confirmed later by other authors. It was also soon demonstrated by Giovanella and Stehlin (16) and confirmed later (6,10) that nude mice, although immunologically crippled, and as such particularly susceptible to infections of every type, if kept under strict pathogen-free conditions can reach the average life span of a normal mouse. Such animals can live for 2 years or more with a mortality during the first year of life of 1 to 3%.

When these animals became available, it was immediately obvious that experimental chemotherapy of human tumors could be attempted outside the patient of origin. Two main approaches have been followed. In the first, individual tumors transplanted into the nude mouse are used to study the effect of different known antitumor drugs. In this way it is possible to find the one drug or group of drugs more effective against the specific tumor of a specific patient in order to choose the chemotherapeutic treatment best suited for this patient when needed. Obviously, such an approach suffers from the inconvenience that, in order to obtain meaningful results, a lapse of time is necessary. However, for certain types of tumors in which the time span between removal of the primary tumor or of a metastasis and relapse can be measured in months, it is possible to establish the sensitivity of the patient's tumor to various drugs before it has to be treated. The results in this type of research are rather long in being evaluated, and few data have been so far published (19,27,31,40), but would undoubtedly offer the capacity to maximize the effectiveness of the chemotherapeutic agents that we possess at the present.

The second approach is to use established human tumors representative of a particular histological type as a testing ground for new drugs. The main limitations of such an approach are three. The first is that we do not yet have proof that human heterotransplanted tumors are better predictors of drugs effective against human tumors than murine tumors. Only further work can solve this question. The second limitation lies in the fact that the nude mouse is a relatively expensive animal, and this increases considerably the expense of the screening itself. The third is that tumors of the same histological type and arising from the same organ nevertheless differ considerably in their sensitivity to the same drug. Let us suppose that tumors heterotransplanted into the nude mouse are identical to the corresponding tumors growing in the human patient as to sensitivity to drugs. In this case, using cancer of the breast, for example, and screening it for potential anticancer chemotherapeutic agents, we will have a 100% probability of picking up such an agent only if this drug is active against 100% of the human breast carcinomas. If we take 5-fluorouracil (5-FU), which is considered one of the best anticancer agents against carcinoma of the breast, we have to keep in mind that 5-FU is active only against approximately 25% of such tumors, i.e., 1 out of 4. Very simple mathematics will tell us that if we use only one breast carcinoma, we have only 25% probability of picking an agent comparable to 5-FU as antitumor activity. Data so far collected with experimental chemotherapy of human tumors heterotransplanted in nude mice fully support such a point (2,19,21,23,28,30,37,38,44). It is equally obvious that, although in theory it would be ideal to have a very large panel of tumors of the same type, such a proposition is not too practical. Compromise can be made using a panel of tumors of the same type small enough to make the expenses not too prohibitive and large enough to allow for finding, with a good probability, drugs that have effectiveness against a good percentage of tumors.

In a recent study, Bellet et al. (3) have shown mathematically that in order to find with 95% probability a drug that is effective against at least 10% of the tumors under study, a panel of 14 tumors is required. Obviously, we should weigh the advantages of such a panel versus the expense encountered and the consequent restriction of the number of drugs that can be tested for activity.

DRUG DOSAGE AND TOXICITY

The doses applied to human tumors growing in the nude mouse are, of course, the maximum tolerated doses, and in this respect it has to be kept in mind that mice do tolerate larger amounts than man of practically all the known anticancer agents. This, however, does not detract from the effectiveness of the test. Drugs in mice are less toxic than in humans because they are metabolized and detoxified faster than in man. Accordingly, the larger dose administered to the mouse does not mean that a larger amount of drug comes in contact with the tumor cell. Nude mice have been found to tolerate even larger doses of anticancer agents than normal mice (29). This is probably because, for reasons not well understood, the liver of the nude mice possesses more active oxidases than the liver of normal mice (14). It has been the constant rule, as in experiments with normal mice, to measure the toxicity of the drug by the weight loss of the animals receiving the drug compared with the constant weight or weight loss of the animals of the control group.

Moreover, the presence of viral infections in many colonies of nude mice which considerably shortens the life span of the animals jeopardizes the results of every experiment that involves long follow-up of the mice, and it is particularly an obstacle in survival experiments, especially of slow-growing tumors. For all of the said reasons, it is obvious that the results obtained with animals that are free from such infections are much more reliable (23).

EFFECT OF DRUGS ON TUMOR GROWTH

Various drugs have been tested against a series of human tumors of various types growing as heterotransplants in nude mice. Drugs have been generally administered subcutaneously or intraperitoneally, whereas the majority of the tumors were grown as subcutaneous transplants. Also, a sizable amount of evidence has been collected using transplants of human tumors under the kidney capsule of host nude mice followed by treatment with the various drugs (4,20).

Some other routes of injection of the tumor have also been attempted, but they are still in the experimental stage, so that for the moment we will consider only the subcutaneous and the subrenal capsule sites. The drugs have been generally given as individual injections with different schedules, and the preferred route of administration has been the intraperitoneal followed by the intravenous, subcutaneous, and intramuscular routes. The notable exception has been the continuous administration of thymidine by subcutaneous infusion (33–35) due to the very short life of such a drug in the blood of the animals so treated. Recently this type of continuous administration has been extended to other drugs.

Human tumors of a certain type heterotransplanted in nude mice have shown a remarkable similarity of response to various chemotherapeutic agents compared with tumors of the same type treated clinically in the patient. Colon carcinomas, for example, have responded rather poorly to any single agent (18,37–40). A Burkitt's lymphoma responded very well to cyclophosphamide (47).

Other tumors studied have been HeLa (1), ovarian carcinomas (7), neuroblastomas (28), melanomas (3,24,33–35,46,50), choriocarcinomas (27,53), carcinomas of the liver (53), brain tumors (57), breast carcinomas (18,19,30), lung carcinomas (30), and others. The sensitivity to known drugs in such trials parallels fairly well the clinical experience, but the number of tumors tested is still too small to give these results statistical significance. Apart from clinically used drugs, experimental drugs such as polyriboinosinic acid and polyribocytidilic acid (8), abrin and ricin (13), DL-amigdalin (41), and diphtheria toxin (48) have also been tested. This last substance is very interesting because it is toxic to human cells but not to mouse cells (52). Accordingly, it can be used as a positive control or when for any reason it is desirable to make a human heterotransplant regress (9). New drugs now being introduced in clinical trials are being investigated on human tumors heterotransplanted in nude mice in a program sponsored by the National Cancer Institute (4,38).

To our knowledge, so far, the only drug which has reached the human treatment stage exclusively through testing in human tumor heterotransplants is thymidine (dThd). dThd was found to have selective antitumor activity *in vitro* against human and murine tumor cells in 1977 (32). *In vivo* tests against human tumors (melanomas, lung carcinomas, breast carcinomas, etc.) heterotransplanted in nude mice confirmed such results (24,33–35), and pharmacokinetic studies conducted in such animals (60) determined the dose to be administered to humans. Human tests after FDA approval of the drug for human experimental use are now under way.

Two of the problems confronting the investigator working with human heterotransplants are the constancy of its material and the way of assessing results. The first problem can be stated thus: Do human tumors, through many passages in the nudes, remain unchanged as to biological characteristics? The results so far obtained are in the affirmative (18); however, not enough studies have been performed on this subject and Bogden et al. (5) have found that rat tumors serially transplanted in nude mice did indeed change their sensitivity to chemotherapy. An additional complication arises from the existence of mixed tumors containing more than one cellular type (22), one of which can prevail over the others during serial transplantation.

The second problem results from the fact that the majority of the studies on the effects of chemotherapy of human tumors in nude mice use as a basis for their calculations the volume of the tumor under study. Unfortunately, such a parameter is far from precise; necrotizing tumors can swell simulating growth and ulcerate. The shape of certain neoplasms makes volume measurements difficult. Finally, such measurements are impossible with tumors growing outside the subcutaneous space (intraperitoneally, intracerebrally, etc.).

Efforts are being made to surmount such difficulties by measuring the amount of human cells present in the mouse by determinations of human lactic dehydrogenase present in the blood of the animal (9,43).

Another approach is to measure the viability of tumor cells in a small fragment of tumor by means of [125]IUDR uptake *in vitro* (49). Both these approaches appear promising.

Also, studies have been initiated to use the human tumors heterotransplanted in nude mice to investigate the mechanism of action of anticancer drugs (11).

The possibility of maintaining alive in the frozen state human heterotransplants (55) favors the accumulation of vast numbers of such tumors which otherwise would require excessive numbers of nudes for maintenance alone.

Finally, the recent finding by Watanabe et al. (58) that human leukemias can be transferred as leukemia in irradiated nude mice opens a new area of investigation for experimental chemotherapy.

CONCLUSIONS

Experimental chemotherapy of human tumors heterotransplanted in nude mice appears to offer an attractive model for human cancer chemotherapy. The vast majority of the data so far accumulated seem to validate the model as an effective predictor of drug actions in humans. However, definite proof is still lacking. This model will acquire full validity when two preconditions are fulfilled. The first is to have a sufficient number of individual human tumors which respond equally to the same drug in the patient and in the nude mouse. The second is to have the same statistic level of response to a drug in a group of tumors of the same type in the nudes and in the patient.

ACKNOWLEDGMENTS

This work was supported by Contract NO1-CM67073 TQ. The authors gratefully acknowledge the invaluable cooperation of Randall C. Shepard, Jan C. Brunn, Dana M. Vardeman, and John T. and Betty J. Mendoza.

REFERENCES

1. Arai, T., Okamoto, K., Ishiguro, K., and Terao, K. (1976): HeLa cell tumor in nude mice and its response to antitumor agents. *Gann*, 67:493–503.
2. Arai, T., Okamoto, K., Terao, K., Tokita, H., Sekimoto, K., Fukushima, T., and Tanaka, N. (1977): Effectiveness of antitumor agents against human tumors in nude mice. In: *Proceedings of the Second International Workshop on Nude Mice*, edited by T. Nomura, N. Ohsawa, N. Tamaoki, and K. Fujiwara, pp. 461–474. University of Tokyo Press, Tokyo.
3. Bellet, R. E., Mastrangelo, J. J., Berd, D., and Danna, V. (1978): Secondary animal tumor screening of chemotherapeutic agents utilizing a human melanoma nude mouse panel. *Proc. Am. Assoc. Cancer Res.*, 19:15.
4. Bogden, A. E., Kelton, D. E., Cobb, W. R., and Esber, H. J. (1978): A rapid screening method for testing chemotherapeutic agents against human tumor xenografts. In: *The Use of Athymic (Nude) Mice in Cancer Research*, edited by D. P. Houchens and A. O. Ovejera, pp. 231–250. G. Fischer, New York.
5. Bogden, A. E., Kelton, D. E., Cobb, W. R., Gulkin, T. A., and Johnson, R. K. (1978): Effect of serial passage in nude athymic mice on the growth characteristics and chemotherapy responsiveness of 13762 and R3230 AC mammary tumor xenografts. *Cancer Res.*, 38:59–64.
6. Committee for the Care and Use of the "Nude" Mouse (1976): Guide for the care and use of the nude (thymus-deficient) mouse. *Biomed. Res. ILAR News*, 19:1–20.
7. Davy, M., Mossige, J., and Johannessen, J. V. (1977): Heterologous growth of human ovarian cancer. A new in vivo testing system. *Acta Obstet. Gynecol. Scand.*, 56:55–59.
8. De Clercq, E. (1977): Effect of mouse interferon and polyriboinosinic acid polyribocytidilic acid on L-cell tumor grown in nude mice. *Cancer Res.*, 37:1502–1506.
9. Di Persio, L., Kyriazis, A. P., Michael, J. G., and Pesce, A. J. (1979): Monitoring the therapy of human tumor xenografts in nude mice by the use of lactate dehydrogenase. *J. Natl. Cancer Inst.*, 62:375–379.
10. Ediger, R., and Giovanella, B. C. (1978): Current knowledge of breeding and mass production of the nude mouse. In: *The Nude Mouse in Experimental and Clinical Research*, edited by J. Fogh and B. C. Giovanella, pp. 16–27. Academic Press, New York.
11. Erickson, L. C., Osieka, R., and Kohn, K. W. (1978): Differential repair of 1-(2-chloroethyl)-3-(4-methylcyclomexyl)-1-nitrosourea-induced DNA damage in two human colon tumor cell lines. *Cancer Res.*, 38:802–808.
12. Flanagan, S. P. (1966): "Nude," a new hairless gene with pleiotropic effects in the mouse. *Genet. Res.*, 8:295–309.
13. Fodstad, O., Olsnes, S., and Pihl, A. (1977): Inhibitory effect of abrin and ricin on the growth of transplantable murine tumors and of abrin on human cancers in nude mice. *Cancer Res.*, 37:4559–4567.
14. Freudenthal, R. I., Leber, A. P., Emmerling, D. C., Kerchner, G. A., and Ovejera, A. A. (1976): Comparisons of the drug metabolizing enzymes in the liver and kidneys, from homozygous nude Swiss, heterozygous normal Swiss, normal Swiss and DBA/2 mice. *Res. Commun. Chem. Pathol. Pharmacol.*, 15:267–278.
15. Giovanella, B. C., and Fogh, J. (1978): Present and future trends in investigations with the nude mouse as a recipient of human tumor transplants. In: *The Nude Mouse in Experimental and Clinical Research*, edited by J. Fogh and B. C. Giovanella, pp. 282–312. Academic Press, New York.
16. Giovanella, B. C., and Stehlin, J. S. (1973): Heterotransplantation of human malignant tumors in "nude" thymusless mice. I. Breeding and maintenance of "nude" mice. *J. Natl. Cancer Inst.*, 51:615–619.
17. Giovanella, B. C., and Stehlin, J. S. (1974): Assessment of the malignant potential of cultured cells by injection in "nude" mice. In: *Proceedings of the First International Workshop on Nude Mice*, edited by J. Rygaard and C. O. Povlsen, pp. 279–284. G. Fischer Verlag, Stuttgart.
18. Giovanella, B. C., Stehlin, J. S., Fogh, J., and Sharkey, F. E. (1978): Serial transplantation of human malignant tumors in nude mice and their use in experimental chemotherapy. In: *The Use of Athymic (Nude) Mice in Cancer Research*, edited by D. P. Houchens and A. O. Ovejera, pp. 163–179. G. Fischer, New York.
19. Giovanella, B. C., Stehlin, J. S., and Shepard, R. C. (1977): Experimental chemotherapy of human breast carcinomas heterotransplanted in nude mice. In: *Proceedings of the Second*

International Workshop on Nude Mice, edited by T. Nomura, N. Ohsawa, N. Tamaoki, and K. Fujiwara, pp. 475–481. University of Tokyo Press, Tokyo.

20. Giovanella, B. C., Stehlin, J. S., and Shepard, R. C. (1978): Experimental chemotherapy of human malignant tumors transplanted subcutaneously and under the kidney capsule of nude mice. *Fed. Proc.,* 37:499.
21. Giovanella, B. C., Stehlin, J. S., Shepard, R. C., and Goldin, A. (1977): Experimental chemotherapy of human malignant tumors serially heterotransplanted in nude mice. *Proc. Am. Assoc. Cancer Res.,* 18:27.
22. Giovanella, B. C., Stehlin, J. S., and Williams, L. J. (1974): Heterotransplantation of human malignant tumors in "nude" thymusless mice. II. Malignant tumors induced by injection of cell cultures derived from human solid tumors. *J. Natl. Cancer Inst.,* 52:921–930.
23. Giovanella, B. C., Stehlin, J. S., Williams, L. J., Lee, S. S., and Shepard, R. C. (1978): Heterotransplantation of human cancers into nude mice—a model for human cancer chemotherapy. *Cancer,* 42:2269–2281.
24. Giovanella, B. C., Williams, L. J., Lee, S. S., and Stehlin, J. S. (1979): Morphological effects of high concentrations of thymidine on normal and neoplastic dividing cells in vitro and in vivo. *Fed. Proc.,* 38:918.
25. Giovanella, B. C., Yim, S. O., Morgan, A. C., Stehlin, J. S., and Williams, L. J. (1973): Metastases of human melanomas transplanted in "nude" mice. *J. Natl. Cancer Inst.,* 50:548–554.
26. Giovanella, B. C., Yim, S. O., Stehlin, J. S., and Williams, L. J. (1972): Development of invasive tumors in the "nude" mouse after injection of cultured human melanoma cells. *J. Natl. Cancer Inst.,* 48:1513–1533.
27. Hayashi, H., Kameya, T., Shimosato, T., and Mukojima, T. (1978): Chemotheraphy of human choriocarcinoma transplanted to nude mice. *Am. J. Obst. Gynecol.,* 131:548–554.
28. Helson, L., Helson, C., Das, S. K., and Rubenstein, R. (1978): Biochemistry and chemotherapy of human neural tumors in nude mice. In: *The Use of Athymic (Nude) Mice in Cancer Research,* edited by D. P. Houchens and A. O. Ovejera, pp. 257–266. G. Fischer, New York.
29. Houchens, D. P., Johnson, R. K., Gaston, M. R., Goldin, A., and Marks, T. (1977): Toxicity of cancer chemotherapeutic agents in athymic (nude) mice. *Cancer Treatment Rep.,* 61:103–104.
30. Houchens, D. P., Ovejera, A. O., and Barker, A. D. (1978): The therapy of human tumors in athymic (nude) mice. In: *The Use of Athymic (Nude) Mice in Cancer Research,* edited by D. P. Houchens and A. O. Ovejera, pp. 267–280. G. Fischer, New York.
31. Kubota, T., Shimosato, Y., and Nagai, K. (1978): Experimental chemotherapy of carcinoma of the human stomach and colon serially transplanted in nude mice. *Gann,* 69:299–309.
32. Lee, S. S., Giovanella, B. C., and Stehlin, J. S. (1977): Selective lethal effect of thymidine on human and mouse tumor cells. *J. Cell. Physiol.,* 92:401–406.
33. Lee, S. S., Giovanella, B. C., and Stehlin, J. S. (1977): Effect of excess thymidine on the growth of human melanoma cells transplanted in thymus-deficient nude mice. *Cancer Lett.,* 3:209–214.
34. Lee, S. S., Giovanella, B. C., Stehlin, J. S., and Brunn, J. C. (1978): Regression of established human tumors in nude mice induced by continuous infusion of thymidine (TdR). *Proc. Am. Assoc. Cancer Res.,* 19:103.
35. Lee, S. S., Giovanella, B. C., Stehlin, J. S., and Brunn, J. C. (1979): Regression of human tumors established in nude mice after continuous infusion of thymidine. *Cancer Res.* 39:2928–2933.
36. Leibovitz, A., Stinson, J. C., McCombs, W. B., McCoy, C. E., Mazur, K. C., and Mabry, N. D. (1976): Classification of human colorectal adenocarcinoma cell lines. *Cancer Res.,* 36:4562–4569.
37. Osieka, R., Houchens, D. P., Goldin, A., and Johnson, R. K. (1977): Chemotherapy of human colon carcinoma xenografts in athymic nude mice. *Cancer,* 40:2640–2650.
38. Osieka, R., and Johnson, R. K. (1978): Evaluation of chemical agents in phase I clinical trials and earlier stages of development against xenografts of human colon carcinoma. In: *The Use of Athymic (Nude) Mice in Cancer Research,* edited by D. P. Houchens and A. O. Ovejera, pp. 217–223. G. Fischer, New York.
39. Ovejera, A. A., Houchens, D. P., and Barker, A. D. (1977): Sensitivity of a human tumor xenograft in nude (athymic) mice to various clinically active drugs. In: *Proceedings of the Second International Workshop on Nude Mice,* edited by T. Nomura, N. Ohsawa, N. Tamaoki, and K. Fujiwara, pp. 451–459. University of Tokyo Press, Tokyo.

Advances in Neuroblastoma Research,
edited by Audrey E. Evans.
Raven Press, New York © 1980.

The Nude Mouse Model for Rational Therapy

Lawrence Helson

Memorial Sloan-Kettering Cancer Center, New York, New York 10021

The capability of determining biological and pharmacological characteristics of neuroblastoma tumors from individual patients has lagged pending the development of cell culture methodology and *in vivo* testing models. Recent innovations with *in vitro* drug testing (4) and *in vivo* testing of tumor heterotransplants in congenitally immune deprived nu/nu mice has permitted such capability (8). Presented here are studies using a nude mouse bearing human neuroblastoma model. These studies of tumors established from treated patients (6) were designed to address selected questions relevant to the treatment of this disease. These include (a) does the tumor retain its original biological and pharmacological activity as a heterotransplant, and (b) can the responses to treatment in nude mice be representative of the responses obtained in the clinical setting. It seems that a rational basis for constructing a treatment program for neuroblastoma would follow if these questions are satisfactorily answered. Some of the construction of our current protocol for the treatment of stage IV neuroblastomas is based on responses obtained in the nude mouse (6), and future modifications of treatment design may follow depending on continued study.

MATERIALS AND METHODS

The nude mice in this study were obtained from the animal facility of the Memorial Sloan-Kettering Cancer Center. The original neuroblastoma tumors were obtained from metastatic sites or from tumor-involved bone marrow.

Tumors were implanted in subcutaneous sites through trocars. Measurements of the two greatest diameters of subcutaneous tumors every other day were made by calipers as soon as growth was detectable. Surgical procedures and irradiation of tumors were always done under sodium pentobarbital anesthesia. Radiation was delivered to selected tumor sites using a lead shield and a cesium 137 source.

Mathematical analysis of the resultant DNA cell number histogram was performed by a curve fitting process using a program developed by Fried (5) on a PDP 11/70 digital computer. Using this process, the fractions of cells in the G0, G1, S, and G2–M compartments could be calculated.

RESULTS

Biological and Pharmacological Studies

Heterotransplanted neuroblastoma continues to maintain its secretory activity in the host animal (7). Dihydroxyphenylalanine (DOPA) is one of the major early metabolites of catecholamine synthesis which is secreted by neuroblastoma cells (9,11). Tumors in nude mice continued to secrete DOPA, and the concentration in mouse blood appeared to be in proportion to the tumor load. The efficiency of secretion, however, appeared to be inversely proportional to tumor size, i.e., the larger tumors produced less serum DOPA on a weight basis than the smaller tumors. These data in nude mice indicate that errors as much as one decade may be made in estimating tumor burden from plasma DOPA levels (Table 1).

Immunological Studies

In children with neuroblastoma, the presence of tumor is usually associated with the development of immune complexes (3). In nude mice, heterotransplanted tumors of 0.5 cm diameter give rise to immune complexes. The level of immune complexes bears a relationship to the total tumor burden which may be linear as the tumor grows in size. When the tumor burden increases to 2.5 to 3 cm (4 g), the level of circulating immune complexes may decrease presumably due to an antigen excess. The changes in complement in serum of mice and patients with tumor are even more complex. When complement levels decrease with increased tumor burden, direct absorption of complement onto tumor cells or immune complexes (2) may be occurring. Although it appears reasonable to study circulating immune complexes as an indicator for tumor antigens and host immunologic reactivity, the degree of sensitivity as determined from the nude mouse model appears to be relatively low. Its utility as a measure of tumor burden is questionable, but its value as a prognostic marker may be of greater interest and it is under current study in a longitudinal trial in patients.

TABLE 1. *Changes in serum DOPA with increasing tumor burden SK-N-Lo in nude mice*

	Weight of tumor, g	Weight mouse	Tumor weight % body weight	Serum DOPA, ng/ml	Specific activity DOPA/g tumor
Control	0	30	—	0.94	—
1	0.183	32	0.5	3.5	7.0
2	1.137	29	3.8	9.37	2.46
3	4.537	39	11.6	15.1	1.30
4	10.31	39	26.4	14.0	0.59
5	17.79	53	33.5	20.5	0.61

Serum DOPA levels were obtained from individual mice and reflect the tumor burden, but specific activity appears to be inversely proportional to size.

Treatment Studies

The tumor-bearing mice lend themselves to studies of the effects of chemotherapy. Since the ratio of surface area to weight is high for mice, the drug dosages administered on a weight basis are relatively low compared to those in patients. Hence, tumor responses obtained with drug dosages equal to, or one or two magnitudes higher than, those given to patients on a dose per weight basis are within a range which may be extrapolated to the human subject. Sensitivities to cyclophosphamide, a standard drug for neuroblastoma, can be used as a yardstick for comparing tumors and drug responses. The responses obtained with different tumors in nude mice appear to correspond with the degree of drug exposure the tumor was subjected to during the patient's lifetime. Tumors of patients treated repeatedly with cyclophosphamide appeared to exhibit proportional degrees of resistance to cyclophosphamide. We currently use tumors in

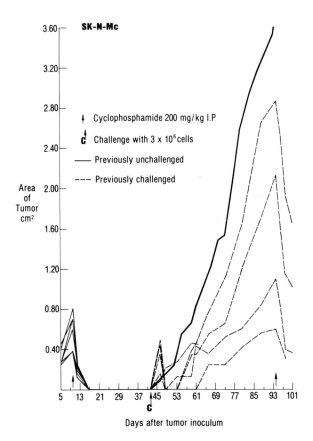

FIG. 1. Prolonged latency occurred on reinoculation of previously cured mice. Re-treatment of same mice bearing rechallenged tumors demonstrated same sensitivity to cyclophosphamide.

our laboratory which have different cyclophosphamide sensitivities; the first was obtained from a patient with little exposure to the drug during her disease course (SK-N-Mc) (10), and the second, with cyclophosphamide resistance (SK-N-Lo) (8), was obtained from a patient treated repeatedly with cyclophosphamide. SK-N-Mc cell line in mice exhibits a dose response curve to cyclophosphamide which is reproducible over any number of transplant generations (8,10) and even in mice which were treated, cured, and rechallenged with tumor and drug. In this particular experiment some degree of resistance to growth (prolonged latency period) of new tumor developed in the nude mice. Mechanisms for this are unknown and do not appear to alter the response to cyclophosphamide in any way (Fig. 1).

By treating tumor-bearing mice with moderately low doses of cyclophosphamide and permitting residual tumor cells to grow, one can induce tumor resistance to cyclophosphamide (Fig. 2). These resistant tumors grow slower than the parental tumor in nude mice, and even after repeated transfer and treatment-free intervals for 6 months retain cyclophosphamide resistance. This would corroborate the clinical observations of cyclophosphamide resistance in patients, and the resistance seen in neuroblastoma tumors obtained from previously treated drug-unresponsive patients. Further understanding of the mechanism of resistance to cyclophosphamide at the cellular level remains to be established.

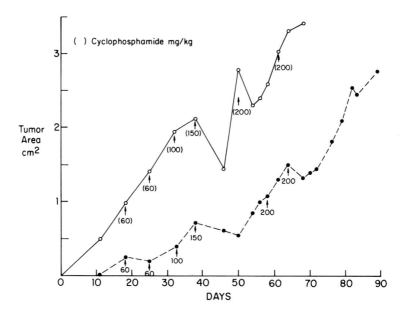

FIG. 2. Effects of graduated doses of cyclophosphamide on the growth of a human neuroblastoma cell line (SK-N-Mc) heterotransplanted to nude (nu/nu) mice reared under specific pathogen-free conditions (SPF). Increasing doses are required to produce antitumor effects and, if administered at long enough intervals, permit resistant cell populations to develop.

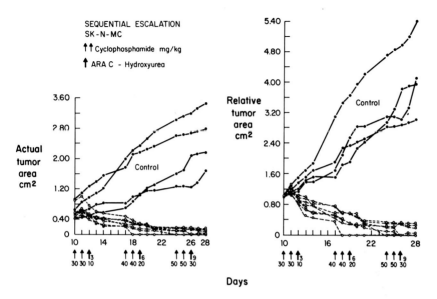

FIG. 3. The combination of cyclophosphamide, cytosine arabinoside (ARA-C), and hydroxyurea on the human neuroblastoma heterograft is effective in tumor control using an escalating dose sequence. These data are displayed as relative tumor area, or actual tumor areas.

Although it appears that increasing the dose of cyclophosphamide can cause regressions in tumors developing resistance, these observations suggest that the intervals between treatments are critical toward obtaining either persistent or complete regressions. This is suggested in the study using cyclophosphamide, cytosine arabinoside, and hydroxyurea (Fig. 3).

This approach has been used in the clinical setting (Table 2) and appears to have some validity (Fig. 4). In this pilot clinical trial, the stage III patients with unresectable tumors appeared to fare well. However, with stage IV patients, even though good responses were universally obtained, complete tumor cell kill was not easily achieved. When these patients relapsed, they generally did so with tumors resistant to cyclophosphamide or had bone marrow reserve which was severely depleted and precluded retreatment with intensive chemo-

TABLE 2. *N-3 sequential escalation (dosages in mg/kg)*

	Cyclophosphamide	Vincristine	F3TdR	Papavarine	Ara-C	Hydroxyurea
I	60	0.05	140	90	9	—
II	80	0.05	175	90	9	—
III	100	0.05	210	90	9	40
IV	120	0.05	210	90	9	80
V	160	0.05	210	90	9	120

The N-3 sequential escalation program includes trifluoromethyl-2-deoxyuridine (F3TdR) and cytosine arabinoside (Ara-C). Courses are given at 21–28-day intervals.

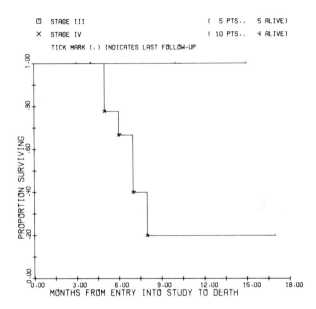

FIG. 4. Kaplan-Meyer survival curve of patients treated with the N-3 SE.

therapy. It should be emphasized that both these patients and the nude mice were treated with chemotherapy alone.

Since tumors compromising the spinal cord, retro-orbital space, or brain require radiation treatment, we studied the effects of radiation alone and with chemotherapy in these mice. It was not known whether radiation and cyclophosphamide given concomitantly or at a few days' interval would have different effects on tumor growth. This question was based on practical problems of administration. Using doses of cyclophosphamide (80 mg/kg) which were less than that expected to achieve total eradication of tumors and single low-dose irradiation (300 rads), we observed that both treatments given concomitantly produced the maximum tumor regression (Fig. 5). At the present time, a pilot study of chemotherapy and 300 rads half-torso irradiation (N-3-SE) is under clinical trial (L. Helson, *unpublished data*). In patients, the additional toxicity encountered from 300 rads half-torso irradiation given 4 days after cyclophosphamide (N3-SE) was 5 to 7 days beyond the generally observed drug-induced suppression. Since improved responses were obtained in nude mice with concomitant chemo-irradiation, a temporally closer administration of the drug and irradiation is now being considered for patients. Possibly the concomitant irradiation prevents repair of sublethal damage induced by cyclophosphamide.

Administration of cyclophosphamide on 2 days in sequence may also prevent repair. Certainly the clearance and probable activation of cyclophosphamide is increased the second day of drug administration (2). Nude mice treated with equivalent doses spread over 2 days had better tumor regressions (Fig. 6). Since

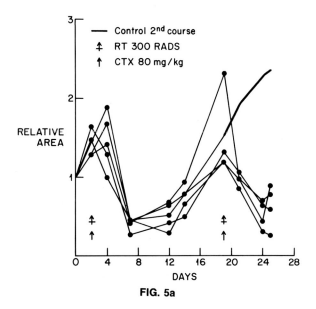

FIG. 5a

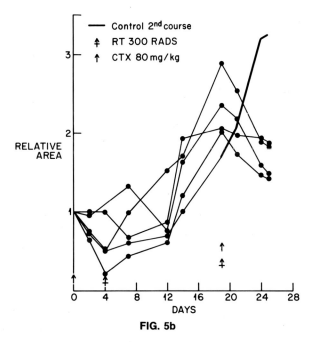

FIG. 5b

FIG. 5. Effects of radiation and cyclophosphamide administered to nude mice bearing human neuroblastoma in combination, at 4-day intervals or individually. Maximal tumor regression was obtained with simultaneous administration.

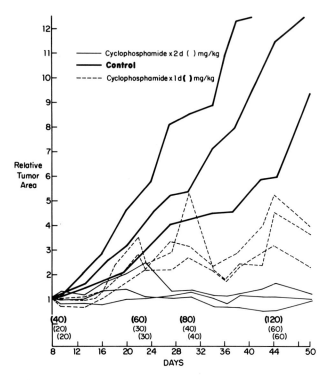

FIG. 6. A comparison of the effects of cyclophosphamide on human neuroblastoma SK-N-Mc given as a single dose or during a 2-day period. The best regressions obtained were from mice treated with the split doses.

the rates of activation of cyclophosphamide are much faster in mice than in man, this is probably not a factor in the enhanced anti-tumor effect (L. Helson, *unpublished data*). The 2-day course of cyclophosphamide continues to be a part of the current clinical program (Table 2). Since the concomitant administration of radiation and cyclophosphamide seems reasonable, it may be clinically advantageous to apply radiotherapy during the second day of the 2-day cyclophosphamide course.

The role of surgery in neuroblastoma has not been carefully defined since most of the experience with good results comes from surgical resections in infants who have a better prognosis and in whom debulking operations appear to be useful. On the other hand, partial tumor resection and delay in administering chemotherapy may add an increased risk of tumor spread. Since the majority of neuroblastomas are not resectable at the time of diagnosis, and in many patients tumors can be only partially excised, we investigated the effects of surgery on the cell kinetics of human neuroblastomas growing subcutaneously in nude mice. The first observations made were that the apparent growth rate and tumor size ranging from 0.5 to 1.5 cm diameter had little relation to the S phase pattern obtained on FMF curves. The S phase histograms for one neuroblastoma heterotransplanted in different mice were essentially identical. Tumors were partially resected, and 24 hr later the residual tumor subjected to FMF analysis. A significant increase in the distribution of cells in early S phase was obtained (13). We interpreted this as recruitment of tumor cells following the partial excision. The implications of this observation are relevant to the clinical setting and suggest that the delay between surgery and administration of chemotherapy should be as short as possible to take advantage of cell recruitment. It is reasonable to administer S phase active drugs such as cytosine arabinoside and hydroxyurea, which probably interfere little with healing during the immediate postoperative period. Apart from the peak at 24 hr, the kinetics of recruitment following surgery are incomplete. In preliminary studies of nude mice treated with cyclophosphamide following surgery, it appears that tumor size may play a role in determining the amount of additional cell kill obtained. This would suggest that the more complete the surgery, the better the results when additional treatment is contemplated, i.e., more complete eradication was obtained with smaller tumors (13). Whether surgery is conducive to the formation of metastases is unknown, since the nude mouse human tumor model in these experiments rarely forms metastases. In a small study, neuroblastomas in 10 animals were partially resected and the animals observed over the next 3 months. Compared to results in control animals which were sham operated, only the growth rate of the operated animals increased over control and there was no evidence of metastases in any of these animals.

CONCLUSIONS

Studies conducted with the human neuroblastoma nude mouse model indicate that it has certain limitations such as failure to develop metastases. Its ease of use in testing for drug and radiation sensitivity compensate for this and indicate its value in helping design more effective clinical treatment schemes. Restrictions such as time for a primary tumor to be established can be circumvented by the use of drug testing with the subrenal capsule assay (1). The difficulties of establishing primary tumors in cell cultures from untreated patients with neuroblastoma can be surmounted by direct inoculation of tumor in the nude mice (8).

ACKNOWLEDGMENTS

This work was supported by the Wahlstrom Foundation, the Ann Marie O'Brien Neuroblastoma Fund, and NCI Grant CA 18856.

REFERENCES

1. Bogden, A. E., Ward, A., Gulkin, T. A., Esber, H. J., and Kelton, D. E. (1979): Ranking the activity of chemotherapeutic (chemo.) agents against individual human tumors: Subrenal

capsule (SRC) assay. In: *Proceedings of the American Society of Clinical Oncology,* New Orleans, Louisiana, Abstract #C-133, p. 323.

2. Brandeis, W. E., Helson, L., Khan, A., and Liu, Y. P. (1978): Circulating immune complexes and complement levels in human neuroblastoma-bearing nude mice. In: *Proceedings of the American Association for Cancer Research,* Washington, D.C., Abstract #319, p. 80.

3. Brandeis, W. E., Helson, L., Wang, Y., Good, R. A., and Day, N. K. (1978): Circulating immune complexes in sera of children with neuroblastoma: Correlation with stage of disease. *J. Clin. Invest.,* 62:1201–1209.

4. Buick, R. N., Frye, S. E., Salmon, S. E., and Stanisic, T. H. (1979): A colony assay for progenitor cells from transitional cell carcinoma of the bladder. In: *Proceedings of the American Association for Cancer Research,* New Orleans, Louisiana, Abstract #792, p. 196.

5. Fried, J. (1977): Analysis of DNA histograms from flow cytofluorometry: estimation of the distribution of cells in S phase. *J. Histochem. Cytochem.,* 25:942–951.

6. Helson, L. (1979): Investigational chemotherapy of neuroblastoma. *J. Fla. Med. Assoc.,* 66:284–287.

7. Helson, L., Das, S. K., and Hajdu, S. I. (1975): Human neuroblastoma in "nude" mice. *Cancer Res.,* 35:2594–2599.

8. Helson, L., Helson, C., Das, S. K., and Rubenstein, R. (1978): Biochemistry and chemotherapy of human neural tumors in nude mice. In: *Proceedings of the Symposium on the Use of Athymic (Nude) Mice in Cancer Research,* edited by David P. Houchens and Artemio A. Ovejera, pp. 257–266. Gustav Fischer, New York.

9. Helson, L., Helson, C., Majeranowski, A., and Johnson, G. A. (1979): Neuroectodermal tumors and 3,4-dihydroxyphenylalanine (DOPA). In: *Proceedings of the American Society of Clinical Oncology,* New Orleans, Louisiana, Abstract #C-37, p. 301.

10. Helson, L., Helson, C., Rubenstein, R., and Hajdu, S. I. (1977): Human neuroblastoma in nude mice. In: *Proceedings of the Second International Workshop on Nude Mice,* edited by Tatsuji Nomura, Nakaaki Ohsawa, Norikazu Tamaoki, and Kosaku Fujiwara, pp. 291–303. University of Tokyo Press, Tokyo.

11. Helson, L., Nisselbaum, J., Helson, C., Majeranowski, A., and Johnson, G. A. (1979): Biological markers in neuroblastoma and other pediatric neoplasias. In: *8th International Symposium on the Biological Characterization of Human Tumors,* Athens, Greece *(in press).*

12. Krivit, W., Sladek, N. E., Doeden, D., Mirocha, C. J., and Pathre, S. (1979): Plasma clearance and urinary excretion of cyclophosphamide in pediatric patients. In: *Proceedings of the American Society of Clinical Oncology,* New Orleans, Louisiana, Abstract #642, p. 159.

13. Sordillo, P., Hansen, H., Helson, L., and Helson, C. (1979): Cytofluorometric analysis of tumors in nude mice. In: *Symposium on Immunodeficient Animals in Cancer Research,* London, England, Feb. 15–16 *(in press).*

Advances in Neuroblastoma Research,
edited by Audrey E. Evans.
Raven Press, New York © 1980.

Antitumor Activity of Chemotherapeutic Agents Alone or in Combination Using a Human Neuroblastoma Model System

Paul J. Harlow, Michael M. Siegel, Stuart E. Siegel, and William F. Benedict

Department of Medicine, Division of Hematology-Oncology, Children's Hospital of Los Angeles, and Department of Pediatrics, University of Southern California School of Medicine, Los Angeles, California 90027

Neuroblastoma is the second most common malignant tumor of childhood, but the treatment results have not significantly improved over the past 25 years (5). Even with intensive chemotherapy, only 30% of patients survive 2 years from diagnosis (3).

The recent availability of established, well-characterized human neuroblastoma cell lines (11,13) as well as athymic nude mice has enabled us to investigate the chemotherapeutic sensitivities of human neuroblastoma both *in vitro* and *in vivo* (12). Our previous studies demonstrated that two human neuroblastoma cell lines, SK-N-MC and LA-N-1, had *in vitro* and *in vivo* chemotherapeutic sensitivities similar to those of the tumors from which they were derived (12). The SK-N-MC cells were sensitive *in vitro* and *in vivo* to cyclophosphamide (CTX) and vincristine (VCR), whereas the LA-N-1 cells were resistant to both agents. In addition, as observed in the patients, both lines showed no response *in vivo* to adriamycin.

Subsequently, we found, unexpectedly, that marked changes occurred in the DNA distribution of the LA-N-1 cells *in vivo* following treatment with CTX, although no significant decrease in tumor weight was observed (2). There was a marked increase in the number of cells in the G2/M phase of the cell cycle with a concomitant decrease in the number of cells in the G1 phase. These changes in cell cycle parameters peaked at 4 days after CTX treatment. In an attempt to overcome the drug resistance of LA-N-1 cells to CTX and VCR and to take advantage of the cell cycle changes produced by CTX, various combinations of CTX and VCR were studied in the nude mouse model (12).

We have been interested also in evaluating new agents in the system. One of the most promising drugs is *cis*-diamminedichloroplatinum (CPDD) (10). Phase II studies of children with neuroblastoma have demonstrated a 30% response rate to this compound. Neither of the patients from whom the SK-

N-MC or LA-N-1 cell lines were obtained received this agent. However, to further examine the usefulness of these cell lines as a screen for new agents, SK-N-MC and LA-N-1 tumor-bearing animals were examined for their response to CPDD. As shown below, both cell lines showed a significant decrease in tumor weight following exposure to CPDD.

MATERIALS AND METHODS

Cell Lines

The human neuroblastoma cell lines LA-N-1 and SK-N-MC have been extensively characterized (1,11,13). LA-N-1 cells were grown in McCoy's 5A medium containing 10% fetal calf serum, glutamine (100 mM), penicillin (100 μg/ml), and streptomycin (100 μg/ml). They were incubated at 37°C in 5% CO_2 in tissue culture flasks (Falcon #3034; Oxnard, Calif.). SK-N-MC cells were grown similarly except Eagle's minimal essential medium was used. Medium, serum, and reagents were obtained from Flow Laboratories, Rockville, Md.

Mice

Eight- to sixteen-week-old Swiss nude mice of both sexes were used for study. They were bred in our animal facilities and housed in autoclaved cages in laminar flow animal stations (Germ Free Inc., Miami, Fla.), fed autoclaved Labblox (Wayne Laboratories, Allied Mills Inc., Chicago, Ill.) and water acidified to pH 2.5 with HCl.

Tumor Growth

SK-N-MC and LA-N-1 cells were grown to subconfluence in tissue culture flasks, removed with 0.25% trypsin-EDTA (Flow Laboratories, Rockville, Md.), washed twice, and resuspended in complete tissue culture medium. SK-N-MC cells (10^7 cells; passage 80) or LA-N-1 cells (3×10^7 cells; passages 88–105) in 0.2 cc of complete medium were injected subcutaneously into the dorsum of each mouse. The mice were observed for the appearance of subcutaneous tumors (minimum of 3 mm diameter), and then tumor diameters were measured twice weekly with Vernier calipers. Tumor weight was calculated by the following formula (4):

$$\text{Weight (mg)} = \frac{\text{Length} \times \text{Width}^2}{2}$$

Chemotherapy

When tumors reached a calculated tumor weight of 400 to 1,200 mg, the mice received chemotherapy consisting of CTX (250 mg/kg), VCR (1.25 mg/

kg), or CPDD (12 mg/kg) as single agents i.p. or various combinations of CTX and VCR at the same dose. Nonlethal drug doses were chosen which would produce an average animal weight loss ≤ 17%. Control animals received an equal volume of normal saline. Toxicity and drug effect were monitored by weighing the mice and measuring their tumors twice weekly. White blood cell counts were obtained on days 0, 4, and 7 of treatment. A significant tumor response was defined as a ≥ 50% reduction in calculated tumor weight from the start of treatment. Following a minimum observation period of 21 days from the start of treatment, the mice were sacrificed and representative animals from each group were autopsied. Tumor weight loss between different groups was analyzed using a Kruskal-Wallis H Test for nonparametric distribution (6).

RESULTS

Treatment with CTX and VCR Alone or in Combinations

LA-N-1 tumors were treated with CTX and VCR alone or in combinations. Both drugs when used singly showed little effect on tumor growth (Table 1), the maximum decrease in tumor size occurring at a mean of 11 and 4 days for CTX and VCR, respectively. All combinations of these drugs were more effective than either one used as a single agent as can be seen in Table 1. Of the combinations, CTX (day 0) VCR (day 0) and CTX (day 0) VCR (day 4) appeared of equal efficacy when analyzed by tumor weight decrease. Both regimens were significantly ($p < 0.001$) more active than the other two combinations used. For all combinations, the nadir of tumor weight was reached 11 to 14 days after initiation of treatment. For all chemotherapy regimens the mean animal weight loss was ≤ 12%; recovery of pretreatment weight occurred by 14 days in all animals. There were no deaths in any group. Myelosuppression followed only regimens containing CTX and was maximal at 4 days post-treatment.

TABLE 1. *Single-agent and combination chemotherapy with cyclophosphamide (CTX) and vincristine (VCR)*

Regimen[a]	Responses[b]	Tumor weight decrease[c]	Animal weight loss[c]
CTX	1/21	19 ± 23	8 ± 3
VCR	0/6	8 ± 9	12 ± 6
CTX(0)VCR(0)	9/18	50 ± 24	10 ± 4
CTX(0)VCR(3)	4/15	38 ± 20	9 ± 5
CTX(0)VCR(4)	10/15	58 ± 13	8 ± 4
CTX(4)VCR(0)	2/14	33 ± 15	13 ± 7

[a] Numbers in parentheses refer to day on which drug was given.
[b] Number of significant tumor responses over number of tumors treated.
[c] Mean % ± 1 SD.

TABLE 2. Cis-*diamminedichloroplatinum (CPDD) treatment of LA-N-1 and SK-N-MC tumors*

Cell line	Treatment	Responses[a]	Tumor weight decrease[b]	Animal weight loss[b]
LA-N-1	CPDD 12 mg/kg	7/9	71 ± 20	15 ± 7
LA-N-1	Normal saline	0/5	0	1.8 ± 2
SK-N-MC	CPDD 12 mg/kg	10/10	71 ± 14	17 ± 4
SK-N-MC	Normal saline	0/6	1 ± 3	0

[a] Number of significant tumor responses over number of tumors treated.
[b] Mean % ± 1 SD.

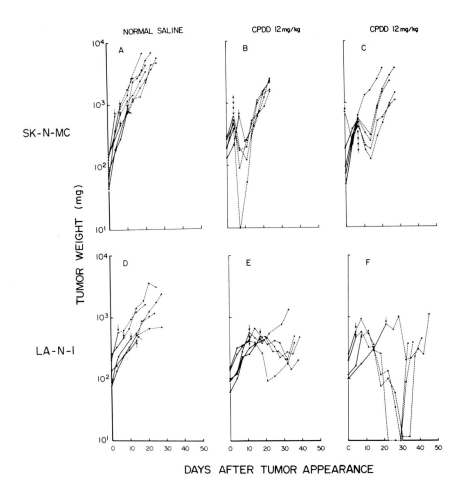

FIG. 1. Response of SK-N-MC and LA-N-1 tumors to normal saline and CPDD. The calculated weight of individual SK-N-MC **(A,B,C)** and LA-N-1 **(D,E,F)** tumors in nude mice is plotted on a semi-logarithmic scale. Each animal was treated with a single dose of normal saline or CPDD (12 mg/kg i.p.). The day of injection is indicated by *arrows.*

Treatment with CPDD

Both LA-N-1 and SK-N-MC tumors treated with CPDD showed a mean tumor weight decrease of approximately 70% (Table 2), whereas those treated with normal saline continued to grow. The nadir of tumor weight for LA-N-1 tumors occurred later after treatment and remained low for a longer time than for SK-N-MC tumors (Fig. 1).

Animal weight loss averaged 15% for LA-N-1 tumors and 18% for SK-N-MC tumors, and was maximal at 6 to 8 days after treatment. Recovery to pretreatment animal weight occurred rapidly in both LA-N-1 and SK-N-MC tumor-bearing mice. Thus, for animals with LA-N-1 tumors, recovery to pretreatment animal weight occurred when tumor weight was still decreasing.

Myelosuppression was minimal in all treated animals and there were no deaths in any groups.

DISCUSSION

Our first group of experiments shows a significant response of LA-N-1 tumors to combinations of CTX and VCR, whereas little or none is observed when either drug is used as a single agent. Previous studies of cytokinetic changes of LA-N-1 tumors following treatment with CTX have shown a marked increase in the number of cells in the G2/M phases of the cell cycle. At the same time, there was no significant decrease in tumor size (2). This change in DNA distribution began at 2 days after treatment and peaked by 4 days. By 8 to 10 days after treatment the DNA distribution had returned to pretreatment patterns.

With these data, we attempted to take advantage of these cell cycle changes by using VCR at different intervals after CTX. Our hypothesis was that the observed cytokinetic changes would enable us to maximize tumor weight decrease if VCR was timed appropriately after CTX. Contrary to our expectations, we found that regimens of CTX (day 0) VCR (day 0) and CTX (day 0) VCR (day 4) were of equal efficacy. Furthermore, both these regimens were significantly more effective than the other two combinations used. We cannot explain this based on our previous data. Additional studies are now being undertaken to examine changes in DNA distributions of LA-N-1 tumor cells following combination chemotherapy with CTX and VCR to determine whether or not there is a cytokinetic basis of these results.

Hayes et al. (7) showed a correlation between changes in mitotic and labeling indices during the first course of therapy with CTX and the clinical response, as evaluated after 4 months of induction chemotherapy. Children with disseminated neuroblastoma were treated with 7 days of CTX followed by adriamycin. The authors demonstrated with sequential bone marrow aspirations that patients with increases in their mitotic and labeling indices during CTX therapy had a better clinical response to treatment than those patients with no increase.

The study of Hayes and co-workers points to the importance of the correct sequencing of agents based on the kinetics of the tumor as well as the pharmacologic actions of the drugs. In humans, obtaining multiple tumor biopsies to assess kinetics is often impossible. Using the nude mouse model with human neuroblastoma cell lines, one can ascertain optimal sequencing of chemotherapy more quickly than in comparable clinical trials.

CPDD is a heavy metal complex found to have significant activity in several animal tumors (10). It has been suggested that its lethal activity is due to interference with DNA crosslinking (10), but its killing effect is similar regardless of the cell cycle phase at which the drug is administered (9). In 1977 Kamalakar et al. (8) reported an objective response in 4 of 16 children with advanced cancer refractory to conventional therapy. One of the responders had neuroblastoma. Nitschke et al. (9) reported a phase II study in which 25 children with advanced neuroblastoma were treated. One complete remission, three partial remissions, and two improvements were observed. In our study, we obtained significant responses in 100% and 78% of SK-N-MC and LA-N-1 tumors, respectively, with tolerable toxicity. Although all SK-N-MC tumors responded, they rapidly regrew. LA-N-1 tumors, however, showed a high response rate with a more prolonged tumor weight decrease. We believe that these results are particularly significant since LA-N-1 tumors have been refractory to all other chemotherapeutic agents studied so far. These data may point to an important role for CPDD in the treatment of resistant neuroblastoma and should suggest its inclusion in first-line combination chemotherapy after further clinical testing.

The results of the experiments with CTX and VCR singly and in combination or CPDD alone emphasize the usefulness of this human neuroblastoma model system. The ability to produce multiple tumors of homogeneous origin for exposure to various therapeutic modalities suggests an increasing applicability for this model in preclinical chemotherapy studies.

ACKNOWLEDGMENTS

This work has been supported by the Stephanie Michelle Milkes Cancer Fund for Children and in part by Grant CA22794 awarded by National Cancer Institute, DHEW. Michael M. Siegel is a recipient of an American Cancer Society Junior Faculty Award 1978–1979. William F. Benedict is the recipient of a Research Career Development Award CA70996. Correspondence should be addressed to William F. Benedict at the Division of Hematology-Oncology, Children's Hospital of Los Angeles, 4650 Sunset Boulevard, Los Angeles, California 90027. We appreciate the secretarial assistance of Ms. Patrice Culbreath.

REFERENCES

1. Biedler, J. L., Helson, L., and Spengler, B. A. (1973): Morphology and growth, tumorigenicity and cytogenetics of human neuroblastoma cells in continuous culture. *Cancer Res.*, 33:2643–2652.

2. Danon, Y. L., Epstein, M. D., Siegel, M. M., Siegel, S. E., Myers, C. P., Benedict, W. F., and Seeger, R. C. (1980): Flow microfluorometric analysis of human DNA distributions. *(This volume).*
3. Evans, A. E., D'Angio, G. J., and Koop, C. E. (1976): Diagnosis and treatment of neuroblastoma. *Pediatr. Clin. North Am.,* 23:161–170.
4. Geran, R. I., Greenberg, N. H., MacDonald, M. M., Schumacher, A. M., and Abbott, B. J. (1972): Protocols for screening chemical agents and natural products against animal tumors and other biological systems. *Cancer Chemother. Rep.,* 3:47–52.
5. Groncy, P., and Finklestein, J. Z. (1978): Neuroblastoma. *Pediatr. Ann.* 7:548–559.
6. Hardyck, C. D., and Petrinovich, L. F. (1969): Distribution free methods. In: *Introduction to Statistics for the Behavioral Sciences,* pp. 173–183. W. B. Saunders Co., Philadelphia.
7. Hayes, F. A., Green, A. A., and Mauer, A. M. (1977): Correlation of cell kinetic and clinical response to chemotherapy in disseminated neuroblastoma. *Cancer Res.,* 37:3766–3770.
8. Kamalakar, P., Freeman, A. I., Higby, D. J., Wallace, H. J., and Sinks, L. F. (1977): Clinical response and toxicity with cis-dichlorodiammineplatinum (II) in children. *Cancer Treatment Rep.,* 61:835–839.
9. Nitschke, R., Starling, K. A., Vats, T., and Bryan, H. (1978): Cis-diamminedichloroplatinum (NSC-119875) in childhood malignancies. A Southwest Oncology Group study. *Med. Pediatr. Oncol.,* 4:127–132.
10. Rozencweig, M., Von Hoff, D. D., Slavik, M., and Muggia, F. M. (1977): Cis-diamminedichloroplatinum: A new anticancer drug. *Ann Intern. Med.,* 86:803–812.
11. Seeger, R. C., Rayner, S. A., Banerjee, A., Chung, H., Laug, W. E., Neustein, H. B., and Benedict, W. F. (1977): Morphology, growth, chromosomal pattern and fibrinolytic activity of two new human neuroblastoma cell lines. *Cancer Res.,* 37:1364–1371.
12. Siegel, M. M., Chung, H. S., Rucker, N., Siegel, S. E., Seeger, R. C., Isaacs, H., and Benedict, W. F. (1979): In vitro/in vivo preclinical chemotherapy studies of human neuroblastoma. *Cancer Treat. Rep. (in press).*
13. West, G. J., Uki, J., Herschman, H. R., and Seeger, R. C. (1977): Adrenergic, cholinergic, and inactive human neuroblastoma cell lines with the action-potential Na^+ ionophore. *Cancer Res.,* 37:1372–1376.

Advances in Neuroblastoma Research,
edited by Audrey E. Evans.
Raven Press, New York © 1980.

Constancy of Cell Cycle Parameters in a Human Neuroblastoma Line in the Nude Mouse

John E. Neely

Children's Hospital Research Foundation, Children's Hospital Medical Center, University of Cincinnati, Cincinnati, Ohio 45229

In preparing for the sequential study of the cellular proliferation kinetics of human neuroblastoma, it becomes important to know the baseline variability between tumors of common kinetic parameters. This is particularly true with respect to variability as a function of tumor size, since mice inoculated with the same tumor at the same time invariably develop a range of tumor sizes.

To evaluate variability in kinetic parameters as a function of tumor size, we studied the SK-N-SH human (2,6) neuroblastoma line—one of six neuroblastomas we currently carry by serial passage in our nude mouse colony. We compared the tritiated thymidine labeling index and DNA histograms by flow cytofluorometry of five groups of tumors classified between 0.01 and 2.50 g weight.

MATERIALS AND METHODS

Eight-week-old male nude mice of NIH Swiss background were used for the experiments. The mice were housed singly in sterilized filter-topped shoe box cages with sterile bedding, laboratory chow, and multivitamin-supplemented water. All manipulations were performed on a laminar flow bench at the same time of day. The animals were housed in a limited access room with a 10 hr–14 hr light-dark cycle.

Twenty-one days prior to usage, the animals were inoculated with bilateral subcutaneous trocar injections of 0.25 cc minced SK-N-SH tumor. Prior to harvesting, the tumors were checked visually for size and were felt to occupy the full range of sizes ordinarily used for experiments. One hour prior to sacrifice by cervical dislocation, each animal was injected with 1.0 μCi tritiated thymidine per gram body weight (1.9 Ci/mmole specific activity). The tumors were then excised and weighed. One-half of each tumor was processed for autoradiography. The remaining half was processed for flow cytofluorometric measurement of DNA.

FACTORS   AFFECTING   LABELLING

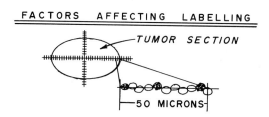

FIG. 1. Tumor sections were analyzed for nuclear labeling by measuring those nuclei lying on a micrometer line horizontally and vertically through the widest diameters of the tumor. Nuclei were scored per 50 μm segment of these lines.

For autoradiography, both methanol-fixed touch preparations and 10% neutral buffered formalin-fixed paraffin-embedded 4 μm thick sections were used. Specimens were placed on cleaned slides, dipped in NTB2 liquid emulsion, and exposed for 2 weeks (touch preparations) or 6 weeks (sections). The autoradiographs were developed with Dektol (Kodak) developer at 20°C for 4 min, and fixed (9). Following development, the specimens were stained with hematoxylin and eosin. The slides were evaluated without knowledge of tumor size or flow cytofluorometry results.

Labeling frequency was determined by sequentially scoring the labeling status of nuclei in a vertical and horizontal line through the center of the section and the widest diameters of the tumor. Nuclei lying on a 50 μm measuring line were counted (Fig. 1). A cell was considered labeled if it was above three standard deviations of the mean background count for that slide. The mean and standard deviation background count was determined by counting four sets of 25 non-nuclear areas of appropriate size. In each case the mean background was less than 1 ± 1 grain/nucleus, thus a nucleus with four or more grains was considered labeled. At least 1,000 nuclei were scored for each tumor.

For the preparation of DNA histograms by flow cytofluorometry, one-half of each tumor sampled was mechanically separated into single cells by gently slicing the tumor and rinsing the fragments through a fine meshed screen and through sequentially smaller hypodermic needles. Cells were then pelleted and stained in propidium iodide (5 mg in 100 cc 0.1% sodium citrate) according to the method of Krishan (7). Cells were checked for staining by fluorescence microscopy. DNA measurements were performed using an Ortho/Biophysics 4802A Cytofluorograf with a 100 channel analyzer.

DNA histograms were dissected into G0-G1, S, and G2-M compartments using the rectangular area of S method of Barfod (1) on a TRS-80 (Radio Shack) minicomputer program kindly provided by Dr. C. E. Donaghey, University of Houston. The histograms were also checked using the computerized dissection method of Fried (4). Both methods concurred.

Twenty-three tumors were studied and the results were grouped into five weight ranges for the purpose of analysis. These results are listed in Table 1. Statistical analyses were performed using Gosset's Student's *t*-test (11).

TABLE 1.

% (1 s.d.)

TUMOR SIZE (GRAMS)	N	LABELLING INDEX	G_0-G_1	S	G_2-M
< 0.05	6	23.3 (4.7)	N.D.	N.D.	N.D.
0.06 - 0.50	7	29.3 (2.4)	57.9 (4.2)	28.7 (3.2)	13.4 (3.9)
0.51 - 0.99	3	32.8 (1.4)	52.5 (3.1)	33.6 (1.2)	14.0 (1.9)
1.00 - 2.00	4	30.9 (3.0)	52.8 (4.9)	32.0 (2.7)	15.2 (2.2)
> 2.00	3	27.1 (2.6)	58.2 (4.6)	27.0 (2.5)	14.8 (2.3)

RESULTS

In determining the labeling indices, factors effecting the sampling errors were first studied. The labeling data were gathered by sequential analysis of 50 μm steps across each tumor in a vertical and horizontal direction so that "maps" of labeling characteristics could be generated. Figure 2 illustrates such a map for one tumor weighing 1.0 g. There was variability in the incidence of nuclei per 200 μm width as well as in the frequency of labeled cells. These variabilities, however, appeared to be randomly distributed in each tumor. No large areas of altered labeling could be found. These characteristics were true of all tumors over the size range tested. We concluded that, as long as an appropriately sized sample was collected to avoid the variability over short areas, any area within the tumor appeared to reflect the labeling status of the entire tumor.

We next examined how many samples within a tumor adequately reflected the true biological variability within the tumor. After we scored at least 3,000 cells in a tumor for labeling status, results were pooled in groups ranging from

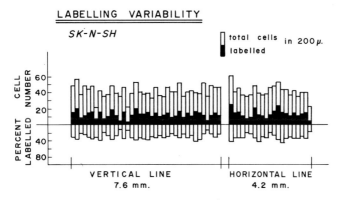

FIG. 2. The bars above the line represent the total number of cells counted per 200 μm segment of lines crossing vertically and horizontally through a tumor measuring 7.6 × 4.2 mm. The dark bars are that portion of the total that were scored as labeled. The bars below the line represent the relative number of labeled cells in each 200 μm step across the tumor.

25 to 1,200 cells per group and the percentage labeled cells for each group was determined. Then groups of similar size were analyzed for mean and standard deviation labeled index. Figure 3 illustrates the changes in the labeling index parameters on the same tumor as a function of sampling size. With small sampling sizes used to determine the percentage of labeled nuclei, there is a large variability reflected in the standard deviation, although the mean labeling index is accurately sampled. With increasing sample size the variability diminishes until it stabilizes when 300 or more cells are used to score the labeling index. This variability reflects the biological variation within this tumor over a reasonable sample size. The lesser sample sizes have an increased sampling error above the biological variability. For the purposes of calculating labeling indices for statistical comparison with other tumors, it is important that the sampling sizes consist of at least 300 cells to adequately describe the true variability within the tumor.

Although 10 samples of 300 cells were used to generate the statistics, it was also determined that three or more such samples appeared to adequately reflect these statistics. Therefore we now routinely score three samples of 300 cells to generate the labeling index for this tumor.

Table 1 compares the labeling indices and DNA histogram analyses for the 23 tumors studied, grouped into five size ranges. We have found that tumors weighing 0.05 g or less are unusable for multiple analyses, such as simultaneous

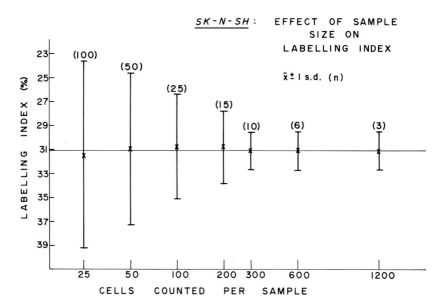

FIG. 3. The mean (X) and SD labeling index as a function of sampling size is shown. The numbers in parentheses are the total numbers of each sample size group used to generate these statistics. At least 3,000 single cells counted across the tumors in two directions were used in each evaluation.

labeling index and flow cytofluorometry, because the cell yield is too small to determine all of these parameters adequately. This group also has the largest variability in its labeling indices and is significantly different from the larger tumors ($p < 0.01$). We therefore do not use tumors weighing less than 0.06 g.

Among the remaining groups, there were no significant differences between labeling indices. The indices also compared favorably with the S compartment determined by flow cytofluorometry. No significant differences were noted between groups with regards to the cell cycle compartments G0-G1, S, or G2-M.

DISCUSSION

We concluded from these studies that, over the useful size range likely to be used for tumor evaluation, no differences could be found in the basic kinetic parameters obtained, and that kinetic data reflecting the entire tumor could be obtained on a small portion of the tumor, provided the sampling was appropriately performed. Thus, for the purposes of sequential sampling of tumors for cell kinetic analysis, this nude mouse model appears to be valid. Caution, however, must be exercised in interpreting changes in the labeling index or flow cytofluorometry data. In spite of appropriate sampling sizes, there was still significant variability in the data (see Table 1). Small changes in percentage label or compartmentalization must not be overinterpreted unless the appropriate statistical analysis permits a high degree of confidence that a real difference is present.

It is interesting that, even with the largest tumors tested, there was homogeneity in nuclear labeling throughout the specimen. The possibility of decreased proliferation in the center of the tumor because of lack of nutrients, blood supply, etc. did not apply. The homogeneity of kinetic parameters throughout the tumor over the size range tested suggests that multiple sequential biopsies or needle aspiration could give accurate kinetic data. We are currently determining whether biopsy itself has any effect on tumor proliferation as has been previously suggested (3). Care was taken in these experiments to manipulate and sample the tumors at the same time of day to control for the possibility of diurnal variations in tumor proliferation. Such variability has been reported in other tissues, such as the hamster cheek pouch (8) or leukemic marrow (10). During a kinetic experiment that will require diurnal sampling, such variability may be important.

In this study, tumors inoculated at the same time grew to different sizes over the same period of time, and yet had similar kinetic parameters suggesting a similar growth pattern. The most likely reason for different sized tumors is variability in initial tumor dose even though inoculum volume was similar. The method of passaging tumors that we have found to be most successful is to mince the tumors in media and to inject 0.25 cc of this product subcutaneously into the flank via trocar. There is likely considerable variability in the cell content of the inocula with this technique. A more uniform technique of passaging tumors might be to inject known quantities of single cells; however, we have encountered problems with this technique. The yield of viable cells obtained by dispersing the tumor is lower than expected. Although the yield is good for the purpose of flow cytofluorometry where the cells are immediately stained, the survival for long enough periods of time to allow successful passaging is apparently unsatisfactory for we have a low yield when passaging tumors this way.

It remains to be seen whether human neuroblastoma grown in the nude mouse reflects a realistic measurement of the true kinetics in humans. Of the six lines we carry in the nude mouse, all have retained a histologic similarity to neuroblastoma. Only one line has, however, shown any tendency to metastasize, a feature that is certainly present in the human. The labeling index of approximately 30% is higher than when directly measured in the human. Wagner and Käser (12) measured an *in vivo* labeling index of 11% in their single-treatment resistant case, whereas Hayes et al. (5) have measured pretreatment labeling indices ranging from 1.6% to 26% in 17 bone marrow specimens containing disseminated neuroblastoma and labeled *in vitro*.

The labeling index of SK-N-SH in the nude mouse is also somewhat higher than that found *in vitro* in the same line. During mid log-phase growth we have found an *in vitro* labeling index of 20% ± 2.6% *(unpublished data)*.

In spite of these differences and precautions, human neuroblastoma grown in solid tumor form in nude mice is a useful model that provides multiple similar samples for sequential analysis that will aid in establishing baseline kinetic parameters on which kinetic responses to various forms of therapy or manipulation can be built.

SUMMARY

The human neuroblastoma line SK-N-SH was grown in the nude mouse and tumors were evaluated for changes in proliferative capacity as a function of varying size by labeling index and flow cytofluorometry. It was found that:

1. These kinetic parameters were the same in tumors over the useful size range tested;
2. The labeling index data were similar throughout the tumor, indicating that a small portion of the tumor could reflect this measurement providing the sample size was appropriate; and
3. The appropriate sampling size for labeling index determination was at least three samples of 300 cells each.

ACKNOWLEDGMENTS

I thank Marianne Brown for her expertise in maintaining the nude mouse colony and her aid in performing these experiments. This work was supported in part by funding from the Phi Beta Psi Sorority and the Children's Hospital Research Foundation Trustee Grant.

REFERENCES

1. Barfod, N. (1977): Flow microfluorometric estimation of G_1 and G_2 chalone inhibition of the JB-1 tumour cell cycle in vitro. *Exp. Cell Res.,* 110:225–236.
2. Biedler, J., Helson, L., and Spengler, B. (1973): Morphology and growth, tumorigenicity, and cytogenetics of human neuroblastoma cells in continuous culture. *Cancer Res.,* 33:2643–2652.
3. Combs, J., and McDougal, D. (1979): Acute kinetic response of residual tumor to partial resection. *Fed. Proc.,* 38:918 (abst.).
4. Fried, J. (1976): Method for the quantitative evaluation of data from flow microfluorometry. *Comput. Biomed. Res.,* 9:263–276.
5. Hayes, F., Green, A., and Mauer, A. (1977): Correlation of cell kinetics and clinical response to chemotherapy in disseminated neuroblastoma. *Cancer Res.,* 37:3766–3770.
6. Helson, L., Das, S., and Hajdu, S. (1975): Human neuroblastoma in nude mice. *Cancer Res.,* 35:2594–2599.
7. Krishan, A. (1975): Rapid flow cytofluorometric analysis of mammalian cell cycle by propidium iodide staining. *J. Cell Biol.,* 66:188–193.
8. Møller, U., Larsen, J., and Faber, M. (1974): The influence of injected tritiated thymidine on the mitotic circadian rhythm in the epithelium of the hamster cheek pouch. *Cell Tissue Kinet.,* 7:231–239.
9. Neely, J., and Combs, J. (1976): Variation in the autoradiographic technique. I. Emulsion-developer combinations assessed by photometric measurement of single silver grains. *J. Histochem. Cytochem.,* 24:1057–1064.
10. Saunders, E. F., Lampkin, B. C., and Mauer, A. M. (1967): Variation of proliferative activity in leukemic cell populations of patients with acute leukemia. *J. Clin. Invest.,* 46:1356–1363.
11. Snedecor, G. (1956): *Statistical Methods.* Iowa State College Press, Ames, Iowa.
12. Wagner, H., and Käser, H. (1970): Cell proliferation in neuroblastoma. *Eur. J. Cancer,* 6:369–372.

Advances in Neuroblastoma Research,
edited by Audrey E. Evans.
Raven Press, New York © 1980.

Discussion: Cytokinetics and Chemotherapy Models

Dr. Nicolini (Philadelphia) explained the difference between Q cells and those in G0 or G1: Cells in Q, G0, and G1 all have the same DNA content, but different amounts of condensation of chromatin; they show three distinct levels of fluorescence on the FMF. The lowest fluorescence occurs with the most condensed chromatin; it corresponds to the G0 state. Physiologically, the differences are that a G0 cell is reversibly out of the cycle whereas a Q cell is irreversibly out of the cycle. The distinction has not yet been established on a vigorous basis.

Discussion turned to the nude mouse model. *Dr. Helson (New York)* pointed out that biochemical activity, such as ornithine decarboxylase activity, was higher at the periphery of large tumors than in the center. The center is necrotic and biochemically inactive. *Dr. Gerson (Bethesda)* then asked about the metastatic potential of neuroblastoma in the nude mouse. Dr. Helson stated that some tumors metastasize and some do not when inoculated subcutaneously. He cited first the Japanese who published on a particular line that metastasized to the ovary and then he quoted *Dr. Sordad (Switzerland)* who found that if tumors are inoculated in mice under 1 week of age, the probability that metastasis will occur increases. In his own experience, Dr. Helson found that only one or two out of several hundred neuroblastomas inoculated subcutaneously metastasized to the liver.

Dr. Casper (Milwaukee) asked why at St. Jude, *cis*-platinum was followed in 48 hr by VM-26 whereas in the Children's Cancer Study Group VM-26 preceded *cis*-platinum by 24 hr. Dr. Hayes stated that the timing of VM-26 and *cis*-platinum was based on preliminary kinetic studies done at St. Jude Children's Research Hospital on *cis*-platinum as a single phase II agent. She argued that although *cis*-platinum has been thought to be non-phase specific, in the bone marrow it appeared to have cycle specificity. At St. Jude, patients on *cis*-platinum showed either killer cells in G2 or a G2 block with increased cells in S phase. Their mitotic index dropped over a 24- to 48-hr period and their labeling index increased at 24 and 48 hr. Based on the G2 block they decided to give VM-26 48 hr after platinum.

Discussion closed with observations about the difficulty of growing neuroblastoma cells in culture. *Dr. Evans (Philadelphia)* commented that primary cultures are established only from untreated patients with aggressive tumors, and early stage tumors rarely, if ever, give rise to established lines. Dr. Benedict requested cells and tissues from patients whose response was known, and Dr. Hayes hypothesized that changes she was observing *in vitro* might be due to selection. It is difficult to be sure that cells derived from patients following treatment represent the original tumor or are simply the residual resistant cells.

Dr. Green (Memphis) stated that since 1974 every primary tumor and every positive bone marrow or lymph node has been placed in culture. The result is 18 lines from 110 patients; only 4 of the 18 lines came from three patients prior to therapy, that is, from three primary tumors and one bone marrow. None of the three patients responded to therapy. He conceded that it is difficult to establish cultures from specimens at diagnosis, but the situation changes after treatment and relapse.

Dr. Seeger (Los Angeles) confirmed these findings. Of four established lines, two were derived from patients who did not respond to therapy. *Dr. D'Angio* added that their experience in Philadelphia was similar: there were no "takes" from tumor stages I, II, or IV-S, nor from the bone marrow except in patients with stage IV disease.

The chairman concluded: the fact that it is impossible now does not mean that it is not going to be possible next week. It is often just a question of finding the proper reagents.

Subject Index

in clonal cell lines, 154–155
and morphological interconversions, 156–158
stability over time, 155
Norepinephrine, inhibiting cell growth in serum-free media, 164
Nude mice, tumor growth in and constancy of cell cycle parameters, 327–332
cyclophosphamide affecting, 289–290, 291
experimental chemotherapy of, 299–303
from hybrid cell lines, 65–67, 104–105, 106, 119
and metastasis, 300, 335
as model for rational therapy, 309–317

O

Oleic acid, inhibiting cell growth in serum-free media, 164
Opsoclonus, with neuroblastoma, 6–7

P

Pancreatic islet cell tumors, pheochromocytoma with, 22
Papaverine, effects on neuroblastoma cells, 139
PHA-stimulated lymphocytes, microfluorometry of, 275–277
Phenylethanolamine-N-methyl transferase (PNMT), activity in neuroblastoma cells, 151–153
Pheochromocytoma, 20–23
tumors with, 19–20, 21
cis-Platinum, response in human neuroblastoma cell lines, 319–324, 335
Polyribocytidilic acid, antitumor activity of, 302
Polyriboinosinic acid, antitumor activity of, 302
Prognosis of neuroblastoma
and age of patients, 5–6
long-term, 18–19
and stage of tumor, 27, 28
and urinary catecholamine metabolites, 25–31
and VMA/HVA ratio, 50

Propidium iodide stain for DNA, 288
Prostaglandins, inhibiting cell growth in serum-free media, 164, 196
Protein kinases, cAMP-dependent, properties in neuroblastoma, 147–149

R

Radiation, chemotherapy with, 314–316
Raji cell lines, recognition by monoclonal antibodies, 224, 229
Recklinghausen's disease, tumors with, 14
Recurrences of neuroblastoma
late, 15
and urinary catecholamine excretion patterns, 29–30
Regression of neuroblastoma, spontaneous, 9, 15, 16, 57, 59, 106
Retinoblastoma, chromosome abnormalities in, 116–117
Ricin
antitumor activity of, 302
endocytosis by murine neuroblastoma, 187–192
RNA, stains for, in microfluorometry, 272–273

S

S-100 protein, in cultured fetal brain cells exposed to EtNU, 131
Second tumor types with neuroblastoma, 18
Selenium, inhibiting cell growth in serum-free media, 164
Sensory-like neuroblastoma cells, 137
Serotonergic neuroblastoma cells, 137
Serum-free culture of neuroblastoma cells, 161–169
for B104 cells, 162–165
and elimination of serum preincubation, 165
and growth response of cells, 165–169
for LA-N-1 cells, 165–169
and substances inhibiting cell growth, 164–165
Sex of neuroblastoma patients, and prognosis, 27
Sites of neuroblastoma, 4–5